Kinesiology

Kinesiology

JOHN M. COOPER, Ed.D.

Professor of Physical Education,
Indiana University,
Bloomington, Indiana

RUTH B. GLASSOW, M.A.

Professor Emeritus of Physical Education,
University of Wisconsin,
Madison, Wisconsin

Fourth edition

with 336 illustrations

The C. V. Mosby Company

Saint Louis   1976

Fourth edition

Copyright © 1976 by The C. V. Mosby Company

All rights reserved. No part of this book may be reproduced
in any manner without written permission of the publisher.

Previous editions copyrighted 1963, 1968, 1972

Printed in the United States of America

Distributed in Great Britain by Henry Kimpton, London

Library of Congress Cataloging in Publication Data

Cooper, John Miller, 1912-
  Kinesiology.

  Bibliography: p.
  Includes index.
  1. Kinesiology. I. Glassow, Ruth Bertha, joint
author. II. Title. [DNLM: 1. Efficiency.
2. Locomotion. 3. Movement. 4. Physical fitness.
WE103 C777k 1976]
QP303.C565 1976   612'.76   75-33991
ISBN 0-8016-1048-6

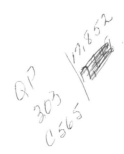

VH/VH/VH 9 8 7 6 5 4 3 2 1

TO OUR STUDENTS

whose hours of film study
and whose data derived from
the use of available equipment have
resulted in new insights and workable
suggestions that have added to our
understanding of human movement

Preface

A decision made some time ago concerning previous editions was adhered to in this one—that is, that a kinesiology text would be most effective if it were written by a man and a woman, since each would have special points of view and understandings considered relevant to students in this area of learning.

This book, although primarily designed for the undergraduate student, should be of value to all those who study human movement. We have organized the material in what we believe to be a logical and meaningful approach to the subject. Once having comprehended the overall organization, students should be able to understand how each detail belongs to the total pattern of the book.

We have kept the previous edition's organizational setup of subject matter unchanged but have attempted to update all material in each of the four parts and in the Appendixes. We have added some new sections in almost all the parts. In a sense this revision is a reorientation to the newest concepts, as well as a rewriting and updating. We have tried to blend the best of the old with the new.

Part I, which is an introduction to the study of kinesiology, contains the concept that human beings have inherited their structure and also a tendency, at least, to execute their motor behavior patterns. Human movement in an action environment is better understood if it is recognized as being influenced by inherited structure functioning for the most part with coordinations that are inherently characteristic of the species. We have included also in this part a condensed history of kinesiology. In the latter part of this particular section, Chapter 2, the emphasis is placed on the contribution of authors of the last 10 years, including those of both national and international stature, as well as on the many new types of equipment that have been designed to make the study of movement more effective.

Part II involves the anatomic bases of movement, relating the skeletal, nervous, and muscular systems to human movement. The skeletal system is the moving portion, containing the action members; the nervous system receives and sends messages; and the muscular system supplies the energy—the motive force.

The skeletal structure is considered first because a movement is described in terms of joint activity and improvement is sought by means of joint action. Since joints in action cause skeletal parts to move, the mechanical aspects of moving segments must be understood if one is to comprehend the value of a joint action in a motor skill. This, then, is our reason for discussing the use of skeletal segments as simple and complex levers.

Next the nervous system is considered. Bones move as levers when muscles contract, and muscles contract only when activated by the nervous system. Any voluntary change in action must be made via the nervous system. Sometimes this change can be directed; at other times, change is activated indirectly by an understanding of inherent patterns of motor behavior. The structure of the nervous system is summarized showing that nerve impulses which originate in the motor cortex may be but a minor portion of those which determine the complex coordinations of a single act. We suggest that the voluntary aspect of a motor act may be a concept of the whole and that the details are involuntary and brought into action by inherited reflexes and behavior patterns. Last in the discussion of anatomic bases of movement, muscle structure and various contributions that muscle contraction makes to skill are described. Muscle action includes more than the moving of body segments: muscles act in combinations by which undesired joint actions that may accompany the desired ones are prevented and bones adjacent to moving segments are stabilized. An understanding of muscle function is not complete when it is limited to the muscles' ability to move a skeletal lever.

Part III, in which the concepts of kinesiology are applied to motor skills, begins with a general plan for studying such skills. This plan presents first a classification of skills: moving external objects, support and movement of the body by itself, and stopping moving objects. Each skill is accomplished by certain basic movement patterns, of which the great majority are inherent.

The mechanics of each pattern are analyzed. With an understanding of these the student is able to analyze any skill, familiar or unfamiliar. Examples of widely used skills are presented to illustrate general underlying principles. Emphasis is given to the concept that at present no known details of coordination are best for all individuals or for any one individual in all situations; however, the basic principles apply to most situations and to normal individuals.

In Part IV and in the Appendixes, general information that is considered to be of value to the instructor and performer is presented: velocity and direction of projectiles, including the angle that will result in their traveling the greatest distance; spin and bounce of balls; information that we have found to be valuable to us about motor behavior; comments on elasticity and friction; and descriptions of muscle attachments for those who wish to study the direction of muscle pull.

The Appendixes include material on principles, patterns, and terminology of movement, which, we believe, will be a valuable aid to teachers. We have added a computer program to the Appendixes.

We thank all our former and present students who read the previous editions and made helpful suggestions for improvement in this fourth edition. We regret that they cannot be mentioned by name: the list is too long. Our thanks are also extended to Charlianna Cooper for helping in the preparation of the revised manuscript and to Robert Sorani for previous drawings and Kela Adams and others for those included in this edition. We thank Wendy Andrews, Kay Flatten, and many others for their thoughtful reading of parts or all of the manuscript.

We also greatly appreciate the permission to use illustrations and advice given by Dr. Anne E. Atwater, Dr. Elizabeth Roberts, and Dr. Joan Waterland and thank Dr. Elizabeth Gardner, Dr. Alice O'Connell, and many others for sharing their publications.

Finally, we appreciate the information made available to us from theses and dissertations written by graduate students from Indiana and Wisconsin universities.

John M. Cooper
Ruth B. Glassow

Contents

PART I

Introduction

CHAPTER 1   Approaches to kinesiology

Kinesiology is a science, an organization of information dealing with motion. The word is not included in the average vocabulary, but observation will show that it is a combination of familiar terms: *ology,* the science of, and *kinesi,* motion. The latter appears in such commonly used words as *kinetic, kinesthetic,* and *cinema* or *cinematography (kinematography).* Even such terms as *kinanthropology* and *human kinetics* have been used in this connection. More recently some universites have begun to use the term *biomechanics* (mechanics as applied to biologic systems). Regardless of the terms used, this text will deal primarily with human motion and will present information that will increase understanding of the purposeful movements of the human body. It is presented with the hope that such understanding will enable the performer to move more skillfully and efficiently and that those persons who attempt to guide others in the improvement of motor skills will gain insight into methods by which their goals can be achieved. The information should be valuable to teachers, coaches, occupational and physical therapists, and persons dealing with problems of human motion at home and in industry.

Fundamental to the understanding of human movement is the realization that the human being is a living organism whose structure and behavior have been shaped by anthropologic ancestors. The backbone was bequeathed by the fish family, who developed that structure when the surface of the earth was covered with water. When part of the earth's surface was raised above the water, animal life, if it was to survive on land, had to develop new structural forms for locomotion. The body needed to be lifted above the earth's surface and yet maintain some contact with it; fins were gradually shaped into legs and feet. Because air does not support the body mass, as does water, the backbone and the newly developed legs needed material to resist gravitational pull better: cartilaginous tissue changed to bone. (See Fig. 1-1.) To escape enemies and to secure food rapid locomotion was needed, and primitive legs lengthened to the thighs and legs of present quadrupeds.

In these changes and in those that followed is seen the capacity of living organisms to adapt structure and behavior to the demands of the environment. A zoologist has expressed this capacity for adjustment as "the creative response of living matter to the challenges of the environment."

As vegetation and trees developed on the land, some kinds of animals escaped ground enemies by choosing an arboreal life. Here a new means of locomotion developed, that of grasping branches and swinging the suspended body from

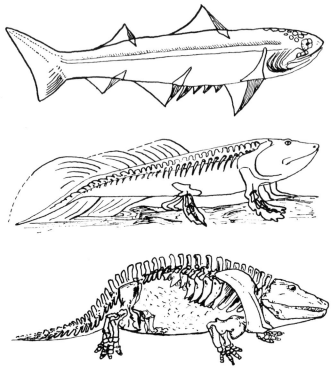

Fig. 1-1. Evolutionary development in resistance to gravitational forces. (Redrawn from Gregory, W. K.: Natural History **51**:222, 1943.)

limb to limb. This type of life modified body structure. The distal ends of the forelimbs were shaped into hands. The proximal end of the forelimb developed a joint capable of great motility. Gravitational force pulled the torso and lower limbs downward, providing a relationship of body segments that would enable descendants to stand on two rather than four feet. Some of these changes have been vividly expressed by Bateman in the phrase "from fin to flinger" (Fig. 1-2).

When some of the tree-dwelling animals returned to ground life and found bipedal locomotion profitable, the human foot was developed. The heels developed and lengthened, providing a rear for the base of support. The forepart of the foot developed to provide the front of the base. According to the anthropologist Howells the structural feature that distinguishes the human being is the foot, "the most peculiar thing about him." The bony structures between the heel and the toes are compactly fitted together to enable them to bear the weight of the body and transmit it to the ball of the foot or to the toes. This compactness allows rotation of weight about the metatarsophalangeal joints, an action that is impossible in animals, such as the ape.

As the foot took over the weight-bearing function, the forelimbs were freed for manipulation of external objects. In such manipulative skills humans sur-

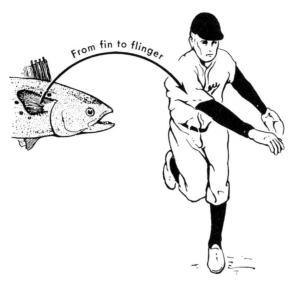

Fig. 1-2. Evolutionary development that resulted from adaptation to changing function; from fin to flinger over millions of years. (From Bateman, J. E.: The shoulder and environs, St. Louis, 1955, The C. V. Mosby Co.)

pass all animals; many believe that the human hand and opposable thumb are unique structural features; yet the primates that live in trees have five digits at the distal ends of the limbs, and the first of these digits can close against the other four as a bough is clasped. The human hand is inherited but the foot was developed.

Each species inherits a basic design that will be modified by its mode of maintaining life. As man's ancestors developed the ability to balance on two feet, they modified also their forms of locomotion—walking, running, leaping, and jumping. The free forelimbs developed the ability to throw and strike, to pull and push, and to lift. The practice of these skills further modified the structure not in basic design but in details.

The influence of environment and function is discussed by Napier in "The Antiquity of Human Walking." He postulates a transitional environment, consisting of forests and open grassland, in which arboreal animals moved in new locomotor forms and that these later developed into the human walking pattern. In this environment, forests were still available for security from enemies and for familiar food; the open areas stimulated the practice of locomotion on the lower limbs. These patterns were further developed when grassland became the major surrounding. The resulting activities modified the skeleton gradually; the pelvis shortened and changed from a horizontal to a vertical position; the lower limbs lengthened; the foot developed. Muscles also changed. The least and middle gluteal muscles became abductors rather than extensors, and the greatest gluteal muscle as an extensor became an important factor in vigorous locomotion.

Not only did bony structures change, but other parts of the body involved in movement—primarily the muscular and nervous systems—were also modified. Structure and function develop simultaneously; they are interrelated and to a great degree inbred. Man does not choose his structure; that is an inheritance from preceding species. The human is, as expressed by Howells, a modified fish. Neither are basic movement patterns chosen; they, too, are inherited. Within limits, structure can be modified by environment, exercise, and nutrition. Movements also have limitations imposed by inheritance of the structure of bone and joints, muscles, and nerve patterns. These can be modified but not basically changed.

Only when survival no longer depended on vigorous movement did humankind begin to think that such activity might be needed for its effect on body, action, and health. Such thinking led to the development of physical education programs and to efforts to understand human movement. Those programs in the United States in the late nineteenth century stressed gymnastics. These were not the vigorous, complex tumbling and apparatus events that comprise the gymnastics of today. They were largely simple movements, consisting of change of body positions, and were artificial forms, as opposed to inherent, /or natural, patterns.

An advocate of the gymnastic program and a student of movement was Dr. William Skarstrom, who published in 1909 *Gymnastic Kinesiology,* a compilation of articles that had appeared in the *Physical Education Review* in 1908 and 1909. This text is an analysis of muscle action and has had a dominant influence on kinesiology in this country. Later publications have not equaled this thorough and detailed description of muscle action in specific movements. A 1963 text, in describing a limited portion of an overarm throw, is probably less explicit in stating that, as the arm moves forward at the shoulder joint, contraction occurs in the greater pectoral, anterior deltoid, and coracobrachial muscles. As the arm rotates outward during the forward movement, the teres minor and the infraspinous muscles contract.

Skarstrom did not limit muscle analysis to naming the muscles that cross the acting joint; consideration was given to other aspects of muscle behavior. For example, he states that contraction of a muscle can cause more than one action at the joint that it crosses; the undesired joint actions must be prevented by opposing contractions; a muscle pulls on all bones to which it is attached, and again undesired movements must be prevented. Movements that Skarstrom analyzes may be simple in joint action but will be complex in muscle action. A simple movement described by Skarstrom is that of complete elbow flexion with the elbows close to the side combined with complete outward rotation of the humerus with hands as far back as possible at the shoulder. The performer will find difficulty in keeping the elbow close to the body. This is due to the abducting pull of the biceps, which has been named as one of the elbow flexors. To prevent shoulder abduction the latissimus dorsi will contract. This muscle will tend to pull the arm back beyond the desired position and to rotate the humerus medially. Other muscles will prevent the undesired actions, and the latissimus will then tend to pull on its other attachments, the pelvis and the lower spine. This may result in a "hollow-back" position, and this too will need counteraction.

Skarstrom's text is not a listing of muscles that cross a joint; it is an analysis of muscle interaction and an explanation of likely faults. It is based on the anatomic knowledge and keen observation of the author. He does not claim that his descriptions are accurate but only that "while personal experience or observation make me fairly confident . . . I . . . wish to disclaim any assumption of finality of judgment." Although gymnastics as advocated by Skarstrom has little or no place in today's physical education program, study of his text should be valuable to any student of kinesiology for its presentation on the complexity of muscle action and for suggestions or explanations of faults observed in present-day motor activities.

More influential in United States kinesiology than Skarstrom's text has been the work of Wilbur Bowen, a professor of physical education at Michigan State Normal College, Ypsilanti, Michigan. Bowen published in 1912 *The Action of Muscles in Bodily Movement and Posture,* a text to be used in teaching anatomy and kinesiology. With an understanding in these subjects one should be able to analyze any movement—in gymnastics, athletics, work, or everyday skills. Included in the text are brief descriptions of the structure of the skeletal, muscular, and nervous systems and a section on the mechanics of joint action, including leverage, direction of pull of a muscle, and the mechanical advantages of two joint muscles, especially in the lower limbs. In presenting the contributions of the nervous system to movement he says that frequently used acts become automatic; these acts consist of a series of reflexes, each one in the chain brought into action by impulses produced by the preceding reflex. The reflexes are built from inherited tendencies, which must be practiced to develop ease of movement.

However, there is little application of this basic information in the procedure recommended to use for analyzing a movement. To do so, said Bowen, one must know the joint actions involved, the bones acting as levers, the contracting muscles, and which of these "have the strongest work." Not many analyses were included in the text—only a few that were presented to illustrate the recommended procedure. Among these was analysis of the overarm throw. A portion of that is summarized as follows:

The humerus is drawn swiftly forward by the pectoral and anterior deltoid muscles; the scapula is moved forward by the serratus and smaller pectoral muscles; the elbow is flexed and then extended by first the flexor and then the triceps muscles. Those chiefly developed are the pectoral, triceps, anterior deltoid, and serratus muscles.

This analysis and others in the text suggest that the purpose was to identify the muscles that would be exercised by the movement. This is indeed the purpose of the text as stated by Bowen—that is, to enable the student to understand how certain types of exercise affect the development and form of the body.

These two pioneer kinesiologists had a common purpose: to develop a harmonious body structure through exercise. Skarstrom advocated achieving this through gymnastic exercises accurately executed in detail. Bowen suggested that any motor activity could be selected to strengthen specific muscles if the kinesiologist could analyze the act to identify the joint actions and the muscles that act strongly in these. The 1912 edition indicates that Bowen expected the student to identify joint actions. He suggested that the student analyze such activities as chopping with an ax, shooting with a bow and arrow, and the movements of the lower limb in climbing a rope. The purpose of the analysis was to identify muscles, not to improve the skill.

In the second quarter of the twentieth century physical education programs in this country gradually decreased the emphasis on gymnastics and increased the proportion of games and athletics used. That may explain why Skarstrom's *Gymnastic Kinesiology* was not published again and Bowen's text with its application to all motor skills was expanded and revised many times. The title was changed to *Applied Anatomy and Kinesiology* and later to *Kinesiology and Applied Anatomy*. For more than half a century the revisd Bowen book has been, and still is, used as a text.

Succeeding editions of Bowen's book added a new content to kinesiology. Whereas the 1912 edition did not include analyses of motor acts except as illustrations of procedure, the sixth edition, published in 1949 (revised by Stone), presents many analyses. These comprise a major portion of the book and include definite statements of occurring joint actions or descriptions from which the acting joints can be determined. This edition stated that to apply kinesiologic principles one must know what constitutes good form in the act to be studied. Included are analyses of posture and many skills used in work, sports, and locomotion. Each includes a description that one can assume represents the author's concept of good form; a section of a motion picture is presented as illustrating "perfect form."

Other differences in this edition are in the statement of kinesiologic purpose and in questioning the soundness of the then current mechanical and muscular analyses. The stated purpose was to improve motor performance through application of kinesiologic principles. Although mechanical analysis was essential for application, Elftman's studies of the kinetics of walking and running had demonstrated that much research of that type was needed before such analysis could be made with confidence. Also muscle analysis was questioned, since electromyographic studies had shown that only through such research could one determine which muscles were acting in what sequence and with what strength. The recommended procedures for 1949 parallel those of 1912: good form (joint action), leverage (mechanical analysis), and acting muscles (muscular analysis). The author (Bowen's revisor) questions the accuracy of mechanical and muscular analyses until substantiated by research but does not question the accuracy of descriptions of good form.

In the 1930s and during the following years the professions concerned with human movement placed increasing emphasis on improving motor skill. Physical educators, occupational and physical therapists, coaches, and dance instructors sought understanding of the human motor mechanism as a means of improving performance. This necessitated knowledge of the "goodness" of each specific skill.

These groups were not satisfied with descriptions of good form, such as those presented in the 1949 Bowen text. Among the objections to such descriptions was the lack of detail in the force-producing phase; usually detailed analyses of the preparatory (backswing) and final (follow-through) phases were presented. These could have many individual characteristics and might not affect the force-producing joint actions. The latter were usually executed too rapidly for the human eye to register adequately. Fortunately by this date, means of recording rapid action were available to supplement visual observation.

Among the methods for studying body movement is photography, which was developed in the middle of the nineteenth century. Early photographic techniques were not capable of registering movement and were used primarily to obtain pictures of landscapes and architectural and other inanimate objects. The exposure time for the first portrait, made in 1839, is reported to have been 30 minutes. Later inventors developed better lenses and chemicals that were more sensitive to light, and exposure time was shortened. In the 1870's the first efforts were made to study motion by means of photography. Leland Stanford, a former governor of California, might be called the first motion-picture producer. The actors were the governor's famous blooded horses. To satisfy his curiosity about foot sequence in the gaits of horses, he secured the services of a photographer, Eadweard Muybridge, and of a mechanical engineer, John Isaacs, who together planned the photographic arrangements that would provide evidence to answer the governor's questions. A series of cameras was spaced along the track on which the animals ran. Muybridge extended his observations to the movements of other animals—goats, cows, and pigs. Later at the University of Pennsylvania with the cooperation of the physical education director, Muybridge photographed men, women, and children as they executed everyday sports and industrial skills. His method required the use of several cameras to photograph one act. Placed side by side, the resulting photographs are like the reproductions of individual frames of present motion pictures. (See Fig. 2-1.)

In the 1880s Thomas Edison and his staff developed a camera that used coated celluloid film and also the equipment for projecting such film. Motion-picture techniques developed rapidly, and today many physical education departments have cameras that take pictures at the rate of 64 per second. Highly specialized equipment that requires exposures of only one thousandth or even one millionth of a second is available. With these higher speeds, the compression and subsequent elongation of tennis and golf balls and footballs as they are impacted may be photographed to show the importance of the follow-through of the racket, the club, and the foot. During recent years, kinesiologists have made increasing use of this photographic equipment and have reported details of motor skill that previously had not been observed. Students of kinesiology in many schools participate in photographing skills and thus become acquainted with details that should be considered and those which should be added to the photographic field to facilitate observation.

If range and speed of joint action are to be measured from film, one frame must be viewed at a time, and for convenience in working, the projector and

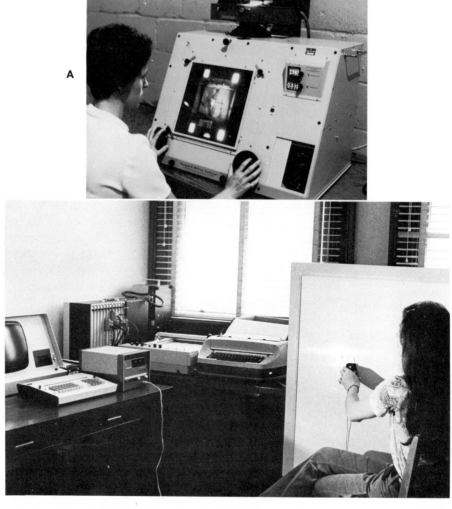

Fig. 1-3. A, Film motion analyzer. **B,** Analog-to-digital conversion equipment used to convert film data to digits. (**A** courtesy Pennsylvania State Biomechanics Laboratory; **B,** special equipment, Biomechanics Laboratory, Indiana University.)

the projected image should be within easy reach of the seated investigator. An apparatus devised by Glassow and Broer in 1938 permitted varying the size of the projection within a limited range. Its use was handicapped by the difficulty of obtaining a projector that could be held on one frame for a long period without burning or buckling the inflammable celluloid roll. Since that time such projectors have become available. One type is like the standard projector, and the image can be projected at distances of 10, to more than 50, feet. This type is valuable for group viewing but is not convenient for detailed measurements. Another type* meets the requirements of having projector and image within easy reach of the observer. The size of the image cannot be changed in this type; however, two models are available, one projecting three frames of 16 mm. film at a time and the other, one frame. With these models the range, speed, and sequence of joint action can be measured in detail.

A decrease in the amount of time involved in obtaining data from film is promised with the use of the Motion Analyzer,† now found in many universities. Fig. 1-3, *A,* shows the vertical projection of one frame within easy reach of the investigator. In successive frames, desired measurements, such as the position of the center of gravity of a body segment or the angle at a joint, can be made. Fig. 1-3, *B,* shows analog-to-digital conversion equipment used to convert film data to digits.

Such measurement is a laborious and time-consuming task and explains in part the limited investigations in which these devices have been used. Also problems arise when movement occurs in planes other than that of the picture; movement can be in three planes, whereas the picture is recorded in one. Side, front, back, and overhead cameras can be used to record movement in three planes. Mathematical procedures can be used to determine action when the angles to the camera are known. Both methods add to the labor and time required for detailed study. However, the recent use of computer and digitizing equipment makes this task much easier to accomplish. Also, during the years in which photographic devices for analyzing movement were developed, techniques for determining muscle action were being improved.

Observation of joint action can be facilitated with the use of the electrogoniometer (elgon), which was devised by Karpovich in the late 1950s. The elgon is essentially a goniometer with a potentiometer substituted for the protractor. The degrees of movement in the joint to which the device has been attached can be read directly from recording paper, thus eliminating laborious measurement. The device has been used with other methods of recording of movement, such as electromyography and cinematography. (An excellent description of the elgon and its application is presented by Adrian in the 1968 *Kinesiology Review.*)

The fallacies of analyzing muscle action on the basis of anatomic position were demonstrated by Duchenne in the middle of the nineteenth century. By electric stimulation of muscles combined with observation of partially paralyzed

---

*Recordak, Recordak Corporation, New York, N.Y.
†Vanguard Instrument Corporation, Melville, L.I., N.Y.

subjects, he described the movements resulting from contraction of specific muscles as they functioned in living subjects. Unfortunately his findings were not widely used in the United States, since they were published in French and were not readily available until translated in 1949 by Kaplan. By that time, investigators in the United States had begun to observe muscle action in living subjects by recording the electric changes that can be observed as muscles contract. The technique of recording, known as *electromyography,* has been greatly refined and, as complex motor acts are studied, will provide valuable information for the kinesiologist. The major current contributor to this development is J. V. Basmajian, a former Canadian, now located at Emory University in Atlanta, Georgia. His book *Muscles Alive* is a classic.

Kinesiologists have made progress in methods of observing participation of bone and muscle in movement; less advance has been made in methods of directly observing nerve participation. However, certain characteristics of nerve action have been observed. Stimulation of a given point of the brain has been shown to result in a pattern of joint action, demonstrating that movement patterns and not contraction of a single muscle are the result of activation of a given brain area. Observation of motor behavior of young children has shown not only reflex behavior but also in purposeful action certain movement patterns.

Since muscles normally contract only when stimulated by nerve impulses, students of movement should be familiar with the gross anatomy of the nervous system. They should know that these impulses arise not only volitionally but also from sources other than the mind. Nature has equipped human mechanisms with many inate neuromuscular responses that combine with voluntarily initiated acts. Information derived from neurophysiology and observations of child development give strength to the comment made by Tuttle, who said that many automatisms enable atheletes to use their bodies to the best advantage and that teachers should not tamper with these but attempt to use them.

Motor skill must be studied with the realization that it is not the result of the experiences of a single life-span. From birth to maturity each individual has at his command motor responses that will to some degree meet the needs of each growth stage. Such responses are the human heritage—gifts from ancestors, who bequeathed to their descendants bone, muscle, and nerve structure and motor behavior patterns that had proved to be valuable. Each bequest has a wise condition: the heir must use and exercise the gift to bring to fulfillment its potential value.

Two outstanding changes have been made in the study of kinesiology in this country since the beginning of this century. One is in the detail of information and means of observation. Today less reliance is placed on personal observation; muscle action can now be determined by electromyography and can show not only which muscles are acting but also the duration, sequence, and comparative strength of contraction. Joint action can be determined by the electrogoniometer and photography and can show range, sequence, and speed. The other change is in the primary purpose of kinesiologic study. Today that purpose is to understand the motor mechanism, its inherent functioning, and the contributions of bone, muscle, and nerve. With understanding, teacher and performer should be able to apply that which will lead to better achievement, whatever the goal.

Desire to understand has led to changes in kinesiologic content. Among these is the recognition that functioning of the nervous system is essential. Reflex and inherent patterns should be identified and their possible involvement in any movement recognized. Another addition is in the field of mechanics. With detailed recording of joint action one can determine acceleration of a body segment and possibly effective joint action in a skill. Skilled performers are not accepted as demonstrating patterns to be copied because of good form, but their actions are presented as those which produce the desired force. This avenue of study has interested mechanical engineers and has led to a study now called *biomechanics*.

With expanded study kinesiologists have become increasingly aware that many areas of study—anatomy, engineering, neurophysiology, physics, and physiology—must be consulted. From these they will select what is pertinent to understanding the motor mechanism, but they will remember that they have the responsibility to observe the mechanism in action. They will apply information derived from other fields of study, and this with knowledge derived from their own observations and calculations will constitute kinesiology.

In summary, kinesiology begins first with the observation of human motor behavior. Such observation includes details of joint action—range, speed, and sequence. Second, the student seeks understanding of these actions. This necessitates recourse to other fields of knowledge: to physics for mechanical and gravitational laws; to anatomy for the structures of bone, muscle, and nerve; and to physiology and neurophysiology for the action of muscle and nerve. From these observations and sources can be accumulated knowledge to guide all persons who attempt to improve motor skills.

SUGGESTED READINGS

Basmajian, J. V.: Muscles alive: their functions as revealed by electromyography, ed. 2, Baltimore, 1967, The Williams & Wilkins Co.

Krogman, W. M.: The scars of human evolution, Sci. Am. **185**:54, Dec., 1951.

Morton, D. J., and Fuller, D. D.: Human locomotion and body form, Baltimore, 1952, The Williams & Wilkins Co.

Napier, J.: The antiquity of human walking, Sci. Am. **216**:56, April, 1967.

See Bibliography for additional references.

CHAPTER 2 Contributions: past and current

In this chapter the origin and development of kinesiology are briefly traced chronologically and logically. The history of kinesiology has been reviewed by many persons (among whom are Braun, Hirt, and Rasch and Burke), and mention of it may be found in treatises and medical histories. Kinesiology reaches back to the first scientific concepts of movement that humanity was able to comprehend, although some of the basic ideas had been known and used since antiquity. Its roots are certainly deep in the beginnings of medical history.

ANCIENT ERA

The Greeks were among the first to practice so-called scientific thinking, as opposed to that based on emotional and spiritual ideas. Hippocrates (460-370 B.C.) advocated the concept that people should base their observations on and draw conclusions from only what they perceived through their senses (particularly those of touch, sight, hearing and smell) without recourse to the supernatural. One of Hippocrates' contemporaries, the Greek scholar Herodicus, was interested in gymnastics (exercise through active volition) as a means of curing disease. In fact, he prescribed it for fever patients and was criticized by Hippocrates for doing so.

Aristotle (384-322 B.C.) has been called *the father of kinesiology*. More than three centuries before Christ, Aristotle wrote, "The animal that moves makes its change of position by pressing against that which is beneath it. Hence, athletes jump farther if they have the weights in their hands than if they have not, and runners run faster if they swing their arms, for in extension of the arms there is a kind of leaning upon the hands and wrists."* Hart said, "From the point of view of mechanics, we may regard Aristotle's work as the starting point of a chain of thought which played an important part in the evolution of the subject up to the days of Leonardo da Vinci."† Hart is of the opinion that many of da Vinci's beliefs were based on Aristotle's principles.

Aristotle made his many observations in almost every field of science. Students of kinesiology are especially impressed with his treatise *Parts of Animals, Move-*

*Aristotle: Parts of animals, movement of animals, and progression of animals, Cambridge, Mass., 1945, Harvard University Press.
†Hart, I.: The mechanical investigations of Leonardo da Vinci, London, 1925, Chapman & Hall, Ltd.

14

ment of Animals, and Progression of Animals. Today's physical education activity teachers, athletic instructors, physical therapists, and industrial engineers, along with all persons who are concerned with the observation and study of human beings in motion, use some of the basic principles of Aristotle. In fact, the good modern teacher of movement makes use of the techniques of close observation as a means of evaluation. Certainly Aristotle's concepts of muscular flexion and the part that it plays in movements such as walking are a good foundation for modern studies on gait and other movements involving the transformation of rotatory motion to translatory motion.

The Greeks love of the perfect mind and body led to participation in athletics and interest in body building (for physical, as well as for therapeutic, development) as a part of the development of the whole being, a concept that has been revived in modern educational philosophy. The ideas expressed by Aristotle were the forerunners of the ideas of Newton, Borelli, and others. His concepts of leverage, gravity, and laws of motion were remarkably accurate.

Archimedes (287-212 B.C.), a renowned mathematician, established the basic principles that undergird the present knowledge of floating bodies—in water, as well as in outer space. Heath has stated that Archimedes' treatise on determining the the center of gravity is the foundation of modern theoretical mechanics. To show his personality and dedication, two stories (even though they probably are not true) are apropos here. As Heath said, "Of the same kind is the well-known story that, when discovered in a bath, the solution of the question referred to him by Hieron as to whether a certain crown supposed to have been made of gold did not in reality contain a certain proportion of silver, he ran through the street to his home shouting 'Eureka! Eureka!' "* The solution that he had arrived at while he was in the bath was that gold was heavier than silver.

Another comment attributed to him is in connection with his solution of the following problem: *to move a given weight by a given force.* He said, "Give me a place to stand on, and I can move the earth."* He was explaining his solution to Hieron. By means of a compound pulley Archimedes moved a ship that many people were unable to launch. Even though the language seems awkward, postulate 1 of Archimedes illustrates his concepts of floating bodies: "Let it be supposed that a fluid is of such a character that, its parts lying evenly and being continuous, that part which is thrust the less is driven along by that which is thrust the more; and each of its parts is thrust by the fluid which is above it in a perpendicular direction if the fluid be sunk in anything and compressed by anything else."* Another comment, proposition 5, is worth repeating: "Any solid lighter than a fluid will, if placed in the fluid, be so far immersed that the weight of the solid will be equal to the weight of the fluid displaced."*

The Romans, who were not averse to recognizing and using the best from the culture of the nations that they conquered, brought home the concepts of Greek medicine. Galen (A.D. 131-201), who was physican to the gladiators of

---

*Heath, T. L.: The works of Archimedes, Cambridge, England, 1897, Cambridge University Press.

Marcus Aurelius some two centuries after the birth of Christ, brought the science of anatomy to Rome. His discoveries and forthright attitude made him the outstanding anatomist and physiologist until the sixteenth century. He dissected many animals, including the ape, to gather information about anatomy and physiology. However, in his capacity as trainer to the gladiators Galen probably offered advice on the proper procedure to use in conditioning for the arena, and he had the opportunity to observe parts of the human body laid open in mortal combat. He used many modern physiologic terms, such as *agonist* and *antagonist,* in reference to muscular contraction. In fact, Galen developed much terminology still in use in certain biologic science fields. However, the basic principle of Galen's physiologic concept was that a spirit drawn from the general "world spirit" entered the body and proceeded through the normal channels to the bloodstream; this spirit constituted the working system of the human body. This idea prevailed until the time of Harvey (1578-1657).

As time went by, the Romans began to neglect the body and even to look with scorn on physical development. They enjoyed watching combats between human beings and animals purely as entertainment, and this attitude influenced Greek culture also. No longer was it believed necessary to develop the body.

EARLY CHRISTIAN ERA

During the Middle Ages in Europe, physical exercise and bodily development were considered to be of little importance, and investigation into the human makeup was neglected. Ludwig Joseph believed that the poor economic situation was another one of the reasons for the declining interest in physical exercise. He stated that during the medieval, as well as the Renaissance, periods people did not have as much material wealth as had the early Greeks and Romans; therefore time for leisure pursuits was not available. As a consequence, during this period little was added to the scientific knowledge of bodily development beyond the contributions of Galen. Hirt gives credit to the Arabs as the true scientists of the Middle Ages because they kept the ancient Greek concepts from perishing. When these concepts were revived, they had to be translated from Arabic into Latin.

RENAISSANCE PERIOD

The scientific awakening known as the *Renaissance* was perhaps initiated and epitomized by the work of Leonardo da Vinci (1452-1519), who is given credit for developing the modern science of anatomy. He studied human structure, especially noting the relation of the center of gravity to balance and motion during different movements. He made these observations while he was developing a treatise on painting. To be sure that his drawings of the body were authentic, da Vinci secured and dissected hundreds of cadavers. Many other great artists of the Renaissance, such as Michelangelo Buonarroti and Raphael, were more than casually interested in the composition and makeup of the human body. They had a great urge to be able to portray the muscular and skeletal portions of the body accurately on canvas in a realistic way. Leonardo da Vinci, one of the world's greatest scientists, was adept in many fields and blended the artistic with the scientific in a way never since duplicated. According to several historians da Vinci was the greatest engineer, biologist, and artist of his time. Robinson stated that da Vinci was one of the first to break away from the acceptance of Galen as the only authority. He was severely criticized by his contemporaries because he did not blindly follow noted authorities. Leonardo da Vinci said, "I do not know how to quote from learned authorities, but it is a much greater and more estimable matter to rely on experience. They scorn me who am a discoverer; yet how much more do they deserve censure who have never found out anything, but only recite and blazen forth other people's works."*

Da Vinci's ability to draw the action of the muscles when the human body was performing a dynamic act was of great value to medical students and to the science of kinesiology. Da Vinci's intelligence and versatility are exemplified in the following quotations from his treatise *On the Flight of Birds,* as translated by Hart.

> When the edge of the point of the wing is opposed to the edge of the wind for an instant, I put this wing under or on this edge of the wind and the same thing happens to the point or sides of the tail, and similarly to the shaft of the shoulders of the wing.
> The descent of a bird will aways be that (part W) extremity which will be nearest to its center of gravity.
> The heaviest part of a bird descending will be always in front of its centre of resistance.
> If the wing and the tail are too much on the wind, lower half of the opposite wing, and therewith receive the force of the wind and equilibruim will be restored.†

Modern pilots use the same method of lowering a wing in righting a plane in flight.

Da Vinci's observations on human action in a specific movement show his insight. He said, "He who descends takes short steps because the weight rests upon the hinder foot. And he who mounts takes long steps because his weight remains on the forward foot."‡

Since da Vinci's scientific contributions were hidden from the world for many years (200 to 300 years after his death) and only recently have been discovered and published, it was left to others to add to human knowledge in this area. Andreas Vesalius (1514-1564), considered to be the developer of the modern concept of anatomy, was one of them. His drawings, which portray muscles in action in a living moving human being, are in keeping with the spirit of the Renaissance.

MODERN ERA

Luigi Galvani (1737-1798), a professor of anatomy at the University of Bologna, Italy, made the discovery that was the forerunner of the concept of the

---

*Robinson, V.: The story of medicine, New York, 1943, Doubleday & Co., Inc.
†Hart, I.: The mechanical investigations of Leonardo da Vinci, London, 1925, Chapman & Hall, Ltd.
‡O'Malley, C. D., and Saunders, J. B. de C. M.: Leonardo da Vinci on the human body, New York, 1952, Henry Schuman, Inc., Publishers.

irritability of muscles. During experiments on muscle and nerve preparations he noted the contraction of muscles when the leg of a frog contacted metal and devised an arc of two metals with which contractions could be induced. Francis Glisson (1597-1677) had earlier demonstrated through plethysmographic experiments that muscles do contract, rather than expand, as Borelli had thought, and that viable tissue had the capacity to react to certain stimuli. The concept of the independent irritability and excitability of muscle tissue was finally brought into clear focus by the Swiss Albrecht von Haller (1708-1777), perhaps the greatest physiologist of the eighteenth century. He first propounded the idea that contractility is an innate property of muscle.

After the discovery of the concept of muscle irritability by Galvani and further clarification and development by von Haller, new information on muscle action became available.

The greatest investigator in this area was Guillaume Benjamin Amand Duchenne (1806-1875), who devoted much of his time and effort to discovering the function of isolated muscles by stimulating them electrically, even though he realized that in actual movement muscles seldom act in isolation. Kaplan considered *Physiologie des Mouvements,* published in 1865 by Duchenne, to be one of the greatest books of all times. The English-speaking world did not have access to this book until it was translated in 1949.

The present theory of resistive exercises is based on the contributions of Adolf Eugen Fick (1829-1901); in his studies of the mechanics of muscular movement he evolved the terms *isotonic* and *isometric*. Wilhelm Roux (1850-1924) published the concept that muscle hypertrophy develops only after muscles have been worked extensively. Later Siebert proved this theory experimentally. Steinhaus gives Morpurgo credit for showing that increased strength and hypertrophy result from an increase in the diameter of the individual fibers, not from an increase in their number.

The development of certain new instruments to study human physical actions greatly aided the field of kinesiology. Particularly significant were such devices as the ergograph, invented by Mosso (1843-1910), and the galvanometer, developed by Einthoven in 1906. The latter opened up the field of electromyography as a means of studying the amplitude and duration of electric impulses generated by muscles in action. By this means it became possible to determine if muscles long thought to be the ones in action during a certain movement were really activated. Some concepts were substantiated, and others were refuted.

A method of determining the presence or absence of muscular tension by the amount of muscle hardening was developed by Stetson and others. This helped in understanding the ballistic concept of muscular contraction.

Many physiologists have contributed to the kinesiologist's background knowledge. Perhaps the name of Archibald Hill should stand out. His work on muscular activity is an outstanding contribution.

Vesalius's publication of *De Humani Corporis Fabrica* (The Fabric of the Human Body) in 1543 marked the beginning of modern science according to many historians. Saunders and O'Malley consider this book the greatest single contribution to the medical sciences, "an exquisite piece of creative art with its perfect blend of format, typography, and illustration."* The drawings give an idea of the magnitude of the work. One of the drawings is a small text figure illustrating the function of particular ligaments, such as the transverse ligament of the ankle, in preventing a tendon from rising out of its bed during the act of contraction. Vesalius was a prodigious investigator and worker, but he needed the help of a good artist and also subjects, and Saunders and O'Malley have quoted him as saying, "Wherefore, if the opportunity of bodies offers, and Jan Stefan (Van Kalkar), outstanding artist of our age, does not refuse his services, I shall by no means evade that labor."*

The basis for the mechanical analysis of movement was established by Galileo (1564-1642) and Newton (1642-1727). Newton's three laws of motion are in use today and, aside from not being applicable in some aspects of space travel, are as valid as they were during his day, as Sullivan has noted. Singer said, "With Newton the universe acquired an independent rationality, and the whole cosmology of Aristotle, of Galen, and of the Middle Ages lay in the dust."†

Galileo, who lived in that era of scientific discoverers, was a noted mathematician and astronomer. Although he is known as one of the exponents of natural law and invented two instruments, the telescope and microscope, his contributions to the field of kinesiology are enormous. According to Cooper, he is credited with "laying firm the foundation of mechanics." Galileo's alleged experiments on the rate of acceleration of falling bodies, supposedly demonstrated in 1590 or 1591 from the leaning tower of Pisa, laid the basis for the present concept about the rate of falling objects in sports and athletics. The possibility that this concept may have been developed in a demonstration some years earlier by a man named Stevin is immaterial. Cooper claimed that in all his writings Galileo never once mentioned the leaning tower of Pisa. On the other hand, Simon Stevin, by his own admission, did drop two weights, one ten times the weight of the other, from a height of 30 feet, and they seemed almost to land with one thump. He and a friend were attempting to show that Aristotle had been mistaken in certain of his concepts of physics. It was J. J. Fahie, a well-known English writer on Galileo, who gave Galileo credit for this experiment. Fahie stated, "Nearly two thousand years before, Aristotle had asserted that if two different weights of the same material were let fall from the same height the heavier would reach the ground sooner than the lighter in the proportion of their weights."‡ Neither Stevin nor Aristotle was talking about objects falling in a vacuum; they both discounted or ignored air resistance.

In search of the reasons that certain physical phenomena occur Galileo turned to the fields of mechanics and mathematics and opened new horizons for scholars who studied human movement. One of Galileo's pupils, Giovanni Alfonso Borelli

---

*Saunders, J. B. de C. M., and O'Malley, C. D., editors: The illustrations from the works of Andreas Vesalius, New York, 1950, World Publishing Co.
†Singer, C.: A short history of medicine, London, 1928, Oxford University Press.
‡Steindler, A.: Kinesiology of the human body under normal and pathological conditions, Springfield, Ill., 1955, Charles C Thomas, Publisher.

(1608-1679), combined the sciences of mathematics, physics, and anatomy in the first treatise on kinesiology, *De Motu Animalium,* published in 1680. He applied Galileo's mathematical principles to movement. Steindler believes that Borelli should be considered the father of modern biomechanics and supports his ideas by saying that "the essential feature of kinesiology is that it treats all motor functions, normal and abnormal, as mechanical events."* Others, among them Singer, regard Borelli as the founder of the physiologic concept that the human muscular system is governed by mechanical laws.

Borelli recognized that bones serve as levers and are moved by muscles in accordance with mathematical laws, and he also believed that the movements of animals are affected by other forces, such as air and water resistance and good or poor mechanical position. Because of these beliefs Hirt called Borelli the father of modern kinesiology. Borelli has even been given credit for discovering the reciprocal action of muscles, a concept that Sherrington is thought to have conceived much later. However, his concept that muscles in action enlarge, instead of contract, did not long prevail. Being an eminent mathematician stirred by Galileo's work, which gave a mathematical expression to mechanical events, Borelli attempted to do the same thing with the movements made by the animal body. Singer says, "He endeavored, with some success, to extend mechanical principles to such movements as the flight of birds and the swimming of fish."†

The Weber brothers investigated the influence of gravity on limb movements in walking and running. Gravity is often the force that propels a walker forward, causing a fall unless balance is reestablished. They were also among the first scholars to study the path of the center of gravity during movement.

Perhaps one of the greatest contributors to the field of kinesiology in the area of efficiency of work and body mechanics was Jules Amar. He wrote *The Human Motor,* which was an attempt to bring to the reader all the known physiologic and kinesiologic principles involved in industrial work and in the performance of certain sports movements. Amar's book was translated into English in 1920 and is now out of print and available to students only on Microcards.‡

Many people then followed in the steps of Amar, making use of the principles of good body mechanics in the performance of tasks. Among those who contributed in this area are Goldthwaite, who wrote on body mechanics in connection with health and disease, and Steindler, who published *Mechanics of Normal and Pathological Locomotion in Man* in 1935 and a larger and more complete volume involving some of the same ideas, *Kinesiology of the Human Body Under Normal and Pathological Conditions,* in 1955. Steindler's works have become classics in the field.

The ideas from the earlier writers were next applied by scientists to the field of human engineering. These persons worked in industry and government. Much

*Steindler, A.: Kinesiology of the human body under normal and pathological conditions, Springfield, Ill., 1955, Charles C Thomas, Publisher.
†Singer, C.: A short history of medicine, London, 1928, Oxford University Press.
‡Microcard Publications, School of Health, Physical Education and Recreation, University of Oregon, Eugene, Ore.

information is available to the student in such publications as those of Woodson and the handbook published by Tufts College. The study of body forms, including those of the lower animals, aided the kinesiologist in the quest for knowledge about human beings. Such investigators as Morton, Darwin, Hooten, Krogman, and Howell made valuable contributions.

Goldthwaite and Steindler's ideas were then transmitted from a static to a dynamic concept. McCloy, Fenn, Cureton, Schwartz, Elftman, Karpovich, and others were interested in the mechanics of human movement and advanced the field of kinesiology into a new era.

How the formation of the bony architecture of the body took place and the influences that helped mold it have been the subject of study by numerous persons throughout the development of kinesiology. For example, Karl Culmann (1821-1881), trained as an engineer, developed a hypothesis that led to the trajectory theory of the architecture of bones. This led Julius Wolff (1836-1902) to develop his famous law: "Bones in their external and internal architecture conform with the intensity and direction of the stresses to which they are habitually subjected."* The Wolff concept that bone is formed through the tension of muscles and pressure of the weight of the body coupled with gravitational pull constitutes the major thesis of current authorities on skeletal development. Such investigators as Kock and Corey refuted some of Wolff's concepts and supported others.

A French physiologist, Étienne Jules Marey (1830-1904), was so interested in human movement that he developed photographic means for use in biologic research. In his works *Du Mouvement dans les Fonctions de la Vie* and *De Mouvement,* he explained and illustrated how this could be accomplished. Some of the translated works include the history of chronophotography and lectures on the phenomenon of flight in the animal world. Marey, as well as Robinson, was convinced that movment was the important human function and affected all other activities.

Eadweard Muybridge (1831-1904), through his photographic skill, brought a new tool to kinesiologic investigation. He was motivated by the work of Janssen, an astronomer who had been successful in taking sequential pictures of stars. Among the numerous Muybridge publications was an eleven-volume work, *Animal Locomotion* (1887). A recent publication called *The Human Figure in Motion* contains much of his original work. Using twenty-four fixed cameras and two portable batteries of twelve cameras each, Muybridge was able to take pictures of animals (Fig. 2-1) and people in action, and by using the zoopraxiscope he could move the pictures fast enough that actual movement was simulated. To illustrate how an idea may be developed Muybridge modified this device by mounting transparencies made from a series of his photographs on a circular glass plate. When the plate was rotated, individual transparencies could be projected by a projection lantern in the usual manner. A major refinement of the device was the addition of a second plate, made of metal and mounted parallel

*Sherrington, C.: Man on his nature, ed. 2, Garden City, N.Y., 1953, Doubleday & Co., Inc.

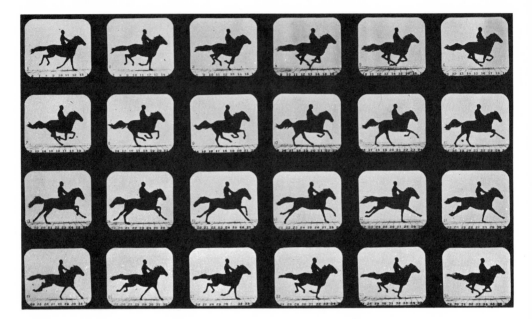

Fig. 2-1. Motion of a running horse. Subject is Phryne L, whose length of stride was reported to be 19 feet 9 inches. (Courtesy Stanford Museum.)

to the glass plate on a concentric axis but turning in the opposite direction. The metal plate was slit at appropriate intervals. When the two plates revolved, the metal plate served as a shutter. The persistence of vision between each slit gave the viewer the illusion of motion as each individual picture in the series was projected. As many as two hundred transparencies could be mounted on a single plate, and the wheels, or plates, could be revolved endlessly, "a period limited only by the patience of the spectators."*

The accomplishments of Marey and Muybridge paved the way for two German scientists, Christian Wilhelm Braune (1831-1892) and Otto Fischer (1861-1917), to study the human gait by means of photographic devices. They also developed an experimental method to determine the center of gravity of the human body. In 1889, these two outstanding German anatomists published a comprehensive paper on an experimental method that they had developed to determine the center of gravity of the human body. Fick, who followed, drew on their work; he eventually became one of the outstanding authorities in the field of joint mechanics. Today's concepts on posture appear to have had their origin in the experiments of Braune and Fischer. Earlier methods of locating the center of gravity of the human body had proved to be ineffective, and Braune and Fischer introduced modifications of some procedures. First, they conceived of a way of freezing a dead body so that it remained unchanged while they made mathematical calculations. Second, they compared the frozen posture of a cadaver

*Muybridge, E.: The human figure in motion, New York, 1955, Dover Publications, Inc.

with the posture of a living person and found the two postures to be markedly similar. They located the center of gravity not only of the body as a whole but also of each component part. They were the first to estimate the percentage of the weights of body segments. After they located the center of gravity of the total body of the frozen cadavers, they cut two of them into body segments and located the center of gravity of each. Much of their work involved the use of photographic apparatus to obtain the evidence that they needed for locating the midpoints of a joint and the axes of rotation, as stated by Hirt and co-workers.

Persons such as Broca (1824-1880), Jackson (1834-1911), and Ferrier did a great deal to localize the functions of the brain, including the motor center, as shown in the work by F. S. Taylor. Beevor gives Jackson credit for the aphorism "Nervous centers know nothing of muscles; they only know of movements."[*] Beevor helped classify muscles into prime movers, synergic muscles, fixators, and antagonists. He believed that the antagonists often relax in strong resistive movements. Beevor used electric stimulation of muscles to help formulate some of his conclusions.

According to Steindler two events had great influence in the field of kinesiology: the development of the theory of the reciprocal innervation of muscles, for which Charles Sherrington (1857-1952) is given credit, and the all-or-none theory of muscular contraction, accredited to Henry P. Bowditch (1814-1911). These men, especially Sherrington in *Man on His Nature,* upheld the value of studying the human body at a time when it was considered a degrading task. His comment on "motor man" is apropos: "The motor individual is driven from two sources. The world around it and its own lesser world within. It can be regarded as a system which in virtue of its arrangement does a number of things and is so constructed that the world outside touches triggers for their doing. But its own internal condition has a say as to which of those things within limits it will do, and how it will do them. Its own internal condition is also initiator of some of its acts."[†]

New devices for studying movement are currently being used by many investigators. Among these are the electron microscope, the higher speeds in photography (thousands up to 1 million frames per second), the electronic stroboscope, the light-tracing system mounted on the subject's limbs, force plates, telemeters, and the electromyograph. Computers are being used to calculate relationships between numerical measurements that are programmed for it. (See Garrett and co-workers.) Nelson of Pennsylvania State University has used a device that makes measurements directly from the film and will feed them directly into the computer.

The search for the answer to why human beings respond as they do in accomplishing movements has intrigued people from numerous disciplines. Weiner

[*]Beevor, C.: The Croonian Lectures on muscular movements, delivered at the Royal College of Physicians of London, London, 1903, Macmillan Publishers, Ltd.
[†]Sherrington, C.: Man on his nature, ed. 2, Garden City, N.Y., 1953, Doubleday & Co., Inc.

has presented many new concepts on how and why humans act as they do under certain conditions and situations. For example, his comparison of the eye and ear in relation to the size of the portion of the brain allotted to their functions helps in understanding reactions to various stimuli. Investigators such as Fay, van der Berg, and Strauss were more interested in mental behavior as it affects the physical or psychosomatic aspects of the field of human movement or both.

Kinesthesis has been explored by many people, but as yet no satisfactory practical application in all situations has been discovered. H'Doubler, Pear, Henry, Mumby, and Scott are but a few of those who contributed to the knowledge of kinesthesis. Much additional research is needed. It is a rich field that invites exploration.

Ellfeldt and Metheny explain their understanding of kinesiology as follows: "a tentative general theory of the meaning of human movement—kinesthesia as a somatic-sensory experience which can be conceptualized by the human mind."* These authors have developed a vocabulary to describe general movements common to all human beings—structural, perceptual, and conceptual movements.

Other vocabularies or notation systems to describe movement have been devised. One of the earliest was that of Laban, whose notation considers time, space, and effort changes in movement primarily for use in teaching dance. Later he extended this system of notation to include the movements of industrial workers. Although such a concept appeals to students of movement, many are not satisfied with the Laban system and have suggested or devised others. Among those published in *Kinesiography,* which is also concerned primarily with dance, by Canna and Loring. Others are attempting to develop a system for dance or to find one that can be applied to sports and especially to gymnastics. A recent article on movement notation systems by Kleinman† mentions three such systems.

Much investigation and research concerning the physiologic and kinesiologic principles of space travel are expected to be forthcoming. One example of a start along these lines is a book by Gartmann, written somewhat in lay language but mentioning many of the principles that are or will be used in space travel.

KINESIOLOGY BOOKS

The textbooks published in the United States in the field of kinesiology include many outstanding contributions. The main sections of Posse's *The Special Kinesiology of Educational Gymnastics* are devoted to descriptions of gymnastic exercises, and the appendix includes a list of the muscles involved in certain joint movements. Skarstrom's *Gymnastic Kinesiology* is a more scientific treatise on kinesiology. Three years later Bowen published *The Action of Muscles in Bodily Movement and Posture,* which was soon expanded by Bowen and Mc-Kenzie into *Applied Anatomy and Kinesiology.* This book, revised many times, was used widely as a text for more than two decades. Wright's *Muscle Function*

---

*Ellfeldt, L., and Metheny, E.: Movement and meaning: development of a general theory, Res. Q. Am. Assoc. Health Phys. Educ. 29:264, 1958.
†Kleinman, S.: Movement notation systems, Quest, p. 33, Jan., 1975.

was widely used at one time by students in the study of the action of muscles. A book by one of us (R. B. G.), *The Fundamentals of Physical Education,* was written to show the relationship of scientific concepts to the understanding of movement.

McKenzie, in a book published in 1933, emphasized the action of muscles. Hawley stressed the action of the muscles in sports movements.

A departure from earlier concepts was Scott's *Analysis of Human Movement,* involving the study of movement to help understand and improve motor performance. Another author, Lipovetz, attempted to analyze many human actions. Anatomic drawings showing the muscles that act in moving body levers in sports and everyday movements were produced by Kranz and later revised by Thompson. Wells, in *Kinesiology,* stressed muscles and joint action, and Morehouse and Cooper (*Kinesiology*) stressed the analysis of sports movements. Morton and Fuller, in *Human Locomotion and Body Form,* made an outstanding contribution toward understanding the why and how of human locomotion. Stone and then Rasch and Burke revised the Bowen and McKenzie text, each emphasizing a slightly different aspect. It is believed that we were the first to harmonize kinesiology in a strict and technical sense with the kinesiology of sports movements, now called *biomechanics* by many.* Duvall related kinesiology to the nursing field. Bunn, Broer, and Dyson stressed the mechanics of sports movements. Recently published books dealing with kinesiology and biomechanics are those by Barham and Thomas; Jensen and Schultz; Karger; Kelly; Logan and McKinney; Plagenhoef; Tricker and Tricker; Barham and Wooten; Hay; Groves and Camaione; Hopper; Lewillie; Miller and Nelson; Nelson and Morehouse; Krause and Barham; Northrip and co-workers; O'Connell and Gardner; Sweigard; Vredenbregt and Wartenweiler; and Wartenweiler and associates. (See Bibliography at end of text.)

Perhaps the richest source of new information is in the proceedings of the Biomechanics Symposia and the best doctoral dissertations, along with the articles found in certain scientific journals.

KINESIOLOGIC AND BIOMECHANICS RESEARCH

The past decade has seen that an outstanding growth in the amount and quality of kinesiologic research and an increase in the variety of equipment used to study human motor behavior. Some equipment has been developed by investigators for problems that they wished to solve; some has been borrowed from other disciplines—sometimes without modification and sometimes adapted to kinesiologic needs. Educational institutions are providing well-equipped laboratories for the study of human movement. Kinesiologists on many campuses are finding colleagues in other departments willing to share their technical skills and equipment; among these have been anatomists, engineers, mathematicians, physicists, physiologists, and psychologists.

---

*Nelson, R. C.: The new world of biomechanics of sport, presented at the 75th Annual Convention of the National College Physical Education Association for Men, New Orleans, Jan. 10, 1972.

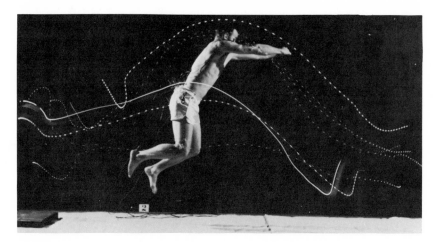

Fig. 2-2. Stroboscopic photography. Film is exposed in semidarkness, while flashing lights record path of lights during action. One instant of illumination of entire field shows position of subject. (Courtesy Motor Learning Research Laboratory, University of Wisconsin.)

The variety of methods and equipment used to study human movement is given in the following outline and in Figs. 2-2 to 2-4.

A. Photography
1. Cinematography is widely used at a speed of 64 frames per second, which is not fast enough to record details of some fast actions, such as those of the hand. Cameras with speeds of up to 10,000 frames or more per second are now available.
2. Stroboscopic photography uses multiple exposures on a single negative, which may be exposed to a brightly lighted or a dark background and subject. In the first case the exposures are determined by the opening of the camera shutter at a set rate. In the second, small electric light bulbs are attached to points on the body. These may be lighted continuously, providing a line of light on the photograph, or they may flash at a set rate, providing a series of dots on the photograph. (See Fig. 2-2.)*
3. X rays, or fluoroscopic rays, are synchronized with a camera, so that bones are filmed in action.

B. Force platforms
The simplest of these is the gravity board, used to find the position of the center-of-gravity line (Fig. 12-1). Starting blocks can be connected with electronic devices for measuring the amount and timing of force applied in the takeoff for a run. Platforms can be connected with strain gauges to measure the force exerted by the subject on the platform in sideward, downward, and forward and backward directions (Figs. 2-3 and 2-5).

*See also Merriman, J. S.: Stroboscopic photography as a research instrument, Res. Q. Am. Assoc. Health Phys. Educ. 46:256, May, 1975.

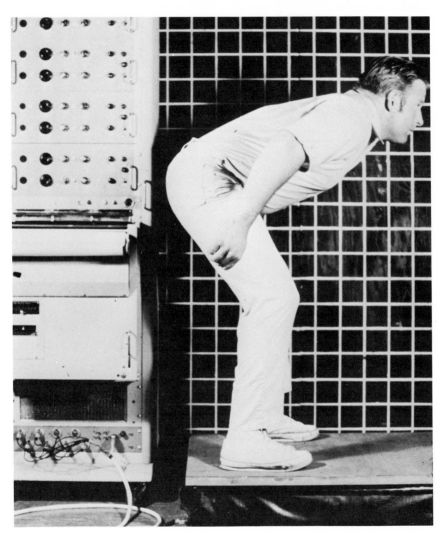

Fig. 2-3. Three-dimensional force platform and eight-channel recorder. This recorder is effective only in slow action. (Courtesy Indiana University Biomechanics Laboratory.)

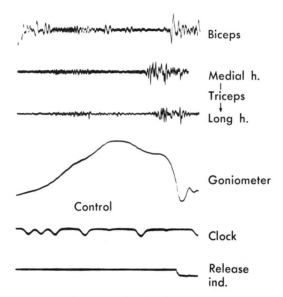

Fig. 2-4. Simultaneous records obtained with four types of equipment show muscle action, joint action, time, and release of ball. (From Dobbins, D. A.: Thesis, University of Wisconsin, 1970.)

C. Electromyography
   Visual records of muscle action derived from electric action in muscles with the use of electrodes attached to the skin or inserted in the muscles (Fig. 2-4)
D. Goniometer
   Device attached to body segments on either side of a joint. Sections moved by joint action, range, and speed are recorded (Fig. 2-4).
E. Aids to photographic study
   1. Motion Analyzer, projection device to facilitate measurements taken from film; measurements may be recorded on program cards for computer processing (Fig. 1-3, *A*). These are now being supplanted by an analog-to-digital conversion system. This enables the investigator to project film onto a digitizing board and with programmable calculator, typewriter, **plotter**, and minicomputer setup get much meaningful data in a short time. (See Fig. 1-3, *B*.)
   2. Mirror to provide for multiple-plane pictures
   3. Timing devices, included in the picture (Fig. 6-1)
F. Tridimensional devices and processes
   1. Three cameras set on the same focal point (Atwater's dissertation and Spray's thesis)
   2. Gamma ray scanner to determine volume
   3. Laser-beam holography to secure tridimensional information (Fig. 2-6)
   4. Computerized axial tomography, or layer-by-layer radiography (The scanner produces three-dimensional information.)
G. Laser beam to measure velocity (Fig. 2-7)

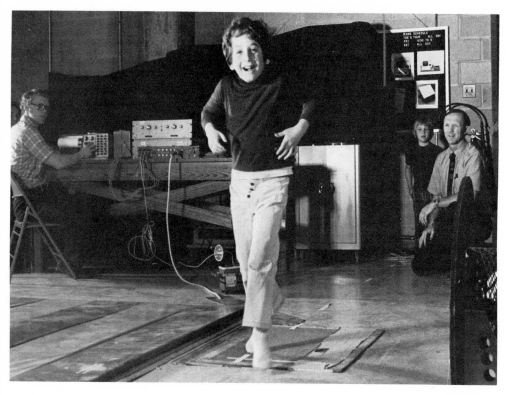

Fig. 2-5. Force platform is in a well. Oscillograph light recorder and accessories shown on the left are used in fast action. Handicapped children were used as subjects in this study.

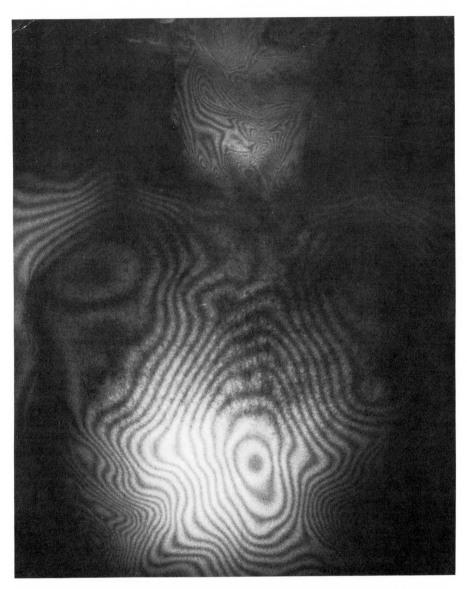

Fig. 2-6. Photograph of motion of a human chest during exhalation. The interferogram was made by ruby laser holography in which the laser was double pulsed while the subject exhaled rapidly into a tube. The image seen is three-dimensional reconstruction of the subject. Interpretation of a photograph of holographic interferogram of a subject requires mathematical analysis involving dark fringe lines in the image, which reveals the amount of movement by representing the displacement of light wavelengths. Future use may include measurements of instantaneous surface velocity distributions in complex motions. (Courtesy S. M. Zivi TRW Instruments, Redondo Beach, Calif.)

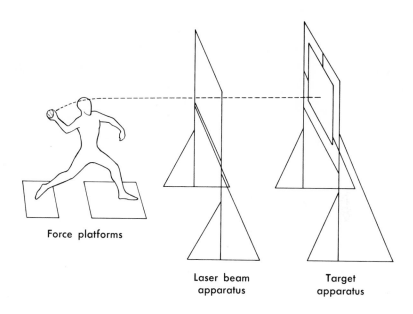

Force platforms

Laser beam
apparatus

Target
apparatus

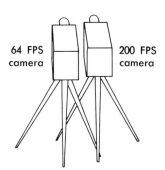

64 FPS
camera

200 FPS
camera

Fig. 2-7. A, Laser beam arrangement for determining velocity of a thrown ball. (Drawing of experimental setup used by Jack Sanders in a study at Indiana University in 1975.)

Continued.

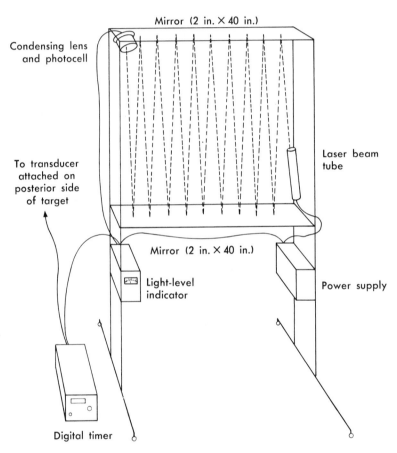

Mirror (2 in. × 40 in.)

Condensing lens
and photocell

To transducer
attached on
posterior side
of target

Laser beam
tube

Mirror (2 in. × 40 in.)

Light-level
indicator

Power supply

Digital timer

Fig. 2-7, cont'd. B, Laser beam arrangement for determining velocity of a thrown ball. (Drawing by Jack Sanders, showing apparatus used in his study at Indiana University in 1975.)

SUGGESTED READINGS

Amar, J.: The human motor, New York, 1920, E. P. Dutton & Co., Inc.

Aristotle: Parts of animals, movements of animals, and progression of animals, Cambridge, Mass., 1945, Harvard University Press.

Atwater, A. E.: Movement characteristics of overarm throw; a kinematic analysis of men and women performers, unpublished doctoral dissertation, 1971, University of Wisconsin.

Beevor, C.: The Croonian Lectures on muscular movements, delivered before the Royal College of Physicians of London, London, 1903, Macmillan Publishers, Ltd.

Braun, G. L.: Kinesiology from Aristotle to the twentieth century, Res. Q. Am. Assoc. Health Phys. Educ. **12:**163, 1941.

Duchenne, G. B.: Physiology of motion, edited and translated by Kaplan, E. B., Philadelphia, 1949, J. B. Lippincott Co.

Hart, I.: The mechanical investigations of Leonardo da Vinci, London, 1925, Chapman & Hall, Ltd.

O'Malley, C. D., and Saunders, J. B. de C. M.: Leonardo da Vinci on the human body, New York, 1952, Henry Schuman, Inc., Publishers.

Spray, J.: Three-dimensional film data validation procedures: a vector approach, unpublished thesis, 1973, University of Arizona.

See Bibliography for additional references.

PART II

Anatomic bases of movement

CHAPTER 3 Role of the skeleton in movement

The earliest kinesiologists recognized that bones serve as part of a lever in motor acts. Since the shape of a bone, its relationship to a joint, and the muscle attachments cannot be changed, one might question whether understanding of body leverage would enable one to make an application that would increase the efficiency of an act. Although anatomic structures cannot be changed voluntarily, adjustments can be made that will affect skill. For example, a lever need not be limited to one bone, since muscles can hold adjoining bones together firmly enough for the two or more to act as a single segment; one relative position of these bones may be of greater advantage than another. Thus voluntarily the length and the shape of a lever may be changed.

Understanding the roles that components of body structure play in human motor acts is essential for students of kinesiology. In any motor act, movement occurs in one or more joints—one or more segments move. Movement, although dependent on neuromuscular activity, is ultimately skeletal. The degree of skill depends on the choice of joint actions, the rate of movement of each, and the sequence of actions and rates. To understand skill one must understand skeletal contributions; to improve motor performance intelligently one must know what skeletal changes should be made.

Observers of motor acts differ on what is perceived, since visual impressions must be interpreted in the light of past experiences. Observing an underarm throw, the average person is likely to see that a right-handed performer steps forward with the left foot as the right arm swings back and that as the weight is transferred to the left foot the right arm swings downward and forward. The observer with anatomic information may see hip flexion in the left limb and extension and abduction in the right shoulder joint, followed by rapid adduction and flexion in the right shoulder. The observer who has a kinesiologic background may see the shoulder joint as the fulcrum of a lever that includes the humerus and ulna and will understand that these bones are parts of a lever transmitting muscular energy to the object to project it into flight. Skeletal segments act as levers in movement, and kinesiologic study should develop the ability to identify body levers in movement and the understanding of the force developed by such levers. Such abilities can be developed through exercises in identifying body levers—first, in the action of single muscles and joints and, second, in identification of levers in complex motor acts.

The ability to recognize and understand lever action frees performer and instructor from imitation. Joint actions in a motor act will be considered desirable because they are mechanically and physiologically sound and not because these actions are included in the good performer's motor pattern. The goal becomes good biomechanics, not "good form," which, says Broer, "has been determined (historically) by analyzing the performance of an individual, or individuals, who have been unusually successful in a particular activity."* This is not to say that the performance of experts should not be studied; however, it should be studied not to provide a model but to gain insight into body mechanics. The performance of less skilled persons should also be studied, and their acting levers should be compared with those of experts. Such study will develop intelligent students of motor skill and free them from blind imitation.

DEFINITION AND DESCRIPTION OF ELEMENTS OF A LEVER

A lever is a machine, a device, for transmitting energy; it is able to do work when energy is transmitted through it. In the human body, energy derived from muscular contraction is transmitted by the bones to move body segments, which may transmit energy to external objects in turn.

The lever is commonly defined as a rigid bar that revolves about a fixed point, the fulcrum. In the body the location of the fulcrum is readily identified as the point within the joint in which the movement occurs. Identification of the rigid bar may be more difficult if the word *bar* suggests a straight mass whose length is considerably greater than its width or thickness. The word *rigid,* too, may present difficulties if it suggests an undivided, continuous mass. One should realize that external levers can vary in shape and in structure. A hammer can be used as a lever in both driving in and pulling out a nail. Yet the hammer is neither a straight bar nor need be an undivided mass; the head need only be securely attached to the handle. Even the common crowbar, often cited as an example of an external lever, although usually one continuous mass, could be an effective device for transmitting energy if it consisted of two or more segments bound together firmly enough to withstand the forces to which it might be subjected.

The student of body mechanics must realize that bony levers may vary in shape from the traditional rigid bar. Bones serve more than one function in the human body. They may support parts, as the pelvis supports abdominal organs; they may protect softer tissues, as the ribs protect the lungs. Yet the same bones can serve as levers when segments are moved. Also one or more bones may be bound together by muscles firmly enough for them to function as a single mass; the bones of the upper and lower arms can be held together by muscles crossing the elbow joint; the bones of the entire arm, the shoulder girdle, the vertebrae, and the pelvis can be held together by muscles crossing all intervening joints. These variations from the common concept of external levers may suggest that lever identification in human movement is difficult. It will be simplified if the following elements of a lever are kept in mind.

*Broer, M. R.: Efficiency of human movement, Philadelphia, 1960, W. B. Saunders Co., pp. 8-9.

1. The *fulcrum* is a point on the axis about which the rigid mass rotates. In the body this axis will pass through the joint in which movement occurs.
2. The *effort arm* includes all parts of the rigid mass between the fulcrum and the point at which the energy is applied to the rigid bar. In the body this point will be that at which the contracting muscle is attached to the moving bone.
3. The *resistance arm* includes all parts of the rigid mass between the fulcrum and the point at which the energy is applied to the object to be moved by the lever. In the body this might be an object held in the hand.

Keep in mind that in a lever the three points—fulcrum (F), point of application of effort (E), and point of application of resistance (R)—may be found in any of three possible space arrangements. Any one of the three may be located between the other two. This relationship is indicated by the terms *first-class, second-class,* and *third-class levers:* E-F-R, first class; E-R-F, second class; F-E-R, third class. These classifications are illustrated in Fig. 3-1.

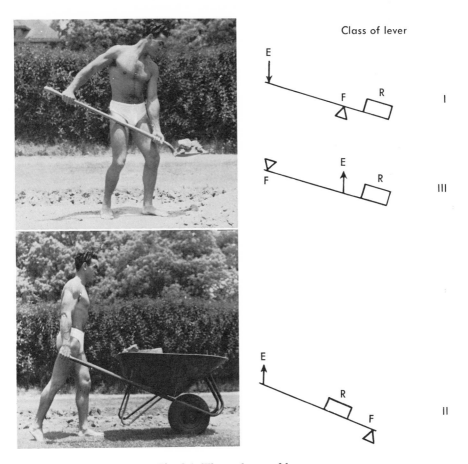

Fig. 3-1. Three classes of levers.

In descriptions of body levers the points E, F, and R will not be exactly located. The attachment of a muscle will necessarily cover more than a point, R may also cover more than a point, and F will be identified as a point on the axis passing through the joint. Located points will therefore be approximations only, but this lack of precision should not hinder the understanding of the lever action in the body.

REFERENCE PLANES FOR BODY MOVEMENTS

Although body movement is rarely the result of contraction of only one muscle, learning to recognize body levers is perhaps best approached through identification of the three parts of a lever as related to the action of a single muscle. To begin such identification, planes of reference to which movement and lines can be related are helpful.

Familiar reference planes are the horizontal and vertical ones. They are defined with reference to the earth's surface. When body movement is described, the following terms, which refer to the body itself, are used (Fig. 3-2):

1. *Sagittal* plane, which divides the body into right and left sections

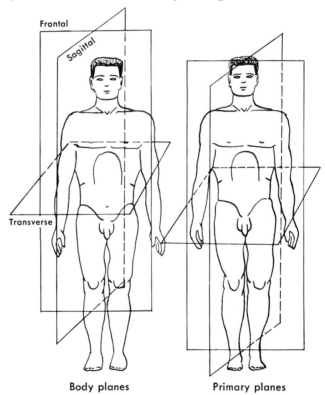

Body planes   Primary planes

Fig. 3-2. Body reference planes. Right, primary planes passing through the center of gravity. Left, transverse plane is higher than the center of gravity; sagittal plane is to the left; frontal plane could be in front of entire body.

2. *Transverse* plane, which divides the body into upper and lower sections

3. *Frontal* plane, which divides the body into front and rear sections

Thus, if the arm of a standing person is abducted, it moves through the frontal plane with reference to the body and the vertical plane with reference to the earth. When the body is in the prone position, the same action moves the arm through the frontal plane with reference to the body but the horizontal plane with reference to the earth. Kinesiologic planes remain the same regardless of the position of the body with reference to the earth.

These imaginary planes, useful in describing body movement, need not divide the body mass into equal sections. However, when half the body weight lies on each side of the dividing plane, the plane is further identified as *primary*. Fig. 3-2 shows the primary planes as well as one additional plane in each category.

SINGLE-MUSCLE LEVERS
Single-muscle levers in the sagittal plane

Action of biceps brachii in forearm flexion. The action of the biceps brachii is illustrated in Fig. 3-3, in which the muscle is shown supporting a weight resting in the hand. The drawing might also be visualized as a "flash" representation of

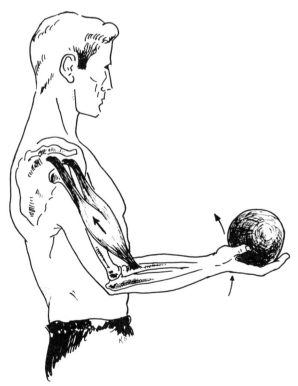

Fig. 3-3. Action of biceps brachii in forearm flexion.

a phase of upward movement of the weight. If the movement starts with the upper arm and forearm at the side and the upper arm is held in that position as the forearm moves forward and upward, the forearm moves through the sagittal plane. The axis of movement will be a line that is perpendicular to the plane of movement and in this situation will be a line that passes through the elbow joint. This line will lie in the transverse and frontal planes, since a line may lie in two planes, and both of them are perpendicular to the plane of movement— the sagittal. The fulcrum will be a point on the axis and in the joint. The rigid bar includes the ulna and radius and the bones of the wrist and hand. The effort arm is that section of the radius and ulna that lies between F and the attachment of the muscle (approximately 1 inch in length). The resistance arm includes the bony mass extending from F to the center of the weight, including the total length of the radius and ulna, the wrist and metacarpals, and a portion of the proximal phalanges, approximately 16 inches in length. The lever is not a simple continuous mass but consists of several bones bound together by muscles, tendons, and ligaments. The weight of the forearm and hand is not included in this analysis. The arrangement is F-E-R, a third-class lever.

Since it is known that to support the weight the length of F-E times the amount of muscular force must equal the length of F-R times the weight of the supported object, the amount of muscular force must be sixteen times the weight of the object. To move the object the force must be even greater (p. 49).

Note that in identifying the lever elements one needs to consider only the muscle attachment to the moving segment. It is the point at which energy is applied to the lever. The muscle must have another point of attachment, but that attachment is not part of the lever, although it is an essential part of the total machine.

Action of psoas muscles in thigh flexion. The attachment of the psoas muscles to the femur is shown in Fig. 3-4. If this illustration is visualized as a phase in hip flexion, the femur is shown moving through the sagittal plane, and the fulcrum of the action is on an axis passing through the hip joint in the transverse and frontal planes. If the weight of the thigh is not considerd, the load to be lifted is that of the lower leg, foot, and shoe, which are attached to the lever (the femur) at its distal end. The femur is the rigid bar; the effort arm includes that section of the femur which extends from the axis to the attachment of the muscle, a length of approximately 3 inches. The resistance arm is that section of the femur which extends from the axis to the point of attachment of the leg, a distance of approximately 15 inches. The lever arrangement is F-E-R, a third-class lever.

Action of brachioradialis in forearm flexion. Flexion of the forearm resulting from contraction of the brachioradialis is illustrated in Fig. 3-5. The forearm moves through the sagittal plane, and the axis, passing through the elbow joint, lies in the frontal and transverse planes; the fulcrum is on that axis and lies within the joint. The lever includes the radius and the ulna; the effort arm includes that length of the bones which extends from the axis to the point of attachment of the muscle, a length of 10 inches. If a weight were suspended at the mid-

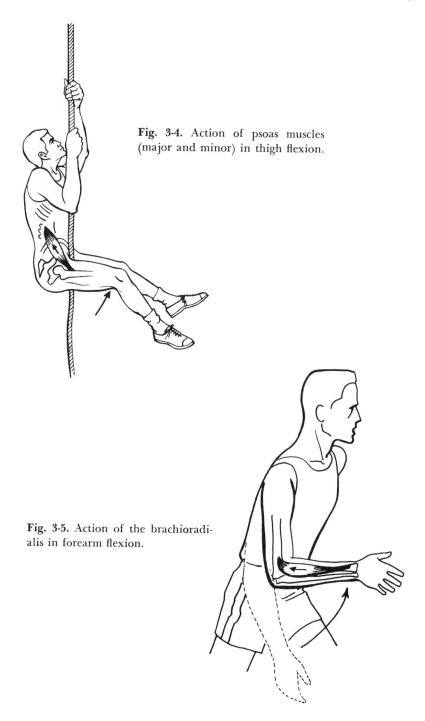

Fig. 3-4. Action of psoas muscles (major and minor) in thigh flexion.

Fig. 3-5. Action of the brachioradialis in forearm flexion.

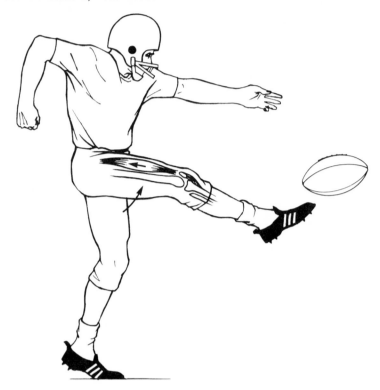

Fig. 3-6. Action of rectus femoris in leg extension. Note position of patella in extension.

point of the forearm, the resistance arm would then include that portion of the radius and ulna which extends from the axis to the weight, a distance of 5 inches. The arrangement is E-R-F—that of a second-class lever. If the weight were moved to the hand, the arrangement would be F-E-R, a third-class lever.

Action of rectus femoris in leg extension. A major joint action in kicking is leg extension. The action of the rectus femoris in kicking is illustrated in Fig. 3-6. The leg is shown moving through the sagittal plane; the fulcrum is in the knee joint on an axis that lies in the frontal and transverse planes. The rigid bar includes the tibia and fibula and those tarsal and metatarsal bones which are held firmly attached to the leg bones from the ankle joint to the point of ball contact. The effort arm is that section of the bones which extends from the axis to the attachment to the tibia, a length of 2 inches, and the resistance arm includes those bones which extend from the axis to the point of ball contact, a length of 16 inches. The arrangement is F-E-R, a third-class lever.

Action of triceps brachii in forearm extension. If the elbow is flexed, as shown in Fig 3-7, and the upper arm is held in a stable position as the triceps muscle contracts to extend the forearm, the latter segment will move in the sagittal plane. The lever includes the ulna, the radius, the wrist and metacarpals, and that portion of the phalanges which extends to a position directly under the

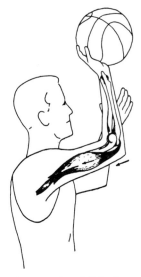

Fig. 3-7. Action of triceps brachii in forearm extension.

center of gravity of the ball. The lever will be 14 to 16 inches in length. The axis passes through the elbow joint in the frontal and transverse planes. The effort arm is very short; it is that portion of the ulna between the attachment of the muscle and the axis and is less than 1 inch in length. The resistance arm includes the bones of the total lever, and that is its length. The arrangement is E-F-R, a first-class lever.

Single-muscle levers in the frontal plane

Action of latissimus dorsi in adduction of the humerus. The humerus in Fig. 3-8 is depicted as starting from 90 degrees of abduction and the forearm from 90 degrees of flexion, pointing directly forward. As the latissimus dorsi contracts, the humerus adducts and moves to the side of the trunk through a frontal plane. This shoulder action moves the forearm, although no action occurs in the elbow joint. The forearm moves through a frontal plane also, a concept that some students find difficult to visualize. Such students have found it helpful to perform the action and in doing so to note that, as the distal end of the upper arm moves through a frontal plane, the proximal end of the forearm moves through a frontal plane parallel to that through which the upper arm moves. The distal end of the forearm and the hand move through frontal planes that are parallel to those through which the upper arm moves.

The fulcrum lies within the shoulder joint on an axis that is in the sagittal and transverse planes. The rigid bar of the lever includes the humerus, the radius, the ulna, the carpals, and the metacarpals. (The handle appears to press against the proximal end of the metacarpals; the phalanges extend beyond this point but are needed only for gripping.) The length of the lever is 20 to 24 inches; the

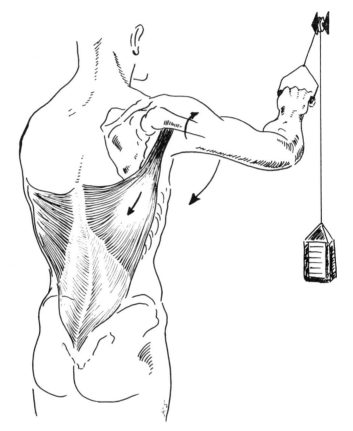

Fig. 3-8. Action of latissimus dorsi in adduction of the humerus.

effort arm is that portion of the humerus between the axis and the attachment of the muscle—2 to 3 inches. The resistance arm includes the same bones and has the same length as the total lever, extending from the axis to the point at which the weight resists the movement at the proximal end of the metacarpals. The arrangement, F-E-R, is that of a third-class lever.

Action of adductors in lower-limb adduction. The action that occurs in moving a soccer ball to the left of the body is shown in Fig. 3-9. As the adductors contract, the lower limb moves through the frontal plane on an axis passing through the hip joint in the sagittal and transverse planes. The lever includes the femur, tibia, fibula, tarsals, metatarsals, and that portion of the phalanges which extends to contact with the ball, a length of 34 to 40 inches. The lever bones and length will be the same for the magnus, longus, and brevis muscles. However, the length of the effort arm will differ for the three. If each muscle is considered separately, each effort arm will include that portion of the femur which extends from the axis to the point of attachment of the muscle under consideration. The effort arm for the magnus is longest, some 14 to 16 inches, and that of the brevis the shortest,

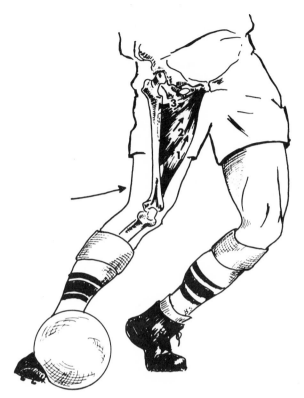

Fig. 3-9. Action of adductors in lower-limb adduction. **1,** Adductor magnus; **2,** adductor longus; **3,** adductor brevis.

some 4 to 6 inches. In all three situations the resistance arm will include the bones and will be the length just mentioned in describing the total lever. All are third-class levers.

Additional examples of barlike levers

The skeletal levers that have been described are those which include the long bones of limbs. They resemble common external levers in that their length is usually greater than their width or thickness. Many such barlike levers, including the following examples, can be found in human movements:

1. Action of the middle deltoid muscle in abduction of the arm resisted by another person's hand placed 8 inches below the shoulder joint
2. Action of the hamstring muscles in leg flexion when resistance is applied 2 inches above the ankle
3. Action of the gastrocnemius muscle when the foot presses against the accelerator in an automobile, with the pressure immediately proximal to the metatarsophalangeal joints

4. Action of the latissimus dorsi in extension of the humerus resisted by pressure 6 inches below the elbow joint

The student of kinesiology should be able to identify the lever and its elements in the actions of any single muscle when long segments of the body are moved.

MUSCLE-GROUP LEVERS
Effort arm for the action of muscle groups

When more than one muscle contracts to move a segment, the point of application of effort is difficult to determine. In Fig. 3-9 three muscles are depicted, and the effort arm for the action of each is described. If the three muscles contract and pull on the femur at the same time, the amount of force that each exerts, as well as the point of attachment of each, must be known to determine the effort arm for the combined action. The amount of force exerted by each is not known, and to describe the effort arm and its length is therefore impossible. This is true for all situations in which the joint action is caused by the contraction of more than one muscle. The descriptions of single-muscle action have been presented only as a means of developing a concept of body levers. Until information regarding the pulling force of individual muscles is available, the kinesiologist will not be able to describe the effort arm for muscle-group action.

This lack of information prevents neither the identification of the other lever elements nor the application of available information to the development of skill. Nothing can be done to change the attachment of muscles; much can be done to change the effectiveness of the resistance arm. In Figs. 3-3 to 3-9 the resistance arm remains the same for the pictured actions whether the action is caused by the contraction of a single muscle or by all forearm or thigh flexors, knee extensors, or shoulder adductors. In those lever actions which result from the contraction of more than one muscle, the effort arm will not and cannot be described.

Movements in transverse plane

Medial rotation of the humerus. If the upper arm is held at the side and the forearm is flexed 90 degrees, medial rotation of the humerus will move the forearm in the transverse plane across the front of the body (no action in the elbow or wrist joint). The action results from contraction of the medial rotators (perhaps the pectoralis major, the latissimus dorsi, and the teres major). If a weight is held in the hand, the lever includes the humerus, the radius and ulna, and the wrist and metacarpals. The axis passes through the shoulder joint and lies in the sagittal and frontal planes. The resistance arm includes the bones of the entire lever; its length is the sum of the lengths of the segments. The arrangement is F-E-R, a third-class lever.

Medial rotation of the pelvis. If the weight is shifted to the left foot with the arms held at the sides and a weight in the right hand, medial rotation of the left hip will rotate the torso, the arms, and the head. These segments will move through the transverse plane; the axis passes through the hip joint and lies in the sagittal and frontal planes. The rigid bar includes the pelvis, spine, clavicle, and bones of the right arm, wrist, and hand. These also comprise the resistance arm, and the sum of their lengths is the length of the resistance arm. The left arm and the head move also but are not a part of the effective lever. The arrangement is E-F-R, a first-class lever.

ADVANTAGE OF THE THIRD-CLASS LEVER

Kinesiologists agree that body levers are mainly third class (F-E-R) with a few first-class levers, but they have not agreed that the body has any of the E-R-F type of levers. Since nature is likely to evolve a structure that is advantageous to a particular species and has equipped the human body with a preponderance of third-class levers, they must have a value that the other types lack. All levers revolve about an axis, and the effectiveness of effort in producing rotation is dependent on the amount of force and its distance from the fulcrum. A lever will balance when E (amount) × EA (length) equals R (amount) × RA (length), as expressed by the following formula:

$$E \times EA = R \times RA$$

Since only in a first-class lever can EA equal RA in length, only when this type is used and the lever arms are equal in length will the amount of effort be equal to the amount of the resistance when balance is desired. In the second-class lever the effort arm is always longer than the resistance, and, if balance is desired, the amount of necessary effort will be less than that of the resistance. In levers of the third class, balance can be achieved only when the amount of effort exceeds that of the resistance. Therefore in body levers, which are predominantly third class, the muscular effort must always be greater than the resistance if balance is to be maintained and still greater if the resistance is to be put in motion. The body structure has adapted to this by developing muscles in which the fibers are arranged in a featherlike structure. This increases the number of fibers in a given bulk, and, since the strength of a muscle depends on the number of contracting fibers, the potential strength is increased. With the increased strength, longer resistance arms can be moved.

The additional length gives the third-class lever an advantage in speed. The resistance arm can be considered the radius of a circle; the longer the radius, the greater the distance its outer end will travel as the radius moves through a specified number of degrees. The length of the circumference of a circle is equal to two times its radius times 3.1416.

$$C = 2 \times r \times 3.1416$$

The effect of the length of r on the distance through which the outer end of the resistance arm moves when r is rotated through a given number of degrees is illustrated in Fig. 3-10. Here the outer end of the shorter radius *r*, if 1 inch in length, as it moves from *A* to *B*, will move through 1.5708 inches [(2 × 1 × 3.1416) ÷ 4], whereas the outer end of the longer radius *r′*, if 2 inches in length, will move through 3.1416 inches [(2 × 2 × 3.1416) ÷ 4]. (NOTE: The division

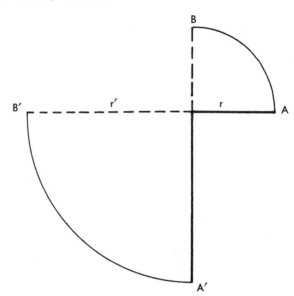

Fig. 3-10. With equal angular velocity the linear velocity of the outer end of **r′** is twice that of the outer end of **r**.

by 4 is made in each case because the illustrated distance is one-fourth of a circle.) If the movements are made in the same length of time, the linear velocity of the end of the longer arm will be twice that of the smaller, whereas the angular velocity is the same.

Human levers are adapted to move objects with speed, and the muscular arrangement and structure have provided the additional force needed to move long resistance arms.

Not only does human structure provide levers in which the length of the resistance arm exceeds that of the effort arm, but it has also provided the ability to lengthen or shorten the skeletal radius. If an object is held in the hand with the arm at the side, the object can be moved by medial rotation of the opposite hip. A line from the hip joint to the hand, approximately 15 inches, or 1.25 feet, is the length of the radius as the hand revolves about the hip. If a rotation of 90 degrees is made in one-fourth of a second, the angular velocity is 360 degrees per second. The linear velocity of the hand in that time is that of the circumference through which the hand would travel—2 × 1.25 × 3.1416, or 7.854 feet per second.

If the arm is abducted 90 degrees, the length of the arm will be added to the length of the radius. If the arm is 2 feet in length, a line from the hand to a vertical line passing through the hip will be 3.25 feet in length. If the hip rotation is the same speed as that just given, the angular velocity will be 360 degrees per second, as it was in the first situation. The speed of the hand, however, will be 20.4204 feet per second, 2 × 3.25 × 3.1416. The linear velocity has increased 2.6 times; the radius was lengthened 2.6 times. Many adjustments can be made to change the length of the radius in body skills; it can be lengthened when greater linear velocity is desired and shortened for greater angular velocity. Nothing can be done to change the length of the effort arm for a given joint action, since that length is determined by the attachments of the muscles.

Individuals differ in length of skeletal parts, as is well known. A child's bones are shorter than those of an adult; those of the average woman are shorter than those of the average man. If all can move segments at the same angular speeds, those with longer limbs will have greater linear velocities. Some authors have suggested that the distance of the muscular attachment from the joint will differ in individuals. The greater this distance, the longer the effort arm, but the advantages of this length depend on the relationship between the length of the effort and resistance arms. If the forearm is 12 inches long and the attachment of the biceps is 1 inch from the fulcrum, the ratio of resistance arm to effort arm is 12:1. If in longer segments the effort arm, although increased in length, remains in the 12:1 ratio, no advantage has been gained. However, if the effort arm increases in greater proportion than the total length of the arm, those individuals, if their muscle strength is the same as those whose ratio is 12:1, will be able to lift heavier weights. Possibly this gain in ability to lift weights because of a proportionately longer effort arm will be accompanied by a decrease in angular velocity. If, when the effort arm is longer, the muscle shortens the same amount in the same time that it does when the effort arm is shorter, the distal end of the bone will be moved a shorter distance in the the same time with a resultant decrease in angular velocity. Little information on individual differences in proportionate length of effort arms is available, but the possibility of such differences suggests the need for investigations that might explain differences in strength and speed of joint actions.

MOMENT ARMS COMPARED TO RESISTANCE ARMS

In the preceding section we showed that for a given angular velocity of medial rotation at the hip joint the linear velocity of the hand was 7.854 feet per second when the arm was held at the side. If the arm position is changed (abducted 90 degrees), the identical hip action moves the hand at a linear velocity of 20.4 feet per second. In the two situations the joint action, the acting muscles, and the bones comprising the resistance arm were identical. The difference in linear velocity resulted from a change in position of part of the resistance arm, that extending from the shoulder to the hand. This change in position changed the length of the radius. This illustrates an important element in body mechanics. The body lever force arm, which is determined by muscle attachments, cannot be changed. The bones comprising the resistance arm cannot be changed. If the resistance arm includes several bones, their positions relative to the axis of rotation can be changed voluntarily. In this lies one of the elements of skill.

A change in the length of the radius is well illustrated by a change in the position of the forearm when the hand is moved by medial rotation of the humerus, a joint action that occurs frequently in throwing and striking skills. To understand these changes better, go through the following movements. First, take a position in which the forearm is fixed in 90 degrees of flexion and the upper arm is abducted 90 degrees and laterally rotated, so that the forearm, pointing directly upward, is vertical. From this starting position rotate the humerus medially so that the forearm is rotated forward and downward in the sagittal plane. The action of the humerus is more difficult to see, but it is also rotating in the same direction and the same plane. The fulcrum, in the shoulder joint, lies on the axis, a line passing through that joint and extending in the same direction as the humerus roughly along its middle. The radius line must pass through the hand (the point of application of force) to the axis, to which it must be perpendicular. This will be at the elbow. The length of the radius will be that of the length of the forearm approximately. Next, take a starting position in which the upper arm is in the same position as in the first movement but the elbow is fully extended and the hand is facing upward. Now rotate the humerus medially so that the hand faces forward and then downward; try to eliminate any pronation of the forearm. The radius will now pass through the hand to the axis line, which must be extended through the forearm and hand as well as through the humerus. The length of the radius from the hand to the axis will be 1 to 2 inches. For the same angular velocity of medial rotation of the humerus the linear velocity of the hand in the first movement will be some ten times greater than in the second because of a change in position of parts of the resistance arm; joint action, acting muscles, and bones comprising the resistance arm are identical. The degree of elbow flexion in this movement can vary from 0 to over 90 degrees. The linear velocity of the hand will be least with no flexion; it will increase as the flexion increases, will be greatest at 90 degrees, and beyond 90 degrees will again decrease.

Because medial rotation of the humerus is an outstanding element in the human overarm pattern, because its angular velocity is one of the fastest of the joint actions, and because beginning kinesiologic students often fail to recognize it, special efforts should be made to develop the ability to identify this action of the humerus in complex skills. To identify relative positions of upper arms and forearms as medial rotation occurs is also important. This rotation of the humerus on its long axis is usually accompanied by pronation of the forearm.

In addition to the length of the radius and its linear velocity, another factor must be considered when one determines the amount of force contributed by a lever. This involves the direction in which the radius is moving at the point of interest. The radius is moving in a circular path, and the direction of its force at any point will be perpendicular to the radius, tangent to the circular path. If this is the desired direction of force application, all the force of the outer end of the moving radius will be used. When a perpendicular to the radius is not in the direction of desired force, only a portion of that force will be effective. Differences in effective force in a rotating radius are illustrated in Fig. 3-11. A radius rotating in a horizonal plane about the fulcrum, *F,* is shown at points *B, A,* and *E.* The desired direction of force is shown by the arrows marked *D.* Perpendiculars to the radius are shown by *BT, AD,* and *ET.* Only at *A* is all available force in the desired direction. To determine the amount of force available at *B* and *E* knowledge of the length of the moment arm at these points is necessary. A moment arm is the length of a line that is perpendicular to the axis and to the

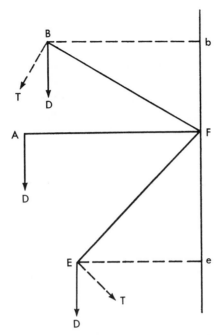

Fig. 3-11. Diagrammatic representation of moment arms. Length of the radius is equal at **A, B,** and **E;** moment arm is longer at **A** than at **B** and at **E.**

desired direction of force. In Fig. 3-11 the length of the moment arm is the length of the radius at *A*. To find the length of the moment arms at *B* one must find a line that is perpendicular to *BD* and to the axis. Since the movement of the radius is in a horizontal plane, the point *F* lies on a line that is in a vertical plane, which is not shown in this one-plane diagram. If the line *BD* is extended to intersect *FA*, the portion of *FA* between the intersection and *F* will be perpendicular to the axis and the desired line of force. This length is equal to that of *Bb*. Likewise, to find the length of the moment arm at *E ED* can be extended to intersect *FA*, and the length of the moment arm at *E* will be seen to equal *Ee*. In many motor skills the length of the moment arm will not equal the length of the resistance arm, and the length of the moment arm must be determined if the velocity in the desired direction is needed for the measurements to be made.

In studies in which the contributions of various body levers to the total force have been measured, the point chosen for observation has been the release in throws and the point of impact in strikes. All segments between that point and a moving joint are parts of the resistance arm. Thus in a throw the resistance arm for hip rotation would include the pelvis, the spine, the shoulder girdle on the right side (for the right-handed performer), the humerus, the bones of the lower arm, wrist, and hand, and the bones of the fingers up to the center of gravity of the projectile. In spinal rotation the resistance arm would include the same segments except for the pelvis; the shoulder joint would include the

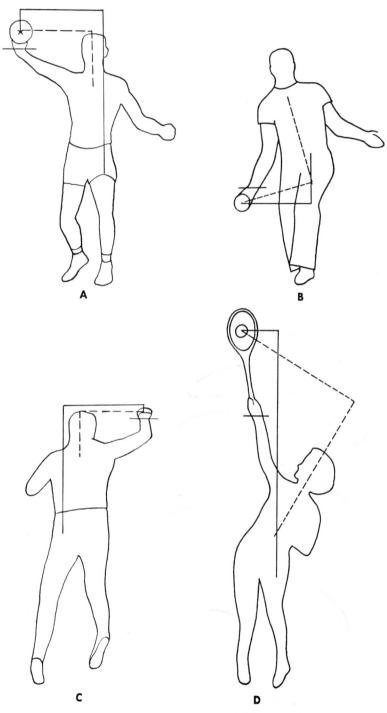

Fig. 3-12. For legend see opposite page.

segments moved by spinal action except for the spine and shoulder girdle. For all joints acting in the throw the point of application of force is the center of gravity of the projectile; for all strikes, it is the point of impact.

The length of the moment arm for any lever and the speed with which it is moving will change during the force-developing phase—in the forward swing in throwing and striking. However, the direct contribution is a result of the length and speed at the time of release. At that instant each acting joint can be considered a separate lever. For example, hip rotation will move the hand, as may spinal rotation and all other joints between the hand and the hip. The linear velocity of each can be determined, and, if the measures are accurate, the sum of these linear velocities should equal the velocity of the object projected. This method of evaluating measures of the contributions of each lever will be illustrated as specific skills are analyzed.

MOMENT ARM MEASURES FOR LEVERS COMMON TO ALL PATTERNS

Moment arm lengths for the hip, spine, and wrist are illustrated in Fig. 3-12 with tracings of the body position at the time of release or impact in (*A*) an overarm throw such as a football pass, (*B*) an underarm throw, (*C*) a push such as the shot put, and (*D*) an overarm pattern such as a tennis serve. These also illustrate changes in body levers because of different relative positions of segments.

On each tracing a vertical line has been drawn through the left hip joint to represent the axis of rotation in that joint. In all four cases that rotation will include in the resistance arm the pelvis, spine, right clavicle, humerus, radius and ulna, and bones of the wrist, hand, and fingers; in the tennis serve the racket, as an extension of the hand, is also included. The moment arm lengths will differ, depending to a minor degree on the length of the individual's segments but much more on the position of the segments at the time of release or impact. Horizontal lines perpendicular to the line of flight have been drawn from the axis to the center of the ball. The line of flight is assumed to be directly forward. Although the picture sizes differ to a small degree, for the illustration here all are assumed to be the same: 1.8/50 inches on the tracing is considered to be equivalent to 1 inch of actual measure.

Fig. 3-12. Length of moment arms in various patterns of joint action. **A,** Football pass. **B,** Underarm throw. **C,** Shot put. **D,** Tennis serve. Hip action is shown by unbroken horizontal line from hip axis to the center of the ball. Spinal action is indicated by broken horizontal or diagonal line from spinal axis to the center of the ball. Wrist action (not indicated here by a line) is the distance from horizontal line through the wrist to the center of the ball.

Table 3-1. Moment arm lengths for hip actions

	Tracing measure in 1/50 inch	Actual measure
Football pass	45.5	25.3 inches, or 2.11 feet
Underarm throw	37.5	20.8 inches, or 1.73 feet
Shot put	43.0	23.9 inches, or 1.99 feet
Tennis serve	20.0	11.1 inches, or 0.92 feet

The moment arm lengths and resulting velocities are presented in Tables 3-1 to 3-3. The tracing measures in fiftieths of an inch are divided by 1.8 to determine the actual measure in inches.

In this illustration all hip joints are assumed to be moving at the same angular velocity—720 degrees per second. If this speed continued for 1 second, each hip action would carry the moment arm through two complete revolutions, a distance that would be equal to twice the length of the circumference that the distal end of each moment arm would inscribe. The speed in feet per second would be as shown in Table 3-2.

The tennis server has lost speed that might be derived from hip rotation by lateral flexion of the spine; the football passer has gained speed by abducting the arm, an advantage that would be increased had that abduction been 90 degrees. In the tennis serve the moment arm of the lever acting at the hip joint is justifiably shortened to add to the height at which the ball is impacted.

The axes for spinal rotation are shown in Fig. 3-12 by broken lines drawn through the upper trunk and extended to the level of the external object (ball or shot). The horizontal or diagonal broken line from the axis to the center of the ball shows the length of the moment arm. If all spinal rotations are assumed to have the same angular velocity of 360 degrees per second, the linear contributions of each will be those shown in Table 3-3.

These illustrations of projections have been those in which the force was applied with one hand. If both hands are used for this purpose, trunk and spinal rotations are not likely to occur in the pattern of movement.

The other joint action common to all patterns is wrist flexion. On each tracing a horizontal line is drawn through the wrist to indicate the axis. A vertical line from the axis to the center of the ball will show the length of each moment arm. Obviously the longest is that in the tennis serve. In the shot put and the football pass, since the ball cannot be carried as close to the distal ends of the fingers as it can when a small object is thrown, the moment arms will be shorter than that of the underarm throw. The speed of wrist action will differ in the pictured events: that of the football pass and the underarm throw might be equal; that in the shot put may well be slowest. Considering angular speed and length of moment arms, one finds that the linear speeds contributed by wrist action would most likely rank in the following order: tennis serve, underarm throw, football pass, and shot put.

Table 3-2. Linear velocities at the time of release and impact because of hip action

Football pass	26.5 feet/sec.
Underarm throw	21.7 feet/sec.
Shot put	25.0 feet/sec.
Tennis serve	11.5 feet/sec.

Table 3-3. Moment arm lengths and linear velocities because of spinal action

	Tracing measure in 1/50 inch	Actual measure		Velocity (feet/sec.)
		Inches	Feet	
Football pass	39	21.7	1.80	11.30
Underarm throw	39	21.7	1.80	11.30
Shot put	34	18.8	1.58	9.92
Tennis serve	71	39.4	3.28	20.61

The linear velocities of the moment arms at the point of application of force reported in Tables 3-2 and 3-3 are based on the following equation:

$$\text{Linear velocity} = \frac{\text{Angular velocity}}{360} \times 2 \times 3.1416 \times \text{Length of moment arm}$$

Another equation that is based on the relationship between the radian and circumference can be used. A radian is an angle whose arc is equal to the radius. A radian subtends 57.2957 degrees. If the angular velocity is divided by 57.2957, the dividend is the number of radians (each equal to the length of the radius), that the moment arm moves in a given time. This equation to determine linear velocity is as follows:

$$\text{Linear velocity} = \frac{\text{Angular velocity}}{57.2957} \times \text{Length of moment arm}$$

SPEED OF BODY SEGMENTS

Little study has been done to indicate the speed with which body segments can be moved. Hill, the English physiologist, has said that in the human body the speed with which each segment moves is related to its length: the longer the segment, the slower its possible speed. This, says Hill, is a safety factor, and he compares these limits to the speeds with which glass rods can be oscillated. A short rod can safely be moved rapidly at a pace that would break a longer one. This relationship of speed to size is seen in the reported number of wingbeats per second of various birds. Hummingbird strokes are as fast as 200/sec.; sparrow, 13; pigeon, 8; parrot, 5; stork, 2. The same relationship is shown in the rate of mastication (contractions per minute) of animals, reported by Amar: ox, 70; human, 90 to 100; cat, 1962; guinea pig, 300; white mouse, 350.

Table 3-4. Speed of various joints in degrees per second

Wrist flexion with empty hand	3000
Wrist flexion with tennis racket in hand	2000
Shoulder flexion in standing broad jump	1600
Ankle, knee, and hip extension in standing broad jump	1480
Rotation of left hip in overhand throw	720

Persons who have observed films of human action know that wrist action is faster than is the action of other joints. Often the hand is not visible as it is moved by wrist flexion. The speed (in degrees per second) of the various joints given in Table 3-4 is that reported in studies made by Froelich, Johnson, and Collins at the University of Wisconsin.

Except for wrist action, the velocities included in Table 3-4 were those observed during a complex act. In such acts the speed of each joint is related to and affected by other acting joints. In the standing broad jump of a skilled performer the speeds of the ankle, knee, and hip were found to be identical. However, the observed speeds indicate that smaller body segments can be moved faster than larger ones.

SUGGESTED READINGS

Bowne, M. E.: The relationship of selected measures of acting body levers to ball throwing velocities, dissertation, 1956, University of Wisconsin.

O'Connell, A. L., and Gardner, E. B.: Understanding the scientific bases of human movement, Baltimore, 1972, The Williams & Wilkins Co.

Steindler, A.: Kinesiology of the human body under normal and pathological conditions, Springfield, Ill., 1955, Charles C Thomas, Publisher.

Thompson, C. W.: Manual of structural kinesiology, ed. 7, St. Louis, 1973, The C. V. Mosby Co.

Williams, M., and Lissner, H. R.: Biomechanics of human motion, Philadelphia, 1962, W. B. Saunders Co.

See Bibliography for additional references.

CHAPTER 4 Role of the nervous system in movement

Understanding of joint actions and the resulting lever actions is only the foundation for improvement of motor skill. The performer, the teacher, the coach, the therapist, and the industrial engineer must seek means by which the desired actions can be woven into behavior. The action of joints depends on muscular contraction, and muscle action depends on nerve impulses. Joint action is the result; nerve action is the means by which the result is achieved. This concept is expressed by Bard: "The problem of behavior is essentially the problem of explaining how the central nervous system distributes messages to the muscles in such quantities and with such dispersion in time and space as to bring about the sequence of integrated motor events which comprise any normal body movement."* Mountcastle, in this same vein, states the following:

> The motor systems of the brain exist to translate thought, sensation, and emotion into movement. . . .
> Movement is the end product of a number of control systems that interact extensively. Their complexity demands that we proceed logically by (1) defining the nature of movement in terms of muscles and joints, (2) presenting an outline of the motor systems so that the relation of the parts to the whole is apparent from the outset, and (3) explaining how "control" is achieved.†

When the details of control of muscles by the nervous system are considered, the general structure of this system should be kept in mind. For convenience in discussion the nervous system is divided into central and peripheral portions. This division does not imply a separation in function, but only in location.

CENTRAL NERVOUS SYSTEM

The central nervous system includes the brain and spinal cord. Both are well protected by the surrounding bones (the skull and the vertebrae).

Brain. The brain, protected by the skull, includes the parts of the nervous system that are the bases of voluntary muscular control, as well as many parts that control reflex behavior. The major portion of the brain consists of the

*Bard, P.: Medical physiology, ed. 11, St. Louis, 1961, The C. V. Mosby Co.
†Mountcastle, V. B., editor: Medical physiology, vol. 1, ed. 13, St. Louis, 1974, The C. V. Mosby Co., p. 603.

59

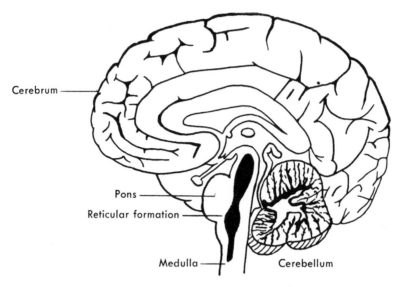

Cerebrum

Pons

Reticular formation

Medulla

Cerebellum

Fig. 4-1. Human brain.

cerebrum, the upper portion (Fig. 4-1). The surface of this portion is composed of gray matter and is mainly cell bodies, rather than nerve fibers. The activity in these cells is the basis of consciousness and thought. Beneath this surface—the cerebral cortex—are nerve fibers and also other groupings of cell bodies, such as the thalamus and hypothalamus, and mixtures of white and gray matter, such as the reticular formation. Connecting these parts of the brain with the cord are the pons and medulla, parts of the *brain stem.*

At the rear of the brain and beneath the cerebrum is the cerebellum, which has an important function in movement. The cortex of this section, like that of the cerebrum, is composed of gray matter, whereas the interior made up mainly of the white matter of nerve fibers.

Spinal cord. Continuous with the medulla, extending through the spinal canal, and terminating at the upper border of the second lumbar vertebra is that portion of the central nervous system known as the *spinal cord.* Unlike the arrangement of the brain the gray matter of the cord is in the interior section, in a configuration resembling the letter H (Fig. 4-2). The ends of the H are referred to as the *anterior* and *posterior horns.* Surrounding the gray matter are the white nerve fibers connecting various parts of the brain with cord cells and connecting cells within the cord. The nerve fibers are grouped into tracts, the names of which often indicate the connected areas and also the direction in which nerve impulses are conducted, such as the spinocerebellar and the corticospinal tracts.

Neurons. Nerve fibers and cell bodies are not separate units, since each fiber arises from a cell body. Each cell body with its fibers is known as a *neuron.* Those fibers which conduct impulses away from the cell body are the efferent fibers, known as *axons;* those which conduct impulses toward the cell body are the afferent fibers, known as *dendrites.* Rarely does a neuron have more than one

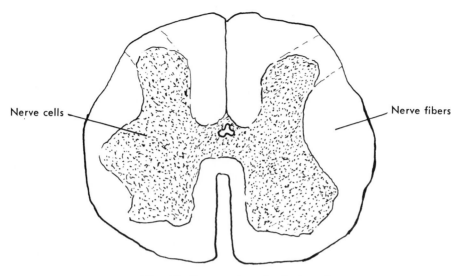

Fig. 4-2. Cross section of spinal cord.

axon, and this one is usually longer than the dendrites; some axons are as long as 3 feet. Often the neuron has several dendrites; near the cell these may be thicker than any axon, but they taper rapidly and branch repeatedly, forming a network of fibers at no great distance from the cell. Impulses do not pass from one neuron to another except at the point where the axon of one cell body is in close contact with the dendrites of another. This contact, known as the *synapse,* is found only within the central nervous system.

PERIPHERAL NERVOUS SYSTEM

The peripheral nervous system includes the cranial and spinal nerves and the peripheral portions of the autonomic nervous system. The latter controls the action of the viscera, glands, heart, blood vessels, and smooth muscles in other parts of the body and is not directly involved in the movement of skeletal parts. The twelve pairs of cranial and thirty-one pairs of spinal nerves control the action of striated muscle and are thus directly involved in joint actions. The cranial nerves connect the muscles of the face and head with the central nervous system and also carry impulses to the central nervous system from the receptors of the special senses—the visual, auditory, olfactory, and gustatory senses—and from the more widely spread receptors of pressure, tension, pain, and temperature located in the face and head.

The spinal nerves are most directly involved in movements of the trunk and limbs. The thirty-one pairs are classified according to the area in which each enters the spinal column: eight cervical, twelve thoracic, five lumbar, five sacral, and one coccygeal. Each group is numbered from the head downward. In general, the shoulders, arms, and hands are connected with the central nervous system by the fifth, sixth, seventh, and eighth cervical nerves and the first thoracic nerve;

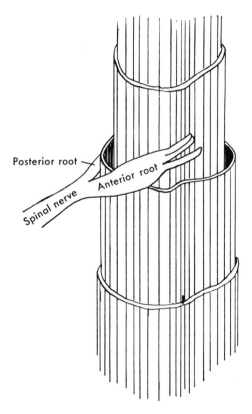

Fig. 4-3. Representation of a spinal nerve and its connections with spinal cord. Anterior root conducts nerve impulses to muscles; posterior root conducts nerve impulses from receptors to central nervous system.

the trunk, by all the thoracic, lumbar, and sacral nerves; the hips, thighs, legs, and feet, by the second, third, fourth and fifth lumbar nerves and the first sacral nerve.

Each spinal nerve connects with the spinal cord by an anterior and a posterior root (Fig. 4-3). The posterior roots (afferent nerves) conduct impulses from the sensory receptors of those parts of the body with which the nerves are connected, and the anterior roots (efferent nerves) conduct impulses to the muscles from the central nervous system.

MOTOR UNITS

Each efferent fiber in the spinal nerve arises from a cell body in the anterior horn and is connected with muscle fiber in some part of the body. The majority of skeletal muscles have thousands of muscle fibers, but each is not supplied with a separate nerve fiber. Instead, the axon divides into many collaterals just before and after entering the muscle; each collateral connects with a single muscle fiber, all of which contract simultaneously when an impulse is sent from the anterior

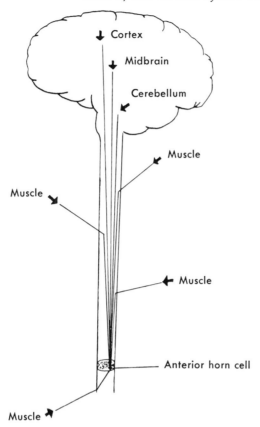

Fig. 4-4. Schematic representation showing the possibility for voluntary control of muscle action from cerebral cortex and for involuntary movements caused by impulses from other parts of the brain and from other muscles.

horn cell. The entire neuron and the muscle fibers that it innervates are called a *motor unit.* By this arrangement part of the fibers in one muscle are able to contract while the remaining ones remain at their relaxed length. This arrangement, for partial contraction of a single muscle, is further facilitated by the different degrees of strength in the stimulus needed to excite a neuron. A stimulus that is just strong enough to excite the most sensitive fiber is called a *threshold stimulus,* whereas one that is just strong enough to excite all the fibers is called a *maximal stimulus.* Thus logically a given muscle should be able to develop as many different degrees of strength (because of the contraction of fibers in a unit) as motor units represented in that muscle. If 100 motor units were present, 100 different degrees of strength would be possible. Since some muscle fibers are innervated by more than one motor unit, the strength of several motor units contracting simultaneously will not equal the sum of the strength of contraction of the individual units. The number of fibers innervated by a single axon varies.

It has been estimated to be 1775 in the medial head of the gastrocnemius, in the tibialis anterior 609, and in the eye muscles from 5 to 8.

Stimulation of motor units. If the muscle fibers in a motor unit are to contract, they must be stimulated by a nerve impulse from the cell body in the anterior horn cell, and this cell, in turn, must be stimulated by impulses that come to it via its short dendrites. The dendrites, in their turn must receive impulses through the synapses that they make with many nerve fibers, both afferent and efferent. These multiple connections make the motor mechanism of the central nervous system highly complex. A concept of this complexity is shown in the simplified diagrammatic illustration of Fig. 4-4, which indicates that, if the intention to move originates in the cerebral cortex, at the time that nerve impulses from the cortex reach the anterior horn cell impulses from the cerebellum, from nerve cells in the brain below the cortex, and from the afferent fibers arising in other muscles and joints are also likely to be received.

Some comprehension of the complexity of the pathways via which a nerve impulse may reach a motor unit can be gained from consideration of the source of impulses. An impulse originates in the endings of nerve fibers that are specialized to be excited by certain changes in the environment. These endings, known as *receptors,* are each specialized to respond to certain changes only: those ending in the eye respond primarily to light; those in the ear, to sound; those in the mouth and nose, to chemical changes; and some near the body surface, to pressure. Impulses resulting from these may reach the cerebral cortex, and the excitations there have become known as *sight, sound, taste, smell,* and *touch.* The average person is unfamiliar with the many other nerve impulses originating in other types of receptors. Sherrington, to whom we owe much of our knowledge of the nervous system, proposed that receptors be classified as: (1) interoceptors, those located in the visceral organs; (2) exteroceptors, those responding to stimuli arising outside the body, such as light, sound, odors, and external pressure; and (3) proprioceptors, those found in muscles, tendons, and joints, which respond to mechanical changes within the body. (The latter are of special interest in the study of movement.)

PROPRIOCEPTORS

Impulses originating in the proprioceptors may travel to the motor unit and be responsible for joint actions that are not consciously directed. They can be the basis for reflex actions, for inherent patterns, for adjustments made during performance, and for learned skills. Several of these receptors have been identified and described; these are discussed in the following paragraphs.

About 1850 it was found that within muscles there are small groupings of fibers that differ in structure from surrounding fibers in the same muscle. These were later given the name *muscle spindle.* Some persons thought that the muscle spindle might be the specialized receptor in which nerve impulses would be initiated by changes in the degree of contraction in the muscle. In 1894 Sherrington demonstrated that a nerve fiber from the spindle carried impulses to the spinal cord.

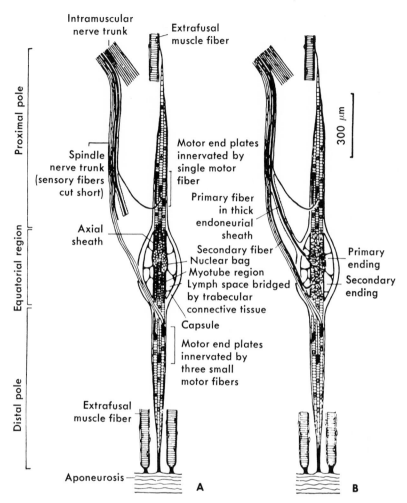

Fig. 4-5. Schematic drawing of the structure and innervation of typical spindle organ from mammalian muscle. **A,** Motor innervation only is shown. **B,** Both sensory and motor innervations are shown. (From Barker, D.: Q. J. Micro. Sc. **89:**156, 1948.)

A representation (schematic drawing) of a muscle spindle is shown in **Fig. 4-5**; this drawing has been widely used since it was first presented. Since that time many investigators have studied the structure and have found details not shown in the drawing. However, it will serve here to give a general idea of the structure and will also serve to increase a realization that there are other receptors, made visible by the microscope, of which the average person is not aware. People have more sense(s) than they realize.

The drawing shows within a connective tissue sheath, or capsule, a number of muscle fibers known as *intrafusal fibers.* Other fibers in the muscle and not within the capsule are known as *extrafusal fibers.* The number of intrafusal fibers shown is not an exact representation. According to Boyd in cat spindle the number varies from 3 to 13, and in humans many more are found. Also not shown in the drawing is the difference in the structure of the fibers. The structure, according to Boyd, differs in several respects, such as length and diameter. The drawing shows in the equatorial region an enlargement known as the *nuclear sac,* or *bag.* It contains a fluid that Boyd says has been referred to as *lymph,* although, as far as he knows, it has not been proved to be lymph. Two types of nerve fibers are connected to the intrafusal ones: one, efferent, carries nerve impulses from the spinal cord to the intrafusal fibers (Fig. 4-5, *A*); the other, afferent, carries impulses from the spindle to the central nervous system (Fig. 4-5, *B*).

The afferent fibers are of two types. They differ in diameter (the larger transmit impulses more rapidly than the smaller) and in type of ending on the intrafusal fiber. The primary, or annulospiral, ending of the larger type rarely branches as it approaches the intrafusal fiber; its ending winds around the fiber in the area of the nuclear sac (Fig. 4-5, *B*). This portion of the fiber does not have contractile ability, as do the outer portions. The secondary, or flower-spray, ending of the smaller afferent fiber also connects with the intrafusal fiber in the region of the nuclear sac, but it is farther from the middle than is the primary ending (Fig. 4-5, *B*). There is only one primary ending on a fiber; there may be as many as five secondary endings, although only one is most commonly found. Whenever the nuclear bag area is stretched, nerve impulses are initiated in primary and secondary endings and transmitted to the spinal cord.

Efferent nerve fibers to the spindle are small in diameter; they connect with the intrafusal fiber, some above the nuclear sac area (Fig. 4-5, *A*), where the muscle fibers have contractile ability. Thus when nerve impulses reach the intrafusal fibers, the latter contract, stretching the nuclear sac area. Since the number of intrafusal fibers as compared to the number of extrafusal fibers in a muscle is small, this contraction appears to make little or no contribution to movement; its function is stimulation of the spindle afferent fibers, which now can be seen as sensory, or at least afferent, receptors. Some of the efferent fibers do connect at the nuclear sac area, according to Boyd; their function is not clear.

When afferent impulses are initiated in the spindle and transmitted to the spinal cord, they have the possibility of reaching many parts of the body via the complex synaptic connections and nerve pathways in the cord. Some may be carried to the extrafusal fibers in the muscle in the spindles of which the impulses originated; some may influence the contraction of other muscles acting on the same joint, bringing into action assisting prime movers and synergistic muscle (Chapter 5); some may inhibit the action of antagonist muscles. Such afferent impulses may also activate anterior horn cells in many parts of the spinal cord and thus affect the movement and position of many segments; some may initiate activity in the nerve cells of the brain stem, subcortical brain areas, and cerebellum. They provide the possibilities for complex reflex acts and movement patterns and for the involuntary joint actions that are a part of voluntarily initiated motor acts. These possibilities support the statement that the mind orders an act and leaves the details of execution to lower levels of the nervous system. Without question the muscle spindle plays a major role in movement; by responding to contraction in the active muscles it serves as a coordinator throughout the action.

Golgi tendon receptors are found in the tendons close to their muscular origin and in the connective tissue of the muscle. The end of an afferent nerve fiber is surrounded by layers of tendon fibers enclosed in a connective sheath. Within this encapsulated mass the nerve ending branches; when the tendon or connective tissue is stretched, the pressure on the nerve ending initiates impulses that will be conducted to the central nervous system.

Pacinian corpuscles are widely distributed in the fascia of muscles, especially beneath the tendinous insertion of muscles at the joints. They are also found in the deeper layers of the skin. The nerve ending is surrounded by concentric layers of fibrous tissue, within which the nerve branches. Pressure will be exerted on the nerve endings when muscles contract or are stretched.

Skin receptors, which respond to touch and pressure, are also activated by changes in joints and muscles, for they change the amount of pressure on the skin and in the area of the movement.

The nerve fibers connected with these receptors reach the spinal cord by way of the posterior branches of the spinal nerves. They branch as they enter the cord, conducting impulses to anterior horn cells at the same level or to higher or lower levels of the cord. These impulses may result in reflex or subconscious movements. Some impulses may be conducted to the cerebellum and influence the coordination of movements that are initiated by efferent impulses originating in this section of the brain.

VOLITIONAL CONTRIBUTION TO MOTOR ACTION

Motor acts are often initiated by a decision (activity in the cerebral cortex). That decision does not include conscious, detailed directions of the joint actions that will be needed. Studying motion pictures of one's own performance demonstrates that many joint actions occurred of which one was not aware at the time. The mind orders a "whole," and the details occur without conscious direction. The neuromuscular system selects its own methods of achieving the goal set. As push-ups are observed, frequently the body is seen to be lifted by trunk extension before the arms take over the task. According to the British neurophysiologist Adrian, "The mind orders a particular movement but leaves its execution to the lower levels of the nervous system."*

A national women's golf champion was asked what she thought about as she prepared to take a shot. She answered, "I see the shot, then feel it, and then I do it." (Further questioning revealed that *seeing* meant visualizing the needed height and distance.) A basketball coach of national repute was asked how he developed skill in shooting from the free throw line. His reply was identical to that of the golfer. He asked the players to visualize the high point of the shot and to feel it before beginning the movement. A British scientist believes that

*Adrian, E. D.: The physical background of perception, London, 1947, Oxford University Press.

it is more important to know *what* to do than *how* to do it and suggests that the less a performer knows about the details of the act, the more efficient it will be.

The lack of cortical control of specific joints and muscles is supported by the investigations of Gellhorn, who reports that stimulation of certain points on the motor cortex results in definite patterns of movement. Among these are such combinations as (1) flexion of the elbow, extension of the wrist, and protraction of the arm, (2) extension of the elbow, flexion of the wrist, and retraction of the shoulder, and (3) flexion of the knee, dorsiflexion of the ankle, and extension of the elbow. Furthermore, Gellhorn found that the same parts of the body could be moved when different cortical points were stimulated: the lips as moved in speaking and in mastication can be activated from different cortical points, as can flexion of the thumb and closure of the hand, which involve the flexors of the thumb. The concept that movements rather than muscles are represented in the cortex has received increasing emphasis in the last decade.

The specific movements activated in the cortex are characteristic of the species: they are not unique for each individual. With the millions of nerve cells in the central nervous system and the millions of muscle fibers in the human body and with the development of independent muscle and nerve in the embryo and during infancy, the fact that connections develop between these which are normally common to all individuals is another miracle of living matter. An explanation for these common connections is given by Sperry, who says that as nerves develop from the central system each has a predestined terminal contact point and that it is guided to this point by a chemical environment. Each nerve fiber as it grows develops numerous ramifications and through these makes contact with numerous cells, but chemical affinity determines which of these will develop into a specialized synapse capable of transmitting a nerve impulse. Among the supporting experiments that Sperry presents is one in which he transposed the nerves connecting the skin of the left and right hind feet of rats. After the nerves regenerated, a mild shock to the sole of the right foot caused the animal to lift the left. During the experiments some of the animals developed a sore on the stimulated foot, and they then hopped about on three feet but raised the uninjured foot. In another series of experiments the optic nerve of the newt was cut, and the eyeball was rotated 180 degrees. After recovery the animal responded to visual stimuli as if they were seen upside down. The severed nerves had evidently grown attachments to those sections of the eye to which they were normally connected.

Observations such as those of Gellhorn and Sperry provide explanations for the common patterns of human action that are observed to occur without conscious control or awareness.

INVOLUNTARY DETAILS OF MOTOR BEHAVIOR

The involuntary details of common human motor behavior can be attributed to reflex action and inherent motor patterns.

Human motor reflexes

The knee jerk is perhaps the most widely recognized human reflex. A sharp blow on the tendon at the knee initiates a nerve impulse in the afferent nerve, which conducts the impulse to the spinal cord and then to the gray matter of the anterior horn, where the afferent fibers synapse with dendrites of anterior horn cells. The impulse is then conducted via the axon of the motor cells to the muscle fibers of the knee extensors, and, as these contract, the leg is rapidly extended. This type of response is also elicited when the pressure on the tendon is a steady pressure, rather than a sharp blow. As stated by Bard, "If the pull on the tendon is steadily exerted, the muscle responds with a steady contraction more than sufficient to balance the force of the pull."*

The voluntary concept and the reflex can be visualized in an act such as holding a weight in the hand with the forearm flexed 90 degrees. The intent of the performer is to maintain this angle with the mind ordering a whole. The stretch on the elbow flexion signals to the muscle the number of motor units needed. If the weight is increased or decreased, reflex information provides the needed adjustment in strength of contraction.

The stretch, or myotatic, reflex is widely distributed in the body and is especially well developed in antigravity muscles. In the description of the mechanical aspects of standing, the center of gravity of the body is known to be normally in front of the ankle joint. Gravitational force would pull the body forward, causing ankle flexion. The resulting stretch on the ankle extensors initiates the nerve impulses that control the amount of contraction needed to maintain the position that the performer intends. If the forward lean approaches the limits of easy ballance, stretch increases and the stimulation to the ankle extensors increases, and the increase in muscle contraction pulls the body back. The intent to stand keeps the ankle joint within a range of flexion that is not consciously controlled.

If the intent is to walk, run, or jump, the degree of ankle flexion is increased, as is shown in Figs. 15-2 to 15-8, which illustrate joint actions. Ankle flexion is permitted to the extent necessary for the specific act. Then the ankle joint may be held stationary as the foot is raised and later extended at an angular rate that exactly parallels that of the metatarsophalangeal action. Basically these joint actions are the same in the unskilled and the skilled. Some mechanism common to both must be in control.

In throwing and striking patterns, the rapid backswing most likely produces by the stretch reflex contraction of muscles needed for the forward swing. Observations of muscle action have shown that the muscles responsible for the forward swing begin their contractions before the limit of the backswing is reached. These contractions not only stop the backswing but also increase the nerve impulses initiated by the stretch and thereby increase the speed of the forward movement.

The myotatic reflex is the simplest of those observed in humans, since often

*Bard, P.: Medical physiology, ed. 11, St. Louis, 1961, The C. V. Mosby Co.

only two neurons are involved. Other, more complex reflex actions that involve action in more than one level of the spinal cord have been observed. These may result in movement of more than one joint and in some cases movement in the contralateral limb. A painful stimulus applied to the foot will result in withdrawal of that limb by flexion of more than one joint (the flexion, or withdrawal, reflex), and this action will initiate impulses that contract extensors in the opposite limb, which are needed to maintain balance (the crossed-extensor reflex). The combination of reflexes that act together to maintain equilibrium is known as the *righting reflexes;* they act in normal standing when the adjustments are barely noticeable and also when there is greater threat to balance. When balance is threatened, many body parts, especially the arms, may be seen moving vigorously and widely. These efforts to bring the body's center of gravity over the feet, needless to say, are not always successful.*

Observers of infant behavior, notably Gesell and McGraw, have reported the age range within which certain reflex acts appear. Their observations suggest that as the infant matures the reflex action comes under voluntary control and appears as part of a volitional act. The stepping actions that an infant 2 to 3 weeks old will make when held upright with the feet contacting a surface continue to operate reflexly in voluntary walking. The weaving of reflex patterns into voluntary movements may (could well) explain the involuntary details of volitionally initiated movement patterns.

An interesting concept can be drawn from observations reported by Hellebrandt and co-workers. When a weight was lifted by wrist flexion and wrist extension, it was observed that under stress other segments of the body were moved and that head movements resembled those of the tonic neck reflex. This has been described in infants by Gesell as a turning of the head to the side, accompanied by movements in the upper and lower limbs. On the side toward which the head is turned there are shoulder abduction and elbow extension in the upper limb and knee flexion in the lower limb. On the opposite side there are shoulder abduction and elbow flexion in the upper limb and knee extension in the lower limb. The resulting position is that seen in the fencing lunge (lower limbs) and thrust (upper limb). After observing the appearance of the head movements Hellebrandt and co-workers found that voluntarily turning the head to the working side increased the work output and turning the head to the opposite side decreased the output. The head position evidently affected the number of nerve impulses sent to the wrist muscles. These findings suggest, as do those of Gellhorn, that the position of segments other than those acting in a given pattern can affect performance.

The neck and labyrinthine reflexes, says Gardner, are among the most import reflex mechanisms in sport and gymnastic skills; divers and tumblers use head movements to facilitate body spin, to flex or extend the limbs and trunk when these are desired in a stunt, and to attain correct position at the finish.

*For a more detailed discussion of reflex actions see O'Connell, A., and Gardner, E.: The scientific bases of human movement, Baltimore, 1972, The Williams & Wilkins Co.

Gardner also states that understanding of these and other reflex mechanisms is valuable when successful performance requires voluntary inhibition of the associated joint actions, such as pivoting in the golf swing without swaying. She makes this point succinctly by saying, "One must inhibit 'what comes naturally'."

Inherent motor patterns

Although reflex actions are inherent patterns, a division is made here to distinguish those which have a conscious purpose from those which are reactions to stimuli that arise in some part of the nervous system other than the cerebral cortex. Thus withdrawal from intense heat occurs without conscious intent; the withdrawal is often said to occur before one is aware of the pain. A reflex response does not vary; a purposeful inherent pattern, characterized by basic similarities, is not stereotyped. If the human overarm throw is an inherent pattern, the details of performance may differ in individuals and in the same individual at various times, but basic similarities will be present. These are not learned responses: they appear without learning. One writer used the term *action or behavior pattern* and defined it as the traditional series of steps by which an objective is achieved. (This is closely related to this text's classification of human patterns according to purpose.) The writer also states that an action pattern is as typical of a particular species as is the structure of the animal and that sometimes species are identified by their action patterns.

Inherent motor patterns in nonhuman vertebrates. According to Lorenz concerted efforts to identify inherent behavior patterns began about 1930. Investigations in this new field of ethology revealed that motor patterns were common not only to the members of one species but also to those of several species. These interspecies patterns reveal a common ancestry, as do similarities of structure; comparative ethology, as well as comparative anatomy, can provide insight into the origin of a species. Lorenz reports that the behavior of a dog scratching with a hind limb crossed over a forelimb is common to most birds, reptiles, and mammals. The dog scratches by reaching over the forelimb to reach a point near the head; the bird, in scratching near the head, lowers a wing, which seems unnecessary. Lorenz believes that before the bird can scratch it must reconstruct the old spatial relationship of the limbs of the four-legged ancestor that it shares with the mammals.

Lorenz has furnished experimental evidence to support observations of innate patterns. By crossbreeding species of ducks he found that genetic factors determine behavior patterns, as well as physical characteristics. The offspring might exhibit movements that were observed in the parents, new combinations of the parents' movements, or even behavior that was exhibited by neither parent.

Evidently the Mendelian law operates in determining behavior.

Inherent human motor patterns. As human throwing, striking, and locomotion patterns are studied, common elements are evident. Of course, these could be learned. However, these elements can be seen in the performance of young children who have had no instruction. We can state with confidence that, even if children had opportunity to observe skilled performers, they would not be

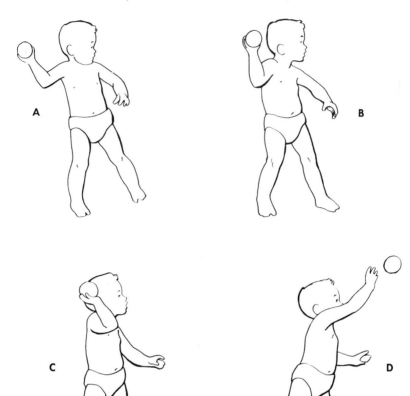

Fig. 4-6. Tracings based on a film showing overarm pattern of a boy 33 months of age who had had no instruction. Joint actions and their sequence resemble those of highly skilled performers and suggest that basic pattern is inherent.

aware of details of action. Fig. 4-6 shows selected tracings taken from a detailed study of the overarm throwing pattern of David, a 33-month-old boy. He had no instruction in throwing; yet the elements of skillful performance are present. In *A* he is seen as forward movement begins. The weight is on the right foot; the left is lifted from the floor; the pelvis is rotated to the right over the supporting foot; the head faces in the direction of the throw. In *B* the left foot has been placed forward to facilitate rotation of the pelvis over that limb; the position of the throwing arm has changed little. In the 0.23 second between *B* and *C*, lateral rotation in the left hip has turned the torso in the direction of the throw, and rotation of the humerus has carried the elbow ahead of the ball. This is an interesting aspect of timing—forward rotation of one segment and simultaneous backward rotation of another. It is interesting to speculate what the actions would be if these were attempted by conscious direction. Two elements that would be seen in a more skillful performer are lacking: (1) no vertebral action is in evidence—the torso acts as a unit—and (2) the humerus has not held its position in the transverse plane but has been adducted. The position at release is shown in *D*, 0.03 second after the action shown in *C*. Rotation of the torso has continued, the humerus has rotated medially, the elbow has extended slightly, and the hand has undoubtedly flexed. The observer can but marvel at the coordinations that result from the intent to throw. Underarm and sidearm patterns were also demonstrated by this boy and other boys of preschool age.

Locomotion patterns—walking, running, jumping, and leaping—can be seen in the performances of the young child. As everyone knows, the complicated coordinations of walking and running develop without instruction. Detailed observation shows that the young child's nervous system controls movements within the limits that ensure balance. As running movements first appear, at no time are both feet off the ground. The forward foot is on the ground before the rear foot leaves. With experience the flight phase develops, and, as skill is improved, the proportion of time of the flight phase increases. In attempting two-footed takeoff for a jump, the nervous system of the young child refuses to allow the center of gravity to move forward unless one foot is moved ahead to receive the weight. This tendency can be seen at all ages perhaps because of lack of experience in attempting a two-footed takeoff. Projecting the body from one foot seems to be the natural, innate pattern.

Another tendency to guard balance has been observed in the use of the arms in the standing broad jump. Effective use would be a forward swing in the sagittal plane on takeoff and a backward swing during flight followed by a forward swing on landing. Film studies at the University of Wisconsin have shown that elementary schoolchildren and college women whose jumps are shorter than those of their peers do not swing the arms in the sagittal plane. Rather they are held at horizontal abduction throughout the jump. This resembles the action patterns of birds, whose wings are stretched to the side as they take off for flight and also at landing as the legs reach forward. Ths brings to mind Lorenz's comment on comparative etholoy. Unlearned joint action can also be observed in young children. A child under 3 years of age was observed as he jumped from a height equal to his own. The hips had been fully extended on takeoff; yet during flight the hips flexed to bring the feet forward for landing. This was not a learned movement; it was the first experience in that situation. What but inherent patterning could be the basis for the action?

Lorenz has stated that undoubtedly animals in general inherit behavioral traits. To suggest that human behavior follows a different pattern would be illogical. It differs only because of the greater human capacity to modify details of motor inheritance.

LEARNING MOTOR PATTERNS

If motor patterns are innate, one may logically question the need for learning. Apparent are at least two reasons for learning experiences. One is that even innate patterns improve with practice, and the possibility is that if not practiced during the time at which they appear naturally they will never be as skillful. Riesen reports that newly hatched chickens kept in darkness for 14 days after hatching failed to peck at spots on the ground when brought into the light; he concludes that prolonged lack of practice can interfere with the development of instinctive reflex behavior. He also reports that vision in chimpanzees will not be normal if the eyes are not exposed to light for an extended period after birth. Hess has shown that the instinctive following of a moving object, characteristic of the young of many animals and known as *imprinting*, is most strongly developed in mallard ducks if the experience occurs within 13 to 16 hours after hatching.

Since children at an early age—certainly before 6 years—have the basic patterns of throwing, striking, and locomotion, it is possible that, if these are not experienced at the time that the nervous system is ready for them to be used, the patterns will never reach their full potentialities. Ransom suggests this possibility when he says that the neurons of the nervous system of an adult human are arranged in a system, the larger outlines of which follow a hereditary pattern but many of the details of which are shaped by the experiences of the individual.

The second reason for learning is that basic human patterns need to and can be modified for specific situations. If the individual is aware of success or failure after performance, the pattern can often be modified without any conscious direction of joint action. This can be illustrated by the experience with the previously mentioned 33-month-old boy. The boy had a running pattern, and an attempt was made to modify the run into a leap. A verbal description of how to do a leap was not attempted; instead a rolled mat was placed in the runway, and the boy was asked to clear it as he ran. In the first attempt he took off from a running step and landed with both feet *on* the mat. No comments were made, and he attempted a second trial. This time he took off from the mat; he had moved the takeoff too far forward. The third trial was successful; he cleared the mat and landed on both feet (Fig. 4-7). He was then asked to continue running after clearing the mat. He then achieved a one-footed landing, which was not balanced but which improved with successive trials. He had in mind a definite purpose as these adjustments were made; that intent was sufficient to modify joint action when he was aware of his failures. His mind had ordered a "whole" but had left the details of execution to those parts of the central nervous system below the level of consciousness.

Also this boy was led from a modification of the walking step into a standing broad jump. When asked to execute a two-footed takeoff, one foot came forward to catch his weight. In an attempt to devise a situation that did not resemble so closely that of walking, he was placed on a platform 8 inches above the floor and asked to jump off. He was able to do this without difficulty, although he had a tendency to lead with one foot. The height was increased to 15, to 20, and to 30 inches. The joint action of the lower limbs as he jumped from these heights took on the pattern of the standing broad jump. After this experience he was able to execute a standing broad jump. Evidently the mind had developed the ability to

First trial

Second trial

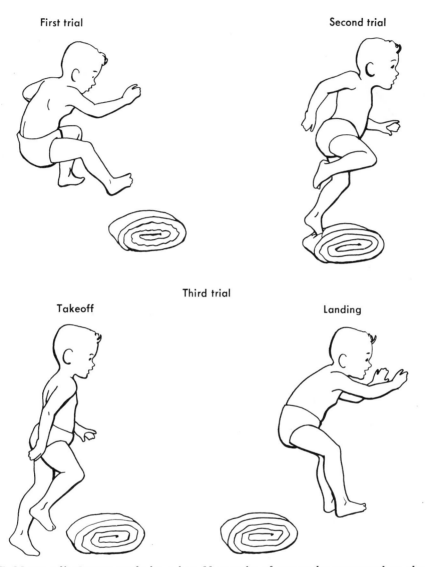

Third trial

Takeoff

Landing

Fig. 4-7. Motor adjustments made by a boy 33 months of age as he attempted to clear an obstacle by a leap. He was given no instructions.

order a given "whole." If the boy were asked to jump toward an object held over his head, he could also perform a standing jump for height. A purposeful intent brings into action the necessary joint movements. The learner can modify the innate patterns if the situation calls for the needed adjustments. The function of the teacher is to set up a situation that calls for the needed response.

Inexperienced jumpers can learn to develop the arm swing more rapidly if verbal suggestions are given. Young children of school age who fall backward on landing can swing their arms forward after verbal direction. After the suggestion to reach forward with the arms is given, this goal often results in a forward loss of balance on landing. Verbal suggestion adds a new goal—that of concentrating on a moving segment while one is executing a basic pattern. This is possible because the mind can be aware of movement.

PERCEPTION OF MOVEMENT AND POSITION

Everyone can describe with substantial accuracy the position of various parts of his body, even with his eyes closed. The skilled basketball player knows as soon as the ball is released whether the free throw movements felt right. As stated previously a skilled performer feels the action before executing it. A number of motor-learning studies have shown that a skill can be improved with mental practice, that is, by recalling the feel of the action and substituting successive recalls for physical practice. These recognitions of position and feel are examples of memory of previous motor experience and of recalling activity in the

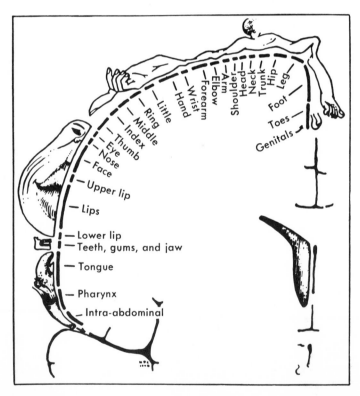

Fig. 4-8. Topographic representation of somatic sensibility in postcentral human gyrus. (From Penfield, W., and Rasmussen, T.: The cerebral cortex in man; a clinical study of localization of function, New York, 1950, Macmillan, Inc.)

cerebral cortex that accompanied motor acts and cerebral activity that was initiated by proprioceptors.

Many kinds of memories are developed from cerebral activity—memories of sounds, sights, smells, touches, and tastes. Each type of memory results from activity that was stimulated by a nerve impulse from a corresponding type of receptor. Memories of sound develop from impulses that were initiated in audioreceptors and visual memories from those initiated in vision receptors. Yet, as far as is known the nerve impulse initiated in one receptor does not differ from that initiated in one of any other type as it travels nerve pathways. The difference in recognition in the cerebral cortex results from the location in which the activity occurs. Cerebral activity initiated by visual receptors is in the lower rear of the cortex. Impulses from proprioceptors arrive in the cortex in a fairly large area that extends from the upper middle surface downward (Fig. 4-8).

The entire body is represented in Fig. 4-8, but the size of representation does not correspond to the size of body parts. The area that receives stimuli from the thumb is as large as that representing the trunk. The cortical representation parallels the density of sensory innervation from the part. When movement occurs, impulses are sent to that part of the cortex which represents the moving segments. The resulting cortical activity becomes associated with a specific movement, is recognized as accompanying the movement, and is the basis for memory of the act.

It is not known that impulses initiated in all types of proprioceptors reach the areas of the cortex shown in Fig. 4-8. When Sherrington demonstrated in 1894 that a nerve fiber from the muscle spindle conducted impulses to the spinal cord, it was thought that these would reach the brain and be the basis for the cerebral activity that resulted in perception of movement and motor memory. Recent investigations agree that impulses from the spindle do go to the spinal cord but question whether they stimulate activity in the cortical area shown in Fig. 4-8. It is thought that on reaching the spinal cord these impulses may be directed to many muscles involved in the act, including the muscle in which they originated. In other words, these impulses coordinate the movement rather than develop memory or awareness.

Memory and awareness develop from impulses that originate in the proprioceptors found in tissue surrounding joints—ligaments, joint capsules, and adjacent connective tissue. As impulses from these receptors enter the spinal cord, they travel on fibers that extend up the posterior portion of the cord and terminate in the medulla, where they synapse with dendrites of cell bodies located in the medulla. The fibers of this second neuron cross to the opposite side of the brain as they ascend, thus conducting impulses originating in the right side of the body to the left side of the brain and vice versa. These fibers terminate in the thalamus and synapse there with a third neuron that conducts the impulses to the brain areas shown in Fig. 4-8.

SUGGESTED READINGS

Gardner, E. B.: Proprioceptive reflexes and their participation in motor skills, Quest **12**:1, 1969.
Hellebrandt, F. A.: The physiology of motor learning, Cereb. Palsy Rev. **10**:9, 1958.

Hellebrandt, F. A., and others: Physiological analysis of basic motor skills, Am. J. Phys. Med. 40:14, 1961.

Moore, J. C.: Neuroanatomy simplified, Dubuque, Iowa, 1969, Kendall/Hunt Publishing Co.

O'Connell, A. L., and Gardner, B.: Understanding the scientific bases of human movement, Baltimore, 1972, The Williams & Wilkens Co.

See Bibliography for additional references.

CHAPTER 5 Role of the muscular system in movement

All animals possess the ability to move in a purposeful manner. In many species purposeful movement is accomplished by means of the movement of bony levers through contraction of the muscles. These muscles are the motive power by which the levers of the bodies of all higher animals, including the human, are moved to accomplish work and play. This contractile function of human muscle is the source of power for the movement of the body and of fluids and solid substances within the body. Stimulation sets off a wave of excitation that causes the muscle to respond.

Approximately 435 voluntary muscles are found in the human body. Schottelius and Schottelius state that the importance of the body musculature is readily appreciated when one learns that it constitutes 43% of the body weight, contains more than one third of all the body proteins, and contributes about one half of the metabolic activity of the resting body. Simple and complex activities are involved when the muscles are activated against the bones that they are attached to and the bony levers are moved. Coordination and organization of these muscles are necessary when movement takes place. This often involves not only individual or a group of muscles but also constituent parts of muscles, as Fulton and Mommaerts have pointed out.

When a muscle contracts, its attachments are normally drawn toward each other. This contraction exerts a tension on whatever is attached to the ends of the muscle. If the muscle fibers are pulling against the tendons or ligaments attached to bones, the muscle will tend to draw the bones closer together.

Remember that outside forces can also bring about movement. The force of gravity, which moves body segments downward unless its pull is resisted, frequently causes movement of the body.

TYPES OF MUSCLE

The three kinds of muscles—cardiac, smooth, and skeletal (striated)—vary in accordance with their function. Cardiac and smooth muscles have similar functions, and both surround hollow organs. Cardiac muscle is that of the heart. It has some characteristics in common with skeletal muscles and is classified as striated. However, single muscle fibers such as those noted in skeletal and smooth muscle are not obvious in cardiac muscle. Smooth muscle is the unit of blood vessels, the digestive tract, and certain other organs of the viscera. Cardiac and smooth muscles contract slowly, rhythmically, and involuntarily. Skeletal muscles are different. They are activated voluntarily as well as reflexively, and their fibers contract with great rapidity. Huxley has stated that striated muscles can shorten at speeds of up to ten times their resting length in a second. Skeletal muscles are usually attached to bones and cartilages. Under an ordinary light microscope these muscles are seen to be crossed by striations, whereas the smooth muscles have none. Most of the discussion in this chapter is concentrated on skeletal muscle and its function.

CHARACTERISTICS OF FIBERS OF SKELETAL MUSCLE

Skeletal (striated) muscle is so named because it is found principally in the muscles moving the skeletal framework. It is also attached to cartilage and is characterized by the cross-striated arrangement within the fibers. Functional characteristics of striated muscle are rapidity and volitional control. Whereas the contraction of cardiac and smooth muscle is mainly reflexive, the striated muscles can be contracted by voluntarily initiated motor nerve impulses.

The individual unit of a skeletal muscle is the long, slender muscle fiber; depending on arrangement within the muscle, it will vary from 1 mm. to 30 cm. in length. The biceps muscle has some 600,000 fibers. Elftman has estimated that 250 million muscle fibers are present in the human body. Each fiber has an elastic connective tissue covering with slender extensions attached to bones.

Huxley states, "Striated muscles are made up of muscle fibers each of which has a diameter of between 10 and 100 microns. [A micron is a thousandth of a millimeter.] The fibers may run the whole length of the muscle and joint with the tendons at its ends. About 20% of the weight of a muscle fiber is represented by protein; the rest is water, plus a small amount of salts and of substances utilized in metabolism. Around each fiber is an electrically polarized membrane the inside of which is about a tenth of a volt negative with respect to the outside."[*]

A muscle consists of many thousands of *fibers* arranged parallel to each other (Fig. 5-1). Each fiber is covered with a connective tissue, or membrane, called *endomysium*. These fibers are arranged together in bundles, 20 to 100 in number, called *primary* bundles. These are often called *fasciculi* and are grouped by connective tissue called *perimysium*. Several bundles wrapped together with perimysium form *secondary* bundles, and several of these bound together form *tertiary* bundles. The entire muscle is covered with connective tissue called *epimysium,* which holds the bundles together as a unit.

The connective tissue makes up the framework of the muscle and becomes the area of attachment either by a tendon or by itself directly to the bony levels. The blood is housed in the capillary beds, which are single-celled, layered structures embedded in the endomysium. Anson states, "The connective tissue sheaths, the larger intramuscular septa and the tendons of the muscles are richly supplied."[†]

[*]Huxley, H. E.: The contraction of muscle, Sci. Am. **199:**67, Nov., 1958.
[†]Anson, B. J.: Morris' human anatomy, New York, 1966, McGraw-Hill Book Co.

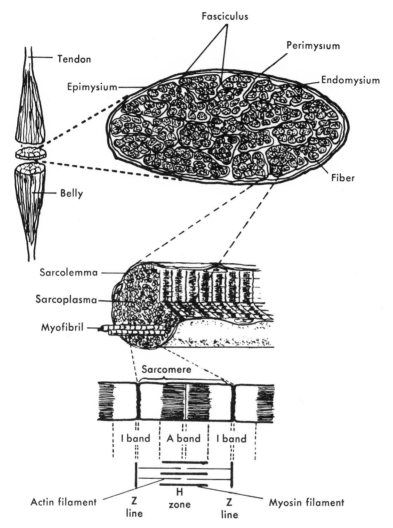

Fig. 5-1. Details of muscle structure. (Adapted from Crouch, J. E.: Functional human anatomy, Philadelphia, 1965, Lea & Febiger, and from Langley, L. L., Telford, I. R., and Christensen, J. B.: Dynamic anatomy and physiology, ed. 3, New York, 1969, McGraw-Hill Book Co.)

Each muscle fiber is cylindrical in shape and tapers toward the ends. Its component parts are myofibrils, sarcoplasm, and sarcolemma. (See Fig. 5-1.)

1. The *myofibrils,* also called *fibrils* or *sarcostyles,* are arranged in columns of several hundred to several thousand in each muscle fiber.
2. The *sarcoplasma* comprises about half the muscle fiber and is the fluid within which the contractile part of the muscle moves.
3. The *sarcolemma* is the membrane that conducts the action potential through the fiber. The endomysium is the covering on the outside of the sarcolemma.

Technically the endomysium acts as the insulator, whereas the sarcolemma functions as a vehicle through which the action potential is carried to all sarcomeres. The sarcolemma also acts to hold the sarcoplasm in place.

The myofibril is the contractile structure of the muscle and is composed of long, thin elements. Myofibrils are arranged longitudinally parallel and are cross-striated. The repeated variations in density, that is, the amount of proteins along the myofibrils, cause this appearance. A myofibril is 0.5 to 1 μm. in diameter. Each myofibril is composed of 400 to 2000 tiny filaments arranged parallel to the length of the myofibril, and each consists of light and dark bands. Mautner has stated, "A more lucid picture of these structures is obtained by observation in polarized light, where only substances that have the property of anisotropism, or birefringence, may be seen to glow. Skeletal muscle possesses this quality. The dark or dense band glows in polarized light, and therefore is called the anisotropic or A band. In polarized light, the light band becomes the dark band and is called the I or isotropic band."*

The proximal end of skeletal muscle is usually attached to a heavier bone than is the distal end. Therefore, when the muscle contracts, the distal bone is the one most likely to move. The effect of contraction on the lever depends on the position of the attachment and also on the length of the muscle fibers and their arrangement within the muscle.

There are two main types of arrangement of muscle fibers: *fusiform* and *penniform*. In the fusiform arrangement the muscle fibers are distributed in longitudinal fashion in the muscle, allowing for maximum range of movement. The sartorius is a good example of fusiform muscle. Its long, slender fibers are stretched between two heavy tendons. It is the longest muscle in the body and has the greatest range of movement in contraction. The sartorius in a man of average size will shorten about 8 inches during the full action of flexing the hip and knee joints and turning the thigh outward. This great range of movement is achieved at the sacrifice of strength. Also parallel arrangement of muscle fibers permits such muscles to move over small distances with great speed.

The penniform arrangement of muscle fibers is similar to that of the barbs of a feather. A tendon is in the position of the quill of a feather. Variations in the penniform arrangement include *demipennate, bipennate, multipennate,* and *circumpennate*. Some of these arrangements are illustrated in Fig. 5-2. In demipennate muscles, such as the adductor magnus, the fibers are arranged diagonally between two tendons and look like a feather cut in two along the quill. Pennate muscles possess a feather-shaped fiber arrangement and include the digitorum longus, peroneus tertius, and flexor pollicis longus. Fibers of bipennate muscles are double feather shaped, as in the vasti medialis and lateralis. Multipennate arrangements of muscle fibers are found in the broad muscles, such as the deltoideus and the pectoralis major. Circumpennate fiber arrangement is noted in circular muscles, such as the orbicularis oris and the levator ani.

---

*Mautner, H. E.: The relationship of function to the microscopic structure of striated muscle: a review, Arch. Phys. Med. Rehabil. **37:**286, 1956.

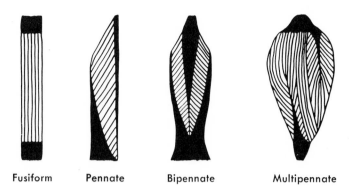

Fusiform   Pennate   Bipennate   Multipennate

Fig. 5-2. Fiber arrangement in skeletal muscle.

The diagonal pulling position of the penniform muscles allows a greater number of fibers to act in a given mass, but there is a loss in the range of movement because these fibers are shorter. As a rule a long sheath of tendon extends nearly the entire length of penniform muscles. In the peroneus longus the tendinous sheath is 18 inches long, whereas the longest muscle fibers measure only 1 inch. The greater number of fibers available for action in the penniform muscles allows only a limited range of movement of the muscle but provides great strength.

The action of the muscle is such that its fibers always contract in a straight line; thus a three-part muscle may actually have discrete and different actions because of the manner in which its fibers are laid. This is evident in large muscles, such as the deltoideus. However, those muscles with tendinous extensions, such as those to the hand and foot, as they cross the wrist or ankle to connect with each finger digit or toe phalanx are able to pull at a changed angle to contract in a straight line. Also in fusiform, as compared to multipennate arrangement, the muscle has the advantage of long fibers but has a narrow origin and insertion. The reverse is true in the multipennate muscle—with broad origin and insertion, there are muscle fibers running parallel to the contracting ones.

Another way of classifying muscles is by their actions. *Shunt* muscles act along the line of a moving bone. They prevent a joint from being pulled apart. *Spurt* muscles are those which give motion to a joint. They act at angles to moving bones.

STIMULATION OF MUSCLE FIBER

The conduction of an electrochemical impulse along the sarcolemma of a muscle fiber causes sufficient shift of ions within the fiber to bring about the formation of an actomyosin complex. Mautner has commented on the importance of the elastic properties of the sarcolemma and its collagenous fibrils in muscle contraction. He contends that the stretching of elastic fibers constitutes a creation of mechanical energy by the chemical process of contraction. He continues, "Implications of these springlike structures are that a bouncing or recoil effect upon reversal of motion exists, making the reversal smoother and faster."*

In the stimulation of a nerve an action potential either travels over the entire neuron or does not travel at all. This is known as the all-or-none law. However, the force of contraction of a muscle fiber may vary in accordance with its contractile state—appropriate nutrients present, fibers not fatigued, and other such conditions. As to the compliance of muscle fibers to the all-or-none law, one should note that "all" must be recognized as subject to a quantitative variation in interpretation. Also a muscle fiber may obey the all-or-none response, but a muscle may not, since it is graded in its response. Muscles may not have a refractory period. It could be called an *"all-or-something response,"* since the force of contraction may vary. Not only does an entire muscle display a graded response, but the same phenomenon can also be exhibited by individual fibers.

One might ask the following questions: (1) Do muscle fibers always obey the all-or-none law? The variation comes in what *all* means. If the stimulus is insufficient, it will be *nothing,* not *something.* (2) Can a muscle fire a second time without a refractory period? Yes, it may be reliably stated that such is the case. (3) Does myelination really come in degrees of thickness? The measure of thickness of myelin sheath has been given as 180 Å. The sheath is described as *lamellar,* and it is suggested that there may be about 100 layers in a mature sheath. It appears that myelination does occur in degrees of thickness.

Afferent nerve fibers are the avenue of communication between the muscle proprioceptors and the central nervous system. The spindles are one type of muscle proprioceptors and are evenly distributed in striated muscle. Mautner has said, "Any pull or stretch exerted on the intrafusal fiber and the spindle will be transmitted via the heavily myelinated nerve fiber, the two motoneurons, and the monosynaptic reflex arc to the muscle fibers, producing a reflex shortening, the myotatic reflex."* This is considered to be the fastest reflex contraction because only one synapse is involved, heavy myelination is present, and a relatively high conduction velocity is possible. The process escapes cortical control for a short time. The small efferent nerve reacts to produce the needed amount of increased discharge volley because of the stretch. This small-nerve and spindle control is considered to be the most important in the control of the maintenance of postural attitudes. When any muscle is placed in a state of readiness, a pull of only 0.05 mm. is needed to activate the annulospiral ending and cause the myotatic reflex to function. Mautner has stated, "Tonus, locostation, and locomotion, which are similar in principle, all being load against gravity, depend on this myotatic reflex. Tonus restores lost balance between agonist and antagonist fiber, locostation maintains standing by restoring somewhat larger loss of balance, and locomotion regains much more obvious loss of balance."* Lifting a heavy load produces a summation of myotatic reflexes for the production of strength. The same would be true for an all-out effort in several sports.

---

*Mautner, H. E.: The relationship of function to the microscopic structure of striated muscle: a review, Arch. Phys. Med. Rehabil. **37:**286, 1956.

Mautner has called adenosine triphosphate (ATP) the master substance in human muscular activity. If this is true, then the myotatic reflex should be the master switch and the muscle spindle the master key.

Some muscles give the appearance of being redder in color than others because in some fibers the sarcoplasm contains relatively more myoglobin than in others. Myoglobin, which is a pigment in muscle similar to hemoglobin, has a greater affinity for oxygen and also disassociates oxygen five times faster than does hemoglobin. The redder muscles are supplied with a red pigment that may serve to store oxygen. They are therefore more suited for performing long, sustained, slow (static) pulls. Thus it is not surprising to find that postural muscles are darker red than are many others. Whiter muscles tend to tire more quickly when subjected to sustained loads over a prolonged time. They are, however, peculiarly adapted to performing fast contractions. A comparison of the muscles of domestic with those of wild fowls illustrates this point. Muscles in the wings and breast as well as in the legs of a wild fowl are usually composed of many red fibers, whereas a domestic bird has more pale fibers in the muscles of the breast and wings from lack of use. In the human body the soleus, as well as most extensor muscles, has a higher percentage of red pigment than do the gastrocnemius and most flexor muscles. The gastrocnemius is fast acting and initiates an action quickly; the soleus moves to sustain the action. The extensor muscles have the task of maintaining posture, whereas the flexors initiate action. In human muscle, however, the distinction between red and white fibers is not as clear as in that of fowl and domesticated birds.

Weiner explains the difference between the finely coordinated function of the central portion of the eye, particularly its concentration on visual information, and that of the periphery of the eye. In the central portion there is often a one-to-one relationship between a motor neuron and the muscle fibers (one-to-one relationship between the rods and cones and the fibers of the optic nerve). On the periphery of the eye the relationship is one optic nerve fiber to ten or more end organs of muscle fibers. Thus the middle of the eye is used to discriminate carefully on movement, and the peripheral fibers are used as pickup mechanisms for centering and focusing, which are necessary in determining the details of an action. A somewhat similar arrangement exists between a motor neuron and the muscle fibers of the fingers as compared to those of postural muscle. Fewer muscle fibers are involved in the relationship with a motor neuron in finger muscles than in postural muscles. Thus finger muscles can perform more coordinated movements.

MUSCLE STRENGTH AND SPEED OF CONTRACTION

The approximately seventy-five pairs of muscles that are directly involved in moving the levers to maintain posture or in activating movement of all or a part of the body are capable of doing a great deal of mechanical work. Schottelius and Schottelius commented on the work of a muscle by saying that the amount of mechanical work done by a muscle is determined by multiplying the grams (or kilograms) of the load lifted by the height to which the load is lifted as measured in millimeters (or meters); the result expresses the work in gram-millimeters (or kilogram-meters). It is possible for a muscle to contract without mechanical work's being involved. If a load is too heavy and is not lifted, the muscle has then accomplished no mechanical work; all the expended energy appears as heat and would have to be measured by the amount of oxygen consumed. The *optimum* load for a muscle to lift is one in which maximum work can be accomplished each time that the muscle contracts. On the other hand, if the muscle can barely lift the load and develops the maximum tension that it can generate in doing so, it lifts the *maximum* load. It has been stated that no muscle can do sustained work when the load that it lifts is greater than one half to one third of its total capacity.

It is generally believed that a given muscle's strength is directly proportional to its physiologic cross section. This means that the cross section is measured in such a way that it is perpendicular to all the fibers of the muscle and not at an angle, as is often the case in an anatomic cross-section measurement. Thus penniform muscles are deemed to be stronger than quadrilateral ones. Evans states, "The force which a muscle can exert when it contracts depends upon the number, length, and arrangement of its fibers, the geometric relations of the muscle fibers to the tendon, the angle of insertion of the tendon on the bone, and the distance the tendon inserts from the joint axis about which movements occur."*

The tension that can be exerted by a muscle becomes less as the muscle becomes shortened. It has been postulated by some writers that this decrease results from internal friction; since a muscle does not liberate more heat as it rapidly shortens, however, this does not appear to be the case. Huxley has said, "When the muscle shortens, it exerts less tension; the tension decreases as the speed of shortening increases. One might suspect that the decrease of tension is due to the internal viscosity or friction in the muscle, but it is not. If it were, a muscle shortening rapidly would liberate more heat than one shortening slowly over the same distance, and this effect is not observed."† Hill has shown that a muscle while shortening does liberate more heat but only in proportion to the distance that it shortens and not to the speed. When a muscle is stretched between two bones in such a fashion that it is elongated, this elongation gives the muscle an advantage, in that the range of contraction is large before tension is significantly reduced. Huxley says, "Such muscles can exert a tension of about 3 kilograms for each square centimeter of their cross section—some 42 pounds per square inch. They exert maximum tension when held at constant length, so that the speed of shortening is zero. Even though a muscle in this state does no external work, it needs energy to maintain its contraction; and since the energy can do no work, it must be dissipated as heat. This so-called 'maintenance heat' slightly warms the muscle."†

---

*Evans, F. G.: Biomechanical implications of anatomy. In Cooper, J. M., editor: Selected topics in biomechanics, Chicago, 1971, The Athletic Institute.
†Huxley, H. E.: The contraction of muscle, Sci. Am. **199:**67, Nov., 1958.

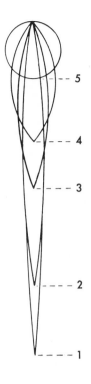

Fig. 5-3. Diagrammatic representation of length of skeletal muscle in five different conditions. 1, Maximum resting length after insertion has been severed; 2, maximum length of intact muscle when elongated by pull of muscles on opposite side (according to Weber-Fick law, twice the length of the condition shown in 4); 3, natural length of noninnervated muscle; 4, maximum shortening of intact muscle in extreme flexion (usually half the length of the condition shown in 2); 5, length of maximally stimulated muscle after insertion has been severed (one fourth to one sixth the length of the condition shown in 2).

Huxley has said that striated muscles can shorten at speeds that are equal to ten times their length in a second. They can also relax in a fraction of a second. This is because each fiber of a muscle is surrounded by an electrically polarized membrane that contains one tenth of a volt negative with respect to the outside portion. When an impulse travels down a nerve to the motor end plate, which is in contact with the muscle fiber, it depolarizes the membrane, and a substance (probably calcium) is released throughout the fiber. Then the process of liberation of energy takes place as mentioned previously, and the fiber contracts.

The behavior of a muscle in regard to shortening and lengthening has been investigated by Fick. He distinguishes between five lengths of a muscle, as shown in Fig. 5-3. The amplitude of a muscle is the range from maximum contraction to maximum stretch. A muscle works through a range somewhat less than its total amplitude, and its greatest contractile power is in the elongated phase.

A muscle that shortens (when contracting) to a greater extent than another has the advantage of contracting through a great distance but would lack strength in lifting a limb. The classic long-fiber arrangement muscle is that of the sartorius, which is reported to be able to contract a maximum of 57% of its resting length. Normally muscles with short fibers contract considerably less than this—some even less than one third their length.

Graduation of contraction. Since an electrically polarized membrane surrounds each fiber, Huxley states, "If the membrane is temporarily depolarized, the muscle fiber contracts; it is by this means that the activity of muscle is controlled by the nervous system. An impulse traveling down a motor nerve is transmitted to the muscle membrane at the motor 'endplate'; then a wave of depolarization (the 'action potential') sweeps down the muscle fiber and in some unknown way causes a single twitch."* He further reports that even when a frog muscle was cooled to the point of freezing the depolarization of the muscle membrane caused it to be activated into action within 0.04 second. The smallest unit of muscular movement is therefore the twitch. A weak contraction is one in which only a few fibers are involved. In *postural tonus* a few fibers are contracting all the time in an alternating fashion. As the volleys of impulses to the muscle through the motor nerve fibers are increased, new fibers are stimulated and thus brought into contraction. The extent of the effort is determined by the number of fibers set into contraction.

Measurement of the increase in the number of active muscle fibers is only one way in which contraction may be graded in strength. The interval between repeated stimuli and the frequency of the responses account for changes in tension. As the interval is shortened and the responses become more frequent, the muscle tension is increased (Fig. 5-4).

A muscle fiber that receives a second stimulus while still responding to the first contracts to a greater degree than to a single stimulation. If the interval between the first and second stimulus is as brief as 25 to 50 msec., the resulting summation of contraction may triple the tension of that of a single twitch.

A continuous series of rapidly repeated stimuli sent to a muscle evokes a prolonged contraction with tension as much as four times as great as that of a simple twitch. The stimuli may arrive in such rapid succession that the muscle

*Huxley, H. E.: The contraction of muscle, Sci. Am. **199**:67, Nov., 1958

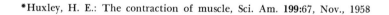

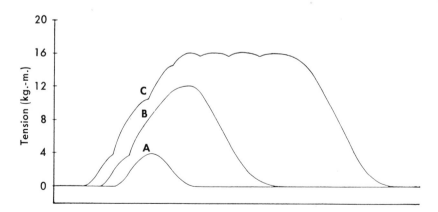

Fig. 5-4. Response of skeletal muscle to successive excitations. **A,** Single twitch; **B,** summation; **C,** tetanus.

remains in contraction as long as the stimulation continues or until the muscle becomes fatigued.

The fibers of separate parts of one muscle may have entirely different actions. Some parts contract, whereas others relax. For example, the actions of the four parts of the trapezius—the clavicular part and the upper, middle, and lower scapular parts—have different actions. The upper part originates at the base of the skull and inserts into the posterior border of the outer third of the clavicle. With the head held erect the upper part of the trapezius acts weakly to lift the clavicle and scapula. With the shoulder fixed, the upper border of the trapezius acts strongly to turn the head and tilt the chin upward. The second part of the trapezius extends from the ligament of the neck to the acromion and pulls the acromion process upward and inward. The second part of the trapezius is used strongly during the recovery of the arm in swimming with both the crawl and the breast stroke. The third part of the trapezius draws the spine of the scapula toward the spinal column. The lowest part of the trapezius draws the vertebral border of the scapula downward, since the origin of this portion of the trapezius extends from the spines of the seventh crevical vertebra downward to the twelfth thoracic vertebra.

TWO-JOINT MUSCLES

Muscles that pass across two joints are called *two-joint muscles*. This arrangement provides another type of human muscular coordination: the use of body levers. The action of these muscles on the levers is similar to that of a pulley; the muscles act at each joint over which they pass. For example, the rectus femoris flexes the hip and extends the knee; the gastrocnemius helps flex the knee and extends the foot; the hamstrings flex the knee and extend the hip. Also the flexors and extensors of the fingers might be called multijoint muscles, since they pass over the wrist and at least two joints of the fingers.

One outstanding characteristic of these muscles is that they are not long enough to permit a complete range of action simultaneously in the joints involved because of their location on two joints, because the antagonist muscles prevent full range of action on these joints, or because antagonistic action occurs in the two joints (flexion in one and extension in the other).

If the rectus femoris contracts, causing flexion at the hip, and at the same time the hamstrings contract to flex the knee, the pull of the rectus is increased at the hip because the muscle does not shorten as much as it would if extension took place at the knee. This is like a pull downward on a rope that passes over an overhead pulley, which in turn transmits tension in a reverse direction to the rope on the other side of the pulley. In the case of the flexors and extensors of the fingers, although the joints move in the same direction, the principle of pulley action is evident. One of the main advantages of using the two-joint muscles is that they maintain tension without complete shortening. This advantage is not enjoyed by one-joint muscles, which lose tension as they shorten.

Two different patterns of action of two-joint muscles have been discussed by Fenn and by Steindler; these patterns are called *concurrent* and *countercur-*

rent. The simultaneous action of flexion (or extension) at the hip and knee is an example of a concurrent pattern. This has been described as follows: as the muscles contract, they do not lose length and therefore are able to maintain tension. In extension of the hip and knee, the rectus femoris muscle's loss of tension at the knee is balanced by an increase in tension at the hip. At the same time the hamstrings gain tension at the knee and lose it at the hip.

During certain phases in the kicking pattern the countercurrent two-joint muscle pattern is seen. If the hip is flexed and the knee extended at the same time, there will be loss of tension in the rectus femoris and gain of tension in the hamstrings. Thus, while one muscle shortens rapidly in an action, the antagonist lengthens to the same degree and maintains tension at both ends of the attachment. This assures an effective and coordinated movement.

This discussion does not minimize the importance of one-joint muscles. In a single-joint action they provide the needed force but expend more energy than do the two-joint muscles in the same action. On the other hand, when two joints are involved in the act, the two-joint muscles are more efficient. In running Elftman found that although one-joint muscles could do the job, two-joint ones were more efficient; the expenditure of 2.61 h.p. by the two-joint muscles could be compared with 3.97 h.p. expenditure if single-joint ones were used.

Energy liberation and muscle contraction. Chemical reactions provide the energy for muscle contraction. This process is controlled by both the change in the length of the muscle and the tension placed on the muscle during the change. The contractile structure of muscle is composed almost entirely of protein, of which 90% is represented by myosin, actin, and tropomyosin. Myosin is the most plentiful, estimated to be about half the dry weight of the contractile part of a muscle. It is now believed that myosin is inseparably associated with the enzyme that catalyzes the reaction $ATP \longrightarrow ADP + PA + E$. However, myosinase must be activated by CaT. Myosin is the catalytic agent by which a phosphate group is removed from adenosine triphosphate (ATP), a substance present in quantity in all muscle as well as in other cells and tissues. This process of energy liberation is believed to be closely connected with the whole process of muscle contraction. Myosin and actin combined form actomyosin. The artificial combination of actomyosin and ATP causes muscle to contract; therefore it is known that these substances (myosin, actin, and ATP) are the essential ingredients for contraction, but it is not known what causes contraction.

According to Szent-Györgyi the actin molecules appear to extend the entire length of the muscle fiber. Myosin molecules lie parallel to the actin in each anisotropic band. A relatively large amount of ATP adheres strongly to the myosin molecules. A chemical reaction between the ATP and myosin molecules causes filament contraction which in turn causes the muscle to contract.

A myofibril is composed of two kinds of filament, one considered to be twice the thickness of the other. Huxley says, "Each filament is arrayed in register with each filament of the same kind, and the two arrays overlap for part of their length. It is this overlapping which gives rise to the cross bands of the myofibril; the dense A band consisting of overlapping thick and thin filaments; the lighter

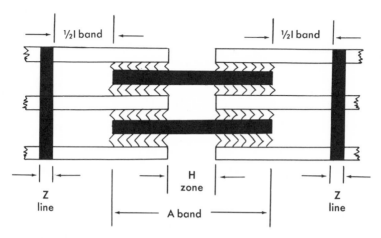

Fig. 5-5. Diagrammatic illustration of Huxley's explanation of muscle contraction.

I band, of thin filaments alone; the H band zone, of thick filaments alone. Half-way along their length the thin filaments pass through a narrow zone of dense material; this comprises the Z line. Where the two kinds of filament overlap, they lie together in a remarkably regular hexagonal array."* These filaments are linked together by specific systems of cross bridges that are believed to have a great deal to do with contraction. (See Fig. 5-5.)

Huxley is of the opinion that the A bands remain constant during both contraction and lengthening, whereas the I bands change in keeping with the length of the muscle. However, the length of the H zone (the lighter region in the middle of the A band) increases and decreases with the length of the I bands, but the total distance from one H zone through the Z line to the beginning of the next H zone remains about the same. The conclusion drawn is that the filaments slide by one another during changes in muscle length. This concept refutes the idea that extensive folding or coiling up of the filaments takes place during contraction. Huxley stated that the advance in the use of the electron microscope and of other techniques has enabled him to substantiate his original hypothesis just mentioned. He has also learned more about the nature of the interaction of the thick and thin filaments. The thick ones are composed of the protein myosin and the thin ones of the protein actin. He believes that at the "site where the proteins of the two kinds of filament are in contact, one of them (probably myosin) acts as an enzyme" to divide "a phosphate group from adenosine triphosphate."† This, he believes, provides the energy for muscle contraction.‡

Furthermore, it is believed that the cross bridges between the filaments mentioned earlier are the places at which the physical combination of actin and myosin takes place. The bridges composed of myosin move back and forth and

*Huxley, H. E.: The contraction of muscle, Sci. Am. **199**:67, Nov., 1958.
†Huxley, H. E.: The mechanism of muscular contraction, Sci. Am. **213**:6, Dec., 1965.
‡See also Cohen, C.: The protein switch of muscle contraction, Sci. Am. **233**:36, Nov., 1975.

hook up with the actin filament. Huxley states, "There is only a certain period of time available for a bridge to become attached to an actin site moving past it and the time decreases as the speed of shortening increases."* If this theory is correct, it would explain how the energy is obtained for contraction; that is, a phosphate group would be split from a single molecule of ATP each time the cross bridge went through its movement cycle and thus supply the energy. Huxley's idea that a ratchetlike device in connection with the cross bridges is responsible for the thick filaments is plausible. This would allow movement at the molecular level to take place without changing the contraction phase. The muscle could do more work during a single contraction. However, the detailed molecular action that takes place within the muscle is as yet unknown.

Where the muscle receives its energy to contract is known. The immediate energy utilized by the actomyosin complex for contraction is derived from ATP, but how it accomplishes this feat is not known.

GROUP ACTION OF MUSCLES

Muscles almost always act in groups rather than individually. In fact, under normal conditions and to all practical purposes, isolated action of any one muscle is impossible. All movement is the result of the combined and coordinated action of groups of muscles operating simultaneously and in various ways.

In kinesiology the student is primarily interested in movement, as Beevor has stated. He mentioned the fact that what a muscle may appear to do and may do under electrical stimulation is not necessarily what it will do in action in sports and in everyday activities. He argued that Duchenne's theory of what a muscle may do when stimulated is only what the particular muscle does singly. Duchenne failed to determine what the action of cooperating and opposing muscles will do. Other muscles almost always contract when one muscle contracts, followed by the contraction of opposing muscles when a natural movement such as walking is accomplished. The resultant action of a group of muscles may be entirely different from the action of a single muscle.

MUSCLE TONE

Muscle tone has been thought to be the condition in which the muscle is in a state of contraction maintained by a low-frequency asynchronous discharge of impulses from the brain stem to a small fraction of motor nerves supplying a muscle. When a muscle is in complete contraction, the condition is known as *tetanus*. Basmajian says that tone is determined by two factors: (1) passive elasticity or turgor of muscular and fibrous tissues and (2) active (although not continuous) contractions of muscle in response to the reaction of the nervous system to stimuli. He states, "In no normal muscle at complete rest has there been any sign of neuromuscular activity."†

Strickholm defines tone as "resistance to deformation." He states that "tone

---

*Huxley, H. E.: The contraction of muscle, Sci. Am. **199:**67, Nov., 1958.
†Basmajian, J. V.: Muscles alive, Baltimore, 1967, The Williams & Wilkins Co.

is a very vague and misleading term. There is no tone at rest."* He believes that tone is accomplished through the muscle spindles and the Golgi sense organs and that tone pertains to posture and movement only.

FRICTIONAL FORCES DURING CONTRACTION

Muscles such as those attached to the limbs are often called on to contract many times in an active person. A baseball pitcher uses the triceps so often in throwing that frictional forces are developed between muscle and bone. The pull can be so strong and so often repeated that the bone to which the muscle is attached may shear off. To some extent runners have a similar situation in the actions of the semitendinous and semimembranous muscles. At points where the muscle slides across a bony structure, tendinous aspects are developed.

HYPERTROPHY OF MUSCLE

A review of the findings of several studies reveals that despite some contradictions striated muscle fibers do not increase as the exercised muscle increases in girth and length. Brouha has said that skeletal muscles are known to increase in size when exposed to repeated muscular work. Individual muscle fibers that are small from disease develop to full size when a greater demand is placed on the muscle through regular bouts of exercise. Then what does take place? Fenn noted the gain in water content in an exercised muscle. Others mentioned the fact that the blood-fluid concentration resulting from the passage of fluids from the blood to the muscles was greater after 2 minutes of contraction than after 10 minutes. Fenn's observation, then, does not seem to be the real answer.

The changes that take place in muscle when it is exercised have been thought to be connected with the number of increased capillaries in exercised muscles. For example, Krogh, in comparing an active muscle on one side of the body with an inactive one on the opposite side, found considerable difference in the number of capillaries in the active muscle. Also the possibility exists that muscle hypertrophy results in opening of vestigial capillaries.

Brouha has stated that through exercise muscles may increase in strength without appreciable increase in girth or length. He says, "The gain in strength is more striking than the hypertrophy of the muscle, and it is possible to increase the power of muscles three times or more without a proportional increase in volume."† This may be caused by a reduction in fat and fluids in the muscle. It is generally accepted now that an increase in the cross-section area of a muscle can be expected to be accompanied by an increase in strength.

During hypertrophy one of the chief factors in the increase appears to result from an addition in the quantity of sarcoplasm that is found in the individual muscle fibers. Sarcoplasm is composed chiefly of protein, and evidence shows that increased amounts of protein are deposited in the muscle during exercise. Other factors are the increase in the number of capillaries and amount of fluids

*Strickholm, A.: Unpublished material, Indiana University, 1970.
†Brouha, L.: Physiology of training, including age and sex differences, J. Sports Med. Phys. Fitness **2:**1, 1962.

concentrated in the muscle as the result of exercise. However, hypertrophy of muscles usually brings about an increase in total body weight. This increased weight may be helpful to an athlete who competes in events such as shot-putting and discus throwing.

CLASSIFICATION OF MUSCLE ACTION

Contraction is commonly thought of as bringing a muscle's proximal and distal ends closer together, but this is not always true. Observation of the muscles of the human body as they contract against a lever soon dispel this concept. Muscular contraction can be thought of as the development of tension within a muscle.

Muscular contraction can be classified generally into three types: concentric, eccentric, and static. *Concentric* contraction occurs when a musle develops sufficient tension to overcome a resistance and shortens. A body lever is moved in opposition to a given resistance. When an individual picks up an object such as a book, some of the muscles of the arm, such as the biceps brachii, shorten as the book is moved (for example, to a table). *Eccentric* contraction occurs when the resistance is not overcome, but the muscle lengthens during the action. Eccentric contractions may occur when muscles are used to oppose a movement but not to stop it, as in the action of the biceps brachii in lowering the arm gradually, whether the weight is greater than can be lifted or a light object is being slowly placed on the floor. The main characteristic is that the muscle lengthens during the action. Both concentric and eccentric contractions are called *isotonic* because the muscle changes length during the movement.

A *static* contraction occurs when a muscle that develops tension is unable to move the load and does not change length. The effort exerted by the muscle is insufficient to move one of the body levers. This condition may occur when the load is too heavy or when opposing muscles contract in opposition to each other, thus preventing movement. This fixation of a muscle's action into a static contraction is termed *isometric* because the muscle develops tension without changing length.

CLASSIFICATION OF MUSCLES ACCORDING TO FUNCTION

For action to take place the muscles of the body develop teamwork through training and practice. However, individually they can do only two things—develop tension to various degrees or relax in various manners.

Since a muscle either develops increased tension within itself or relaxes (in varying degrees), it performs various roles as action of the skeletal levers takes place. The shape, arrangement, size, and location, including whether it is a one- or two-joint muscle, the length and nature of the tendons at either or both the origin and insertion, the type and mechanical advantage (s) of the bone (s) to which it is attached, and the insertion's angle with and distance from the fulcrum of the action bones are all factors in determining how the muscle functions in moving its bony lever. Some method of classifying these roles and functions of muscles and giving them names is needed by the student of kinesiology. However, muscles are normally classified with regard to their direction of pull on the joint and the subsequent skeletal movement. Such actions as extension, flexion, adduction, abduction, and lateral and medial rotation are classified according to the direction of the movement produced in the limb. In the following pages descriptive terms are used in a more or less arbitrary manner to defend and describe these roles and functions.

It has been mentioned previously that muscles seldom operate singly; rather, they act in cooperation with one or more other muscles or as members of a team (sometimes involving most of the major muscles of the body) in a variety of combinations and patterns. Muscular contraction is not always for the purpose of causing the levers to move. It may involve contraction to help steady or support the lever, to stabilize a body part, or even to neutralize the undesired action of some other muscles. Primarily then muscles are *movers, stabilizers,* and *neutralizers.*

Mover, or agonist. A muscle that is known to be the principal mover or one of the principal movers of a lever is called a *mover.* This muscle, which contracts concentrically, may be along with one or more other muscles directly responsible for movement of a lever. This is known as a *prime mover* when it has or shares primary responsibility for a joint action. When a muscle aids the prime mover in its action, it is known as an *assistant mover.* The biceps brachii is known as a prime mover of both the elbow in flexion and of the forearm in supination. In addition, because of the position of its two-headed origin on the scapula, it aids in action of the shoulder joint. For example, the long head of the biceps brachii, although not often involved in shoulder abduction, becomes involved under certain circumstances. Brunnstrom claims that patients have been taught by therapists to use this muscle to abduct the shoulder when the deltoideus and supraspinatus have been paralyzed.

Reversed action. Although, as previously stated, a contracting muscle usually moves the lighter of the bones to which it is attached, when the feet (or the hands) are fixed and supporting the body weight, the proximal (heavier) segment is moved. In running and jumping when the foot is on the ground, contraction of the ankle extensors moves the leg, not the foot; contraction of the knee extensors moves the thigh, not the leg. When the hands are supporting the body weight in a hanging position, contraction of the elbow flexors moves the upper arm, rather than the forearm.

Fixator, stabilizer, or supporter. A muscle that steadys, fixes, or anchors a bone or body part against contracting muscles is known as a *fixator,* or *supporter.* The support may also be used to combat the pull of gravity and the effects of momentum and interaction. For action to take place one end of a muscle must be free to move and the other end firmly anchored.

A stabilizing muscle is rarely in static contraction because the part being stabilized is in motion. Actually the anchoring part may be gradually moved to direct or guide the moving part as it performs its task.

The hip flexors stabilize when the rectus abdominis and other muscles flex the thoracic and lumbar spine (from the supine position). On the other hand, the abdominal muscles and lumbar spine extensors stabilize when the thigh is being extended by the gluteus maximus, hamstrings, and adductor magnus (especially when the knee is extended and the thigh is flexed beyond a 45-degree angle). However, when the foot is fixed and supports the weight, knee action extends the thigh (reversed muscle action). The parallel pull along the long axis of the bone that is accomplished by certain muscles makes them better suited for stabilizing a joint than others. Thus shunt muscles are considered better stabilizers than spurt muscles. This is a convenient arrangement, since the slower, stronger muscles help support the limbs, whereas the weaker, faster ones produce the limb movement.

Antagonist. A muscle that acts as an *antagonist* is one that in contracting tends to produce movement opposite to that of the mover. In extension, the extensors are the movers and the flexors are the antagonists. After studies of muscle action. Elftman concluded that antagonists play a strong role in walking and running. In such actions when the limbs are about to complete a movement, the pull of the antagonists aids in the deceleration of the limb.

Neutralizer. A muscle that acts to prevent an undesired action of a mover is call a *neutralizer.* Rasch and Burke use this term to avoid the difficulty with the term *synergist.* If a muscle both extends and adducts but the performer wishes to extend only, the abductors are activated to prevent adduction. They are neutralizers preventing the undesired action of the agonist.

Synergist. Authors have presented many different meanings for this term. Morris has stated that writers in this field show little agreement, but the term continues to be used. Some call a muscle that functions as a neutralizer a *synergist,* and others use this to mean a muscle that aids and abets the action of other muscles. Wright classifies muscles in this category as *true* synergists and *helping* synergists. The *true* synergist is a muscle that acts to prevent an undesired action of an agonist but has no effect on its desired action. The *helping* synergist is one that helps another muscle to move a lever in a desired way and at the same time prevents an undesired action.

CLASSIFICATION OF MOVEMENT

Studies of the electrical activity and the changes in tension in the various muscles involved in a voluntary movement have illustrated that a close cooperation between anatomically antagonistic muscles. The adjustment of the time relations and the magnitude of the responses to degrees of resistance and velocity of movement are infinitely variable. Nevertheless, rather fixed patterns of responses to different movements have encouraged systems of classification of movement. Some of these systems have been reviewed and summarized by Hill. A classification along these lines is as follows: (1) slow tension movements, (2) rapid tension movements, and (3) rapid ballistic movements.

Slow tension movements. Slow movements of body parts and objects that offer a large resistance are phasic in character. A phasic movement is indicated by moderate to strong cocontraction of antagonists. The cocontraction serves to fix the joints involved in the action and to aid in accurate positioning of the body part or object being moved.

In the slow, controlled forms of movement the antagonistic muscle groups are continuously contracted against each other, giving rise to tension. Tremors occur when antagonistic muscles are in contraction and balanced against each other in fixation.

Voluntary movement has been observed by Travis and Hunter to be a continuation of a tremor without interruption of the tremor rhythm. The elementary unit of a slow, controlled movement is the *tremor*. If a short movement is attempted, its amplitude is determined by that of the tremor. Ability to make movements more and more minute is limited not by sensory methods of control but by the fundamental tremor element. Stetson and McDill have determined that the magnification of the visual field does not improve the delicacy of minute movement.

Slow, controlled movements result from a slight increase in the algebraic sum of the number of muscle fibers contracting the positive muscle as against the number of fibers contracting in the antagonist muscle group. The limb moves in the direction of the group exerting the stronger pull, and tension of the two groups of antagonistic muscles is continually readjusted.

Rapid tension movements. A movement in which tension is present in all the opposing muscle groups throughout the motion may be considered a movement of translation superimposed on fixation. Rapid shaking may develop from tremors of fixation with one group of contracting muscles suddenly initiating the movement, followed by contraction of the antagonistic group to stop the movement. Control of these faster movements cannot be attained more often than ten times in a second, since modifying the course of a movement is possible only at the tremor terminations and not at other points in the movement. If the tremor cycles average ten each second, then no modification of the movement could occur in less than one tenth of a second. This limitation is imposed on the maximum rate of tapping. If the rate of tremor is ten a second, then the rate of tapping cannot exceed that value. Travis has shown that a majority of movements of the faster type synchronize with the tremor cycle.

Rapid ballistic movements. A ballistic movement, begun by a rapid initial contraction of the prime mover, proceeds relatively unhindered by antagonistic contractions and is followed by a relaxation of the protagonist while the movement is still in progress. During a movement such as throwing a baseball, the antagonist progressively decreases in activity during the throw, indicating cocontraction. In comparison with the activity of the prime movers, however, the tension in the antagonists is slight during the ballistic type of movement. There is some question whether true ballistic movements occur in sport skills.

One of the greatest differences between skilled and unskilled movements centers around changing tension movements to ballistic movements. Attempts to make ballistic movements with muscles that are already fixed are fatiguing. Tension in one group of muscles necessitates an increase in the intensity of contraction of other sets. The spread of intensity results in rigidity, which is wasteful and restrictive.

In a ballistic movement such as a golf swing the moving limb swings rapidly about a joint, and the movement is terminated by cocontraction of the opposing

muscles and the loss of momentum. If a movement is arrested by a strong contraction of the antagonistic group of muscles and as a result moves in the opposite direction, the movement is said to be *oscillatory*. Movements of great
amplitude are more economical than those of small amplitude because of the
intensity and continuity of muscular activity required to stop and start each
phase of oscillation. A fast, shallow kick in swimming requires more effort to
gain the same propulsive force as a slower, deeper kick. Hubbard has stated that
fast action of a limb involves muscular contraction that acts as an impulse (Fr,
same force for same time). A limb once set in action by an impulse will continue
to move by virtue of its own momentum until acted on by an outside force. The
muscle, having developed energy in the limb, then tends to relax.

MUSCLE ANALYSIS OF MOTOR SKILLS

Analysis of muscular participation in a motor act is complex because muscles
as they contract serve several different purposes, all contributing to the efficiency
of the skill. The primary purpose is, of course, to move a lever in a certain direction. The muscles that do this are known as *prime movers*. Yet few muscles are
so attached that when contracting they move the bone in one plane only; they
tend to move it in two or more planes, only one of which may be desired. The
pectoralis major, for example, flexes, adducts, and medially rotates the upper
arm. It moves the humerus in the sagittal, frontal, and transverse planes. A
counter force must be available to prevent the undesired actions. The muscles
that contract to provide the counter force are known as *synergists* or *neutralizers*.

Also the prime movers (and the synergists and neutralizers) pull not only on
the bone to be moved but also with equal force on the other bony segment to
which they are attached. That bone must be stabilized if the prime mover's pull
on the lever is to be effective; this will be done by muscles that pull the bone in
a direction opposite to that of the pull of the prime movers. For example, if the
pectoralis is a prime mover of the humerus, it tends to pull the shoulder girdle
forward. Some muscular contraction must prevent this. Those muscles that contract to prevent such movements are known as *fixators*.

Other factors add to the complexity of muscle participation. As stated previously some muscles pass over more than one joint and, when they contract, they
tend to cause movements in all the joints over which they pass. However, if
Wright's statement that "the two-joint muscles do not usually contract when the
intention is to move the upper joint only" is true, such muscles would not be
considered prime movers for the upper joint. Yet when such muscles do contract
as prime movers of the lower joint, they "exert power on the upper joint also"
according to Wright. Two-joint muscle participation as explained by Wright
would be efficient. If two-joint muscles acted as prime movers of the upper joint,
when lower-joint actions were not desired, additional synergists would be needed
to prevent them. This would not be the case if the two-joint muscles did not act
as prime movers of the upper joint. Until evidence to the contrary is found, it is
logical to accept Wright's statements because everything that is known about the
inherent responses of the neuromuscular mechanism suggests that they are likely
to be efficient.

Another complicating factor in naming the participating muscles in any act is the constantly changing position of bony segments in relation to each other; this is especially true in the many-levered skills. The change in position changes the direction of pull of the muscles, and as the position and the direction of pull change, the needed muscle group may change. For example, when the arm is raised in the sagittal plane above the horizontal, the action is flexion at the shoulder joint. An anatomy text will list the pectoralis as a flexor for this action; there is justification for naming it as a participating muscle in the action. Yet when the arm is lowered vigorously from the vertical, the pectoralis, by virtue of the position of its attachments, is also capable of participating in the movement, which is now extension. The direction of pull must be considered as the position of the segments changes.

This discussion has been included to present the difficulties in naming accurately the participating muscles in a skill, especially in those skills in which many levers are acting. When acting muscles are named, the listing has often been based on the anatomic position—on the actions listed for a muscle in an anatomy text—and not on observation of contraction in a muscle as the skill is performed. Also efforts have been made to observe muscle action in living moving human beings. Kinesiology class experiences have included observations of actions by individuals with small amounts of subcutaneous fat. As these subjects move (usually slowly) or assume certain positions, vision and palpation reveal bulging or hardening of a given muscle as it contracts. These methods of observing were employed by Beevor and by Wright, who attempted to show characteristics of muscle action. They have provided insights not shown by analysis based on anatomic position only. Useful and valuable as visual inspection and palpation are in studying muscle action, the observations that can be made with them are limited. Among these are the difficulties in observing action that is rapidly executed, in observing more than one part of the body at the same time in complex actions, and in observing small degrees of muscle action, in which the amount of bulging or hardening is slight. These limitations are not found in the method of observing muscle action currently used—electromyography.

ELECTROMYOGRAPHY

Electromyography* is the process of recording electrical changes that occur in a muscle during or immediately prior to contraction. Necessary equipment includes a device for picking up the electrical activity, a means for conducting the electric impulses, and a device for translating them to visual form. The pickup devices are metal disks placed on the skin over the muscle or fine wires inserted into the muscle to be observed. Insulated wires conduct impulses from the pickup to the translating devices. Among the latter are ink writers, electro-

---

*For detailed descriptions of electromyography see Basmajian, J. B.: Electromyographic analysis, Proceedings of Biomechanics Symposium at Indiana University, Chicago, 1971, The Athletic Institute; O'Connell, A. L., and Gardner, E. B.: The use of electromyography in kinesiological research, Res. Q. Am. Assoc. Health Phys. Educ. **34:**166, 1963; and Waterland, J. C., and Shambes, G. M.: Electromyography; one link in the experimental chain of kinesiological research, J. Am. Phys. Ther. Assoc. **49:**1351, 1969.

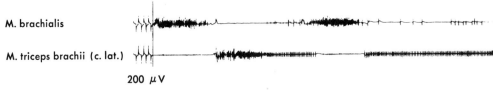

M. brachialis

M. triceps brachii (c. lat.)

200 μV

Fig. 5-6. Simple electromyogram. (From Waterland, J. C.: Aspects of motor learning. In Proceedings of Biomechanics Symposium, Chicago, 1969, The Athletic Institute.)

magnetic tape recorders, and oscilloscopes, from which photographs are made during the activity. The final form is a record, an electromyogram, similar to that shown in Fig. 5-6.

This brief, simplified statement concerning electromyography does not convey one essential concept—that the competent, trustworthy investigator must have special technical skills. Such skills include the ability to select the best equipment for each study, to use the equipment, and to interpret the electromyograms intelligently. This last skill is illustrated by one investigator's analysis of the simple record shown in Fig. 5-6: "To the far right of the lower line the evenly spaced vertical lines indicate that the electrodes have picked up contractions of a single motor unit; the heavy black recordings at the left and the middle of the upper line and at the second fourth of the lower line are overlapping recordings of motor unit contractions; the vertical lines at the right of the upper line are due to artifacts, such as slipping of the electrode on the skin."

To interpret an electromyogram it is necessary to know which body segments have moved; in which joints actions have occurred, at what rates, and in what sequence; which muscles pass over these joints; and to which bones these muscles are attached. It is also necessary to know whether other forces were acting on body segments, especially gravitational force. Since electromyograms do not provide such information, other records of the action are made at the same time, for example, with photography (biplane is recommended) and electrogoniometry.

THEORETICAL ANALYSIS OF MUSCLE ACTION

Muscle analysis based on anatomic position of muscles cannot be accepted as definitive of the action that occurs in the living, moving body; however, such analysis can aid in understanding the complexity of muscle action and can be undertaken as a worthwhile kinesiologic experience. Analysis begins with naming the joint actions that occur in a given activity. Next, the muscles that are prime movers for these actions are listed and with them the joint actions (other than those desired in the action) that will accompany shortening of each muscle. Perhaps these actions would neutralize each other; if not, other muscles could be named that would act as synergists to the undesired actions. Also the bones (other than the acting levers) to which the prime movers are attached could be viewed as needing stabilization, and fixator muscles could be added to the list. Remember that, although prime, synergistic, and fixator actions are essential, one cannot with equal confidence be sure that the muscles which might be named as contracting for the needed actions are the ones that contract. Yet naming of the muscles is valuable in understanding the complexity of muscle participation.

Tables 5-1 and 5-2 can aid in studying muscle action. Table 5-1 lists the muscles of the upper limb, and Table 5-2 those of the lower limb. In each table the muscles are grouped alphabetically according to the body segment on which each exerts primary action. Following Wright's explanation of the action of two-joint muscles, these muscles are listed with the distal rather than the proximal segment that the muscle can move. Thus the flexor carpi ulnaris is listed with the movers of the hand, although it tends to flex the forearm when it contracts; the biceps is listed with the muscles of the forearm rather than with those of the upper arm, although it does act at the shoulder joint when it contracts.

Opposite each muscle an X shows the movements that, according to one standard anatomy text, occur when the muscle contracts. (These movements differ in some cases from those reported by other texts.)

As an example of the use that can be made of the charts, a one-joint action will be analyzed—that of upper-arm flexion. According to the chart the prime movers for this action are the coracobrachialis, the anterior deltoideus, and the pectoralis major. The biceps is not included in the list even though it can act as a shoulder flexor because it is a two-joint muscle and the shoulder is the proximal joint over which it passes. The chart shows that, as the three muscles contract, they tend to produce besides the desired shoulder flexion the following movements:

> Coracobrachialis—adduction
> Anterior deltoideus—abduction
> Pectoralis major—adduction and medial rotation

Perhaps the undesired adduction and abduction will neutralize each other. Since medial rotation is not desired, some synergist must be found. The chart shows that the lateral rotators are the infraspinatus, the supraspinatus, and the teres minor. The infraspinatus and the teres minor also extend the arm; the supraspinatus abducts it. Without some observation such as that made with electromyography it is impossible to know which muscle will act. However, with confidence in the wisdom of the body one could reasonably guess that the supraspinatus will act, since it aids in neutralizing the adducting of the coracobrachialis and the pectoralis major. The other two possible lateral rotators would pull against the desired flexion.

The prime movers are attached to the shoulder girdle and, if the flexion is a strong movement, tend to protract the shoulder girdle. In such cases the girdle should be stabilized by the action of muscles acting as fixators. Reasonable choices would be the levator scapula and the inferior trapezius, since the elevating pull of the first would be neutralized by the depressing pull of the second.

· · ·

Discussion of specific skills in the following chapters will include no muscular analysis. The foregoing discussion explains the reason for this omission. However, joint action will be described, and such description means that the related muscle

Text continued on p. 108.

Table 5-1. Muscle actions of the upper limb*

Muscle	Shoulder girdle						Upper arm						Lower arm			
	El.	Dep.	Pro.	Ret.	Rot. up	Rot. down	Fl.	Ext.	Abd.	Add.	Med. rot.	Lat. rot.	Fl.	Ext.	Sup.	Pro.
Levator scapulae	X															
Pectoralis minor		X	X			X										
Rhomboideus major		X		X		X										
Rhomboideus minor		X		X		X										
Serratus anterior			X		X											
Subclavius		X														
Trapezius	Superior	Inferior		X		Middle and inferior										
Coracobrachialis							X			X						
Deltoideus							Anterior	Posterior	X							
Infraspinatus								X				X				
Latissimus dorsi								X		X	X					
Pectoralis major							X			X	X					
Subscapularis										X	X					
Supraspinatus									X			X				
Teres major								X		X	X					
Teres minor								X		X		X				
Anconeus													-	X		
Biceps									Long	Short			X		X	
Brachialis													X			

Muscle	Lower arm				Hand				Thumb				Fingers			
	Fl.	Ext.	Sup.	Pro.	Fl.	Ext.	Abd.	Add.	Fl.	Ext.	Abd.	Add.	Fl.	Ext.	Abd.	Add.
Brachioradialis	X															
Triceps		X														
Pronator quadratus				X					Long							X
Pronator teres		X		X									Long			X
Supinator			X												X	
Flexor carpi ulnaris	X				X			X								
Flexor carpi radialis	X			X	X		X									
Extensor carpi radialis brevis						X	X									
Extensor carpi radialis longus	X					X	X									
Extensor carpi ulnaris		X				X		X								
Palmaris longus	X				X											
Abductor digiti quinti manus													Proximal finger phalanges		Little finger	
Abductor pollicis brevis											Draws thumb to plane at right angles to palm					
Abductor pollicis longus						X	X				Carries thumb laterally from palm					

*Information based on Goss, C. M., editor: Gray's anatomy of the human body, ed. 29, Philadelphia, 1973, Lea & Febiger.
Key: Abd.—abducts; Add.—adducts; Dep.—depresses; El.—elevates; Ext.—extends or extension; Fl.—flexes; Lat.—lateral; Med.—medial; Pro.—pronates or protracts; Ret.—retracts; Rot.—rotates or rotation; Sup.—supinates.

Continued.

Table 5-1. Muscle actions of the upper limb—cont'd

Muscle	Lower arm				Hand				Thumb				Fingers			
	Fl.	Ext.	Sup.	Pro.	Fl.	Ext.	Abd.	Add.	Fl.	Ext.	Abd.	Add.	Fl.	Ext.	Abd.	Add.
Adductor pollicis									Approximates thumb to palm							
Extensor digiti quinti proprius						X								Little finger		
Extensor digitorum communis		X				X								X	In ext.	
Extensor indicis proprius						X								Index finger		
Extensor pollicis brevis						X				X						
Extensor pollicis longus						X				X						
Flexor digiti quinti brevis manus													Little finger			
Flexor digitorum profundus					X				X							
Flexor digitorum sublimis	X				X								Middle and proximal phalanges			

Muscle	Proximal	Proximal phalanx			
Flexor pollicis brevis					X
Flexor pollicis longus					X
Interossei dorsales manus	X		First finger	Second and third phalanges	X
Interossei volares			First finger	Second and third phalanges	X
Lumbricales manus	X		First finger	Second and third phalanges	
Palmaris brevis			Corrugates skin on ulnar side of hand		
Opponens pollicis	X	X			
Opponens digiti quinti manus		X	Deepens hollow of palm		

Table 5-2. Muscle actions of the lower limb*

Muscle	Thigh						Lower leg			
	Fl.	Ext.	Abd.	Add.	Rot. med.	Rot. lat.	Fl.	Ext.	Rot. med.	Rot. lat.
Adductor brevis	X			X		X				
Adductor longus	X			X		X				
Adductor magnus	Upper part	Lower part		X	Lower part	Upper part				
Gemelli			In flexion			X				
Gluteus maximus		X		Lower part		Lower part				
Gluteus medius			In extension		Anterior fibers					
Gluteus minimus			In extension		Anterior fibers					
Gracilis	X			X	X				X	
Iliacus	X				Slight					
Obturator externus			In flexion			X				
Obturator internus			In flexion			X				
Pectineus	X			X		X				
Piriformis			X			X				
Psoas major	X				Slight					
Psoas minor			Tensor of iliac fascia							
Quadratus femoris				X		X		X		
Sartorius	X			X		X	X			
Tensor fasciae latae			X		X					
Biceps femoris		X					X			In flexion

*Information based on Goss, C. M., editor: Gray's anatomy of the human body, ed. 29, Philadelphia, 1973, Lea & Febiger.
Key: Abd.—abducts; Add.—adducts; Ever.—everts; Ext.—extends; Fl.—flexes; Inv.—inverts; Lat.—laterally; Med.—medially; Pro.—pronates; Rot.—rotates; Sup.—supinates.

Table 5-2. Muscle actions of the lower limb—cont'd

Muscle	Thigh						Lower leg			
	Fl.	Ext.	Abd.	Add.	Rot. med.	Rot. lat.	Fl.	Ext.	Rot. med.	Rot. lat.
Semimembranosus		X					X		Slight	
Semitendinosus		X					X		X	
Popliteus							X		In flexion	
Rectus femoris	X							X		
Vastus medialis								X		
Vastus internus								X		
Vastus lateralis								X		
Articularis genu					Occasionally blended with vastus intermedius					

Muscle	Lower leg				Foot				Toes			
	Fl.	Ext.	Rot. med.	Rot. lat.	Plantar fl.	Dorsi-fl.	Inv.	Ever.	Fl.	Ext.	Abd.	Add.
Gastrocnemius	X				X							
Peroneus brevis					X			X				
Peroneus longus					X			X				
Peroneus tertius						X		X				
Plantaris	X				X							
Soleus					X							
Tibialis anterior						X	X					
Tibialis posterior					X		X					
Abductor digiti quinti									X		X	
Abductor hallucis									X		X	
Adductor hallucis									X			X
Extensor digitorum brevis										X	X	

Continued.

Table 5-2. Muscle actions of the lower limb—cont'd

Muscle	Foot				Toes			
	Plantar fl.	Dorsi- fl.	Inv.	Ever.	Fl.	Ext.	Abd.	Add.
Extensor digitorum longus		X				X		
Extensor hallucis longus		X				X		
Flexor digitorum longus	X				X			
Flexor digitorum brevis					X Little toe		X Little toe	
Flexor digitorum quinti					X			X
Flexor hallucis brevis					X			
Flexor hallucis longus	X				X			
Interossei dorsales pedis					X	X	X	
Interossei plantares					X	X		X
Lumbricales pedis					X	X		
Quadratus plantae					X			

group must have been contracting. If the joint action was flexion, the flexors (or at least some of them) contracted to provide the energy for the action. If the joint action was supination, the supinators supplied the energy. Present knowledge does not warrant naming specific muscles.

SUGGESTED READINGS

Basmajian, J. V.: Muscles alive; their functions as revealed by electromyography, ed. 2, Baltimore, 1967, The Williams & Wilkins Co.

Huxley, H. E.: The contraction of muscle, Sci. Am. **199**:67, Nov., 1958.

Huxley, H. E.: The mechanics of muscular contraction, Sci. Am. **213**:6, Dec., 1965.

Johnson, T. B., editor: Gray's Anatomy of the human body, ed. 35, London, 1972, W. B. Saunders Co., Ltd.

O'Connell, A. L., and Gardner, E. B.: Understanding the scientific bases of human movement, Baltimore, 1972, The Williams & Wilkins Co., Chap. 2.

Skarstrom, W.: Gymnastic kinesiology, Springfield, Mass., 1909, F. H. Bassette Co.

Steindler, A.: Kinesiology of the human body under normal and pathological conditions, Springfield, Ill., 1955, Charles C Thomas, Publisher.

Thompson, C. W.: Manual of structural kinesiology, ed. 7, St. Louis, 1973, The C. V. Mosby Co.

Wright, W.: Muscle function, New York, 1928, Paul B. Hoeber, Inc.

See Bibliography for additional references.

PART III

Application of kinesiology to motor skills

CHAPTER 6 General plan for studying
motor skill

Three body systems that are the primary components of the human motor mechanism were discussed in preceding chapters. To summarize with extreme brevity, movement initiated within the body was said to require first that nerve impulses reach muscle fibers. In the fibers the impulses start a chemical reaction that results in contraction of the fibers. As the muscle shortens during contraction, it tends to pull its bony attachments toward each other. The moving bones act as levers, transmitting energy from the muscle to a body part or an external object.

Students of motor skill reverse this process; they begin with the final phase— the levers and the joint actions, which determine the degree of skill. If the levers are not producing the desired amount of force in the desired direction, they know that lever and joint action should be changed. If they are well versed in kinesiology, they will know a good deal about what the changes should be.

However, changes must be made through the nerve-muscle chain. Little is known about that chain except in a general way. Sometimes nerve action can be started in a simple way: a decision may be made to move or not to move a joint that is part of a complex pattern. What occurs between decision and muscle contraction is not known in detail; when such knowledge is available, the teaching of motor skill should be more effective. Meanwhile efforts should be made to apply present knowledge.

It is logical to begin the study of motor skill with a consideration of human levers and their efficient use. This is not a simple task. First, it is complicated by the number of directions in which each lever can be moved. Every segment can be moved in at least two directions from its anatomic position. If flexion, medial rotation, or adduction is a possible action for a segment, the opposing action— extension, lateral rotation, or abduction—is possible also. Also a segment can be moved in two directions simultaneously; for example, the humerus can adduct and rotate at the same time.

Second, in most skills more than one lever is moving at the same time; as many as five or six levers may be involved. This feature, combined with the number of directions in which a segment can move, provides thousands of possible combinations. Suppose that only two levers are moving at the same time. Lever A can move in a, b, c, d, e, and f directions and lever B in a, b, c, and d directions. Theoretically each A action could be combined with each B action—

AaBa, AaBb, AaBc, AaBd. Also Ab, Ac, Ad, Ae, and Af might act with each B action. The thousands of possibilities are evident.

If the study of human movement warrants the title *kinesiology*, pertinent information, like that in every science, should be systematically organized. One kinesiologic grouping is widely used—the grouping of joint action: flexion, extension, rotations, abduction, and adduction. The definition of each term in this classification should be such that it could be applied to movements of any body segment. Application of this classification based on description is limited to the action of a single joint. Since the great majority of motor acts are complex, involving several segments and joint actions, there should be some type of grouping that could be applied to the many possible combinations.

An outstanding student of human movement has said, "Voluntary movement is goal-oriented."* This statement suggests that voluntary actions could be classified on the basis of purpose. Such grouping was recommended by one of us (Glassow) in 1932, by Wells in the several editions of her kinesiology text, and by Broer in *Efficiency of human movement*. Although originally it was based on voluntary acts, it is now evident that it applies to inherent movement patterns also.

Major divisions in the recommended classification include moving external objects, moving and balancing the body itself, and stopping moving objects. These represent types of activities that have for centuries been essential for man's survival and he, like all living organisms, developed structure and motor behavior that enabled him to cope with his environment. Motor patterns, unique combinations of nerve-muscle-bone actions, were developed to accomplish certain purposes. (See Chapter 1.) Today these patterns are the foundations of human motor skills. They need not be learned; coordinations related to purpose are inherent. Children as young as 3 years of age, when in situations not encountered previously, respond with effective movements. Basically these movements are those which would be used by skilled performers; the child needs no instruction to bring forth the fundamental pattern. (See Chapter 4.)

However, a purpose is not always accomplished with the same movement pattern. An external object can be moved with a throw, strike, pull, or push. A throw can be made with an overarm, an underarm, or a sidearm pattern; a strike may also be made with these patterns. The human body moves itself by a run, walk, and jump. Similar patterns can be identified by even the casual observer in a general way, but for identification of details other methods of observation are needed. Broer has presented similarities with film sequences of skills in which she shows that an underarm throw, an underarm volleyball serve, and a badminton serve have the same basic pattern; an overarm throw, a badminton clear, and a tennis serve are basically the same, as are a sidearm basketball throw, a tennis drive, and a baseball batting action. She also shows the similarity in the pattern of the lower limbs in a one-footed takeoff in the basketball lay-up, the volleyball spike, and the hurdle for the running dive.

---

*Gardner, E. B.: Proprioceptive reflexes and their participation in motor skills, Quest 12:1, 1969.

Another means of identifying similarities has employed detailed analysis of film. From photographs such as those shown in Fig. 6-1 each acting joint can be identified. The number of degrees that each segment moves from frame to frame can be measured, and, since the clock in the picture gives the time per frame, the angular velocity can be determined. If the change in degrees is plotted against the time, the graph of all joints presents a picture of what is occurring during the total performance. Here can be seen the sequence and range of joint actions in relationship to each other. The joints acting in the final phase, such as the release in a throw, the impact in a strike, and the takeoff in a jump, can be identified.

In this final phase the length of the moment arm of each acting joint can be measured from the view best suited to provide the length (side, front or back, or overhead). When the length of the moment arm and the angular velocity of the joint are known, the linear velocity of each moment arm can be calculated. The contribution made by each acting joint to the final application of force can then be determined.

The use of triplane photography (Fig. 6-1) has been helpful in the development of research technique. The earliest film studies were based on views taken with one camera usually from a side view. From those, only joint actions that occurred in the picture plane could be measured directly. As research progressed, cameras were added to obtain overhead and rear (or front) views. The overhead camera is likely to present the most difficulty in the filming situation. The distance between that camera and the subject must be great enough to include the field to be photographed and so that the photographed size of an object in the sides of the field will not differ significantly from its size when photographed in the middle of the field.

Another development in research devices is seen in the cone-shaped clock in Fig. 6-1. When film studies were based on one-plane views, a flat-faced clock could be used; with biplane photography, the clock could be placed at an angle and be seen in both views. When three cameras were used, the cone-shaped clock, which can be read in all three views, was suggested. Roberts has recently added an electric device to the cone that permits recording of time intervals and eliminates the necessity of reading the clock. The velocity of thrown balls and the forces made by the feet in a throw may be determined by the use of a laser beam and force platforms, as shown in Fig. 2-7. The accuracy of recording is improved with this device.

Tracings from a film study are shown in Fig. 6-2. A primary purpose of the investigator was to observe the path of the ball before release when the subject used the overarm throwing pattern. The tracings are from the side and over-head views and illustrate the value of biplane photography. The circles are tracings of the ball in successive frames and represent the same points of time in the two views. (Note the lettering and numbering.) The time relationship is more easily identified by the blackened circles. With reference to the performer the circles show the ball progress from the back toward the front. Only the side view shows the downward and upward progress (vertical plane), and only the

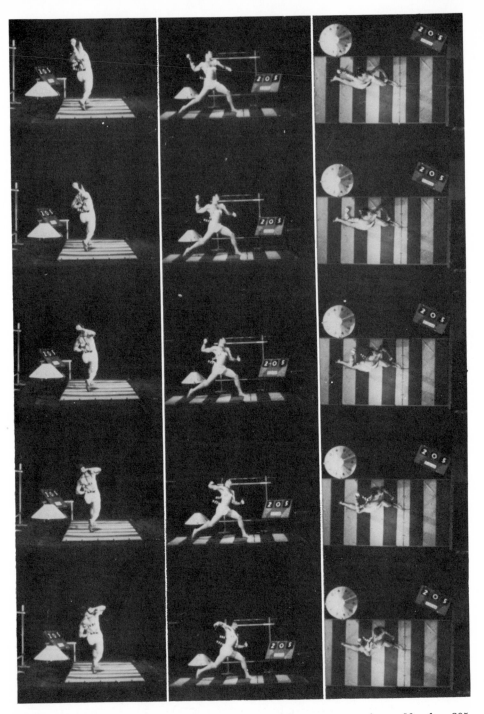

Fig. 6-1. Rear, side, and overhead views taken to study an overarm throw. Number 205 identifies subject and trial in a series; note presence of cone-shaped timing device and uprights and crossbars that establish vertical and horizontal lines to aid in measurement. (Courtesy Kinesiology Research Laboratories, University of Wisconsin, and A. E. Atwater, University of Arizona.)

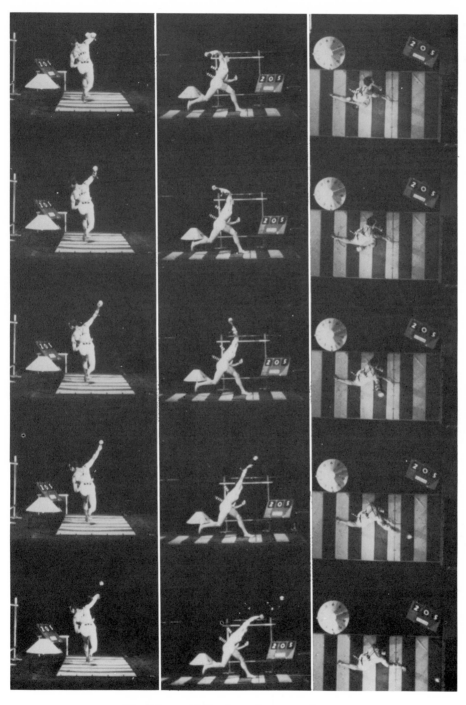

Fig. 6-1, cont'd. For legend see opposite page.

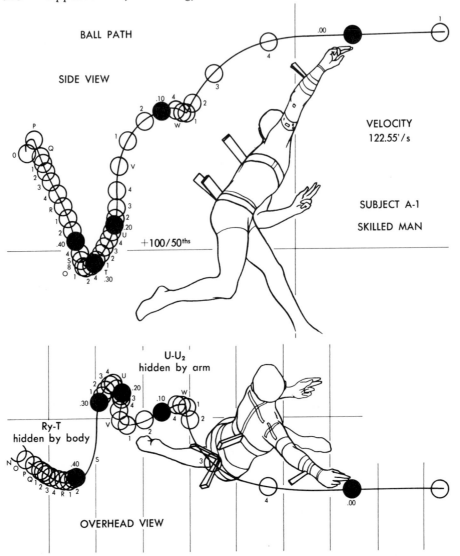

BALL PATH

SIDE VIEW

VELOCITY
122.55'/s

SUBJECT A-1

SKILLED MAN

$+100/50^{ths}$

U-U$_2$
hidden by arm

Ry-T
hidden by body

OVERHEAD VIEW

Fig. 6-2. Tracings from film to show path of ball. Circles represent equal time intervals. (From Atwater, A. E.: Movement characteristics of the overarm throw, dissertation, University of Wisconsin, 1970.)

overhead view shows the right to left to right movement (horizontal plane). This investigator chose to trace the performer when the ball had been released. A similar tracing could be made to accompany any ball position.

This type of detailed observation and measurement shows similarities and differences in movement patterns. Equally important is the understanding of the mechanics of body action that it provides. With such understanding students of movement are freed from imitation of the expert. If a joint action is recommended in a pattern, they should ask, "What will it contribute?" They should not be satisfied with developing a pattern because they are told that it is "good form," the pattern of some well-known skilled performer. If reference is made to the pattern of an expert, the mechanical advantages of the expert's joint actions should be understood. Students should not strive to develop a description of expert performance; they should strive to develop an understanding of a pattern that is mechanically and physiologically efficient.

Insight into the mechanics of a skill can be gained from studying film of poor performers and comparing it with film of good performers. For example, the graph of the moving segments of a highly skilled girl as she executes the standing broad jump shows that in the final phase most of the power is derived from the movements of the thigh and the foot. Since the thigh is moved by extension at the knee joint, study of the graph suggests that knee extension is a major factor in attaining power in the standing broad jump. This concept is given support by a comparison of knee action in observations made by Felton. Five college women whose jumps averaged 85 inches were extending the knee at takeoff at an average velocity of 729 degrees per second, whereas five women whose jumps averaged 48 inches extended the knee at an average velocity of 183 degrees per second.

Knee action has been shown to be an important factor in producing power in another form of locomotion—the run. Knee action of a skilled performer was compared with that of an unskilled runner. Measurements from film showed the range of knee extension to be 32 degrees in the skilled and 6 degrees in the unskilled and the velocity of knee extension to be 711 degrees per second in the skilled and 80 degrees in the unskilled.

The similarity in the mechanics of jumping and running, as described in the preceding paragraphs, and of other activities that will be discussed later in the text, suggests that these skills are modifications of the same basic pattern. Running and jumping have a common purpose—to move the body. For any given purpose, the human mechanism is likely to have inherent patterns that to some degree will achieve the desired end. By recognizing these patterns in attempts to improve skill, the student can utilize the nerve-muscle chains that move the body levers. Each situation will require its own modifications of the basic pattern. The modifications should be made to improve the mechanics.

This text will follow a general plan in discussing motor skill. Specific skills will be discussed, since they are the primary concern of the performer, student, instructor, and therapist. Skills will be grouped according to the basic pattern of which each is a modification. Patterns will be grouped according to purpose. Pattern and purpose recognize inherent coordinations; the discussion of each skill will be concerned with the mechanics, an understanding of which is essential to intelligent modification of a pattern.

Not every skill that people are likely to perform will be discussed. It is hoped that with understanding of the content of the text, students of movement will be able to classify any skill according to purpose and also in most cases according to pattern. In addition, they should have some understanding of the mechanical modifications that are necessary in any pattern for skilled performance.

Frequent comments have suggested that greater detail concerning procedures used in studying film should be included in this text. We agree that publication of such procedures is needed but do not agree that they would be properly included in this text. Those desiring this type of information will find Atwater's 1970 dissertation valuable.

SUGGESTED READINGS

Atwater, A. E.: Movement characteristics of the overarm throw; a kinematic analysis of men and women performers, dissertation, University of Wisconsin, 1970.

Broer, M. R.: Efficiency of human movement, Philadelphia, 1966, W. B. Saunders Co.

Glassow, R. B.: Fundamentals of physical education, Philadelphia, 1932, Lea & Febiger.

Miller, D. I., and Petak, K. L.: Three dimensional cinematography. In Kinesiology III, Washington, D.C., 1973, AAHPER, p. 14.

Wells, K. F.: Kinesiology, Philadelphia, 1950, W. B. Saunders Co.

See Bibliography for additional references.

MOVING
EXTERNAL
OBJECTS

CHAPTER 7 Underarm patterns

MECHANICS OF UNDERARM PATTERN

The underarm pattern is most frequently seen in skills that project an object by a throw or strike. Its outstanding characteristic is movement of the arm, usually with extended elbow, by shoulder joint action. At the height of the backswing the arm is approximately shoulder height; during the force-producing phase, the arm is moved rapidly downward and at release or impact it reaches a position that is usually parallel with or slightly beyond the line of the trunk.

The lever of this shoulder action includes the bones of the upper arm and forearm, the wrist and hand, and in the throw the portion of the phalanges up to the center of gravity of the projectile. If an implement is used, all the phalanges will be included, in addition to the length of the implement from grasp to point of impact. The resistance arm includes the same rigid masses as does the entire lever; the fulcrum is in the shoulder joint. The length of the moment arm at the time that the object is started on its flight will be that of a line from the proximal end of the humerus to the point of impact or the center of gravity of the projectile. This line will be perpendicular to the axis and to the line of the applied force.

Various levers can be added to this primary action to increase the amount of applied force. Among the most common is that which moves the pelvis by rotation at the hip joint. This lever will include the pelvis, the spine, the right side of the shoulder girdle, and the rigid masses included in the shoulder-action lever. (This description and that which follows refer to a right-handed performer.) The resistance arm will include the same masses as does the entire lever. At release or impact the length of the moment arm will be the distance from the axis (a line passing through the hip joint that is rotating) to the point of release or impact. This line, perpendicular to the axis and to the direction of applied force, can be changed in length by the positions of the trunk and the arm. If the trunk is flexed to the right, the moment arm will be lengthened; if flexed to the left, it will be shortened. If the arm is abducted, the moment arm will be lengthened. In some underarm patterns that have been studied, although pelvic rotation occurred during the force-producing phase, it was not found to occur at the time of application of force. Thus if the linear velocities of moment arms acting at release or impact are determined and if the velocity of pelvic rotation is not one of them, it makes no direct contribution to the force at that time. Most likely its contribution, made before the final phase, is reflected in the actions of the other joints.

Pelvic rotation is facilitated by a transfer of weight of the total body. In the preparatory phase the weight is transferred to the right foot, and the pelvis is rotated to the right; rotation can be more than 90 degrees from the intended direction of flight of the projectile. This range of rotation is not possible unless the weight is taken from the left foot. Pelvic rotation facilitates arm action. As the pelvis turns, it carries the torso with it until it, too, is at right angles to the intended line of flight. As the arm is raised upward and backward, it is abducting, instead of extending, as it would be if the torso were facing forward. The shoulder joint's abduction range is greater than its hyperextension range, and according to present knowledge a segment can be moved faster if its range of action is increased.

While the weight is on the right foot, the left foot can be lifted in preparation for a forward step. No evidence is available to indicate the most advantageous exact length of this step. Studies do show that good performers take longer steps than those who are less skilled and that the length of the step is a feature that distinguishes between good and poor performers. As the forward step is taken, some forward movement of the whole body occurs. This adds to the force that can be imparted to the projectile, but compared to that developed by hip and shoulder action it is small. The step alone is not an important factor in increasing force; the step accompanied by increased range of hip and shoulder action is important.

Rotation of the spine can add another lever to the pattern. In comparison to other possible levers that may be a part of the pattern, the contribution of the spine is small. Although the action occurs in many vertebral joints, the fulcrum can be considered as that acting at the level of the sternoclavicular joint. The lever will include the right clavicle and the masses included in the shoulder lever; the resistance arm will include the masses of the entire lever. The length of the moment arm will be the perpendicular distance from the axis; it will pass through the upper spine, to the point of release or impact. The length of the moment arm can be altered by changes of trunk or arm position, as described for the moment arm of pelvic rotation.

An important lever is that acting at the wrist joint because this action can be the fastest of the acting joints and because the length of the moment arm can be greatly increased by an implement. For the throw the lever arm and the resistance arm include the bones of the hand and fingers to the center of gravity of the projectile; for the strike, they include the bones of the hand and fingers and the implement if one is used to the point of impact. In a throw, depending on the size of the hand, the moment arm from the wrist to the center of gravity of the projectile could be 3 or 4 inches in a child and 8 or 9 inches in an adult; in a strike it would be increased by the length of the implement from grasp to point of impact.

The levers described in the preceding paragraphs, acting at shoulder, hip, spine, and wrist joints, are those most commonly used in a variety of underarm patterns. Whether more than one is used in the pattern will depend on the demands of the situation. Shoulder action will always be used, since it is the basis for the classification *underarm*. It is possible that in some situations other joint actions can be used efficiently, but such additions will not change the classification when the shoulder action is that described here.

In the following section the underarm pattern as it is used in specific skills will be described. This is not intended as a description of the one best pattern. There is not sufficient evidence at present for anyone to describe in detail the joint actions that should be used by everyone performing a certain skill. However, every performer who wishes to improve a skill should strive to employ the levers that are the major contributors. It can confidently be said that, when great force is desired, the fundamental mechanics used by all individuals in a particular skill should be similar. There are likely to be individual differences, but, as Morton and Dudley said in discussing differences in walking, "they represent only superficial modifications of the essentially uniform characteristics."*

BOWLING

Among the least complex of the underarm patterns is the bowling delivery at the time of release. Obviously the major contribution to the velocity of the ball is the force derived from shoulder action. It is also apparent that hip and spinal rotation will be limited, since the bowler tends to keep the upper torso facing the lane, and the weight of the ball will limit wrist action.

Although the details of each bowler's performance differs from that of others, a general idea of the contribution of each acting lever can be gained from the following analysis. From a film showing the delivery of a man physical education major observations disclosed that at the time of release spinal rotation and shoulder flexion occurred but no hip rotation or wrist flexion. An unexpected action was elbow flexion.

To determine the contribution of each acting joint, the following measurements were made for the two frames preceding release: (1) the range of action of each joint (Table 7-1) and (2) the time during which this action occurred. The time per frame was 0.0158 second and for 2 frames was 0.0316 second, or approximately 64 frames per second. The length of each moment arm at the time of release was measured from a side view. These were (1) for shoulder action (from shoulder to center of the ball), (2) for the elbow (from elbow to center of the ball), and (3) for the spine (a horizontal line from the upper spine to a vertical line passing through the center of the ball).

The sum of the linear velocities of the three levers is 25.60 feet per second. The velocity of the ball as it moved away from the hand was measured and calculated as 29.11 feet per second. The difference suggests that a contributing fac-

*Morton, D. J., and Dudley, D. F.: Human locomotion and body form, Baltimore, 1952, The Williams & Wilkins Co.

Table 7-1. Lever contributions to ball velocity in bowling

	Range	Angular velocity	Moment arm length	Linear velocity
Shoulder	14	443	2.45	18.94
Spine	6	190	1.04	3.45
Elbow	4	127	1.45	3.21

Table 7-2. Lever contributions to ball velocity in bowling

	Range	Angular velocity	Moment arm length	Linear velocity
Shoulder	12	400.00	2.480	17.31
Elbow	2	66.66	1.530	1.78
Wrist	11	366.66	0.425	2.72

tor was not included or that errors were made in measurements. Further study of the films showed that the torso moved forward during the two frames because of sliding on the left foot and flexion in the left ankle. The distance that the shoulder moved forward was measured as 0.144 foot. The linear velocity of this movement would be 4.56 feet per second. The summed velocities were now 30.16 feet per second, or 1.05 feet more than the measured velocity of the ball. The discrepancy is less than the 3.51 feet before the forward movement of the body was observed; however, better techniques are needed to provide greater accuracy.

The film of a highly skilled woman bowler, whose season's average score in three leagues was 182, was studied by Anhalt; results are shown in Table 7-2. Measurements were made from a side view.

As shown in Table 7-2 the moving joints at release were the shoulder, elbow, and wrist. The sum of their linear velocities is 21.81 feet per second. The film showed that the body was moving forward at the same time at a rate of 4.72 feet per second. This added to the lever velocities totals 26.53 feet per second. The measured velocity of the ball in the film was 26.74 feet per second after release. The degree to which the summed velocities agree with the ball velocity indicates the accuracy of the measurements.

In Tables 7-1 and 7-2 range refers to degrees, angular velocity to degrees per second, moment arm to length in feet, and linear velocity to feet per second. The linear velocities were calculated using the formula given in Chapter 3.

Increased velocity of the ball should be a goal for beginning bowlers; observations have now been extensive enough to set such goals with confidence. Casady and Liba recommend that women bowlers should impart to the ball a velocity that would send it from the foul line to the head pin in 2.5 to 2.75 seconds (24 to 21.9 feet per second) and men bowlers in 2.0 to 2.5 seconds (30 to 24 feet per second). Randomly selected league bowlers, five from each of the following classifications, had the following average scores for the season: skilled men, above 190;

average men, 150 to 160; skilled women, above 180; average women, 120 to 130. The velocity scores for these groups were as follows: skilled men, 28.38 feet per second (2.11 seconds for 60 feet); average men, 28.26 feet per second (2.12 seconds for 60 feet); skilled women, 29.12 feet per second (2.06 seconds for 60 feet); average women, 23.94 feet per second (2.50 seconds for 60 feet). Since the expert does not deliver the ball with the greatest possible velocity but with only enough to make effective impact with the pins, the velocity of the highly skilled performer is one that the beginner can attain.

Both the man and the woman discussed in Tables 7-1 and 7-2 derived over 60% of their velocity from the lever acting at the shoulder joint. The bowler should strive to use this action effectively. It is frequently said that the arm should reach the horizontal at the height of the backswing. Shoulder hyperextension, when the body is erect, will not carry the arm to this height. By flexing at the hips therefore the bowler inclines the trunk forward. In this position, although the range of shoulder hyperextension is not increased, the arm, depending on the degree of trunk inclination, can approach, reach, or pass the horizontal. Widule found that, in the groups that she observed, the upper arms reached the following positions; skilled men, 185 degrees; average men, 180 degrees; skilled women, 199 degrees; average women, 163 degrees. (The horizontal is represented by 180 degrees, more than that means higher than the horizontal.) Inclinations of the trunk for these groups were skilled men 35 degrees, average men 51 degrees, skilled women 41 degrees, and average women 54 degrees. (If the trunk were erect, the inclination would be 90 degrees; the greater the forward inclination of the trunk, the smaller will be the inclination measure.) The height of the arm on the backswing depends on the degree of trunk inclination and the degree of shoulder hyperextension at the shoulder joint. At the height of the backswing Widule found the following measures: skilled men 40 degrees, average men 52 degrees, skilled women 59 degrees, and average women 37 degrees. (The greater the measure, the greater the degree of hyperextension.)

The length of the bowler's arm will also affect the linear velocity of that lever. In the measurements shown in Table 7-1, had the moment arm for shoulder action been 2.2 feet instead of 2.45 and had the angular velocity been the same (443 degrees per second), the linear velocity would have been 17.01 feet per second. A difference of 3 inches in length decreased the velocity almost 2 feet per second (1.93).

The strength of grip has been shown by two studies (Curtis and Sabol) to be related to the speed of the swing. The nervous system evidently controls the speed, limiting it to the ability to hold the ball as it moves through the backward and forward arcs. The difference in strength of grip enables men to use a heavier ball than women normally use.

The contribution of the approach steps is not entirely shown in the forward movement of the torso at the time of release. As the ball is moved backward past the right leg by the arm, the approach steps are moving it forward. In the film study the ball was observed to move forward faster than it moved backward, so that during the backswing the ball was moving forward. This may be more easily visualized when compared to a person walking toward the rear of a railway car as the train moves forward. The person is walking backward but moving forward. As the bowling swing begins its downward, forward action, the ball already has a forward velocity, and the body levers add to this, rather than beginning from a zero velocity. The velocity of the approach increases with each step; the speed of the steps is usually kept constant, but the length of each increases over that of the preceding one.

If the velocity derived from body levers is to be fully used, there should be no downward direction in the ball's movement as it touches the floor. The arm should be a degree or 2 past the perpendicular at release, even if this means that the ball is released an inch or 2 above the alley. The impact with the floor from this height will be slight and will be decreased by the roll given to the ball at release. Widule found that the upper arm had passed the perpendicular at release and also that the elbow was flexing. This action not only raises the ball slightly but adds to the velocity. (See Tables 7-1 and 7-2.)

The analysis of the swing thus far has dealt with factors affecting the speed of the ball. The direction given to the ball is an important factor in the number of pins knocked down. In the distance that the ball travels from release to the pins, approximately 60 feet, a slight deviation from the exact line to the point of aim can result in a marked deviation as pin contact is made. For every 0.25 degree in direction the ball will miss the point of aim by 3 inches (approximately). A variation of 1 degree in direction would miss the point of aim by 1 foot; a ball started at the midpoint of the alley, if it deviated by 2 degrees from a perpendicular to the foul line, would end up in the gutter. Since slight deviations in direction have this marked effect on point of contact, the bowler must give careful attention to factors affecting accuracy.

Among these factors is the point at which the ball crosses the foul line. The starting position should be carefully determined with reference to this line, and the approach should be consistently straight forward. From the point on the foul line the ball should be directed along the selected line of direction. That line should be clearly visualized, and the arm should swing along this line even after the ball is released. (For additional details in achieving accuracy see Casady and Liba.)

UNDERARM THROW AND PITCH

In the basic underhand pattern the joints that move levers in the direction of the throw normally occur in the following sequence: hip rotation, spinal rotation, shoulder adduction and flexion, and wrist flexion. As the trunk is rotated backward, the arm is raised to the rear in a combined abducting and extending shoulder joint action; as the arm is moved forward, it is kept in the sagittal plane by a combination of shoulder adduction and flexion. The underarm throw and pitch are much alike in joint and lever actions. The moment arm lengths for this form of throwing were described at the beginning of this chapter. However, observers will find many individual modifications of the basic joint actions.

Normally the first forward movement is a step with the left foot. This necessitates first putting the weight on the right foot, facilitates pelvic rotation over that support, carries the left side of the pelvis forward, and increases the length of the step. As the left foot contacts the ground, the right arm usually reaches a horizontal position and is ready to begin its forward swing. For most effective action the upper torso, at this time, would, be facing to the right with the shoulders in line with the direction of the throw. Women often fail to take advantage of this position. Instead they tend to keep the upper torso facing the direction of the throw and thereby decrease both hip and spinal actions sometimes with complete loss of the latter. The major forward movement of the body is made as the left foot moves forward; there is rarely a slide on the left foot such as in bowling. At the time of release, forward movement of the body contributes little to the force of the throw.

A skilled woman's underarm throw is shown in Fig. 7-1. This performer takes a longer step than do most women; the step moves the total body except the right foot forward. The greatest part of that forward movement is seen to occur before the release phase; note the distance in which the head and upper trunk move with reference to the right foot from *C* to *F* and that these segments move a short distance with reference to the left heel from *F* to release, which occurs between *G* and *H*.

The pelvis is rotated on the right femur when the right foot carries the weight *(C and D)*. The range of pelvic rotation is limited somewhat by the position of the right foot, which is not turned 90 degrees from the intended flight of the ball. The right arm position, which is almost horizontal as the weight is taken by the left foot *(E)*, is typical of most performers.

At release the contributing joint actions are left hip rotation, right shoulder and wrist flexion, and left ankle flexion. Note the hyperextension of the wrist in *F* and the flexion in *H*. The increasing speed of the ball can be seen in the change of the pictured image from *E* to *H*. Note that it is a circle in *E* and that in the succeeding pictures it becomes an oval that increases in length.

Medial rotation of the humerus and supination of the forearm will impart rotation to the ball. Film observations have shown that men frequently flex the elbow and use either lateral or medial rotation of the humerus to develop speed. In doing so they they decrease the amount of shoulder flexion. Present information does not indicate whether rotation of the humerus develops more speed than does greater flexion of the shoulder with the elbow extended.

Measurements of the basic pattern provide insight into the potential contributions of each lever. Observations were made of the film of the skilled college woman pitcher. The measurements were made for two frames, including that showing the release; the time for all joint actions except the wrist was 0.03 second. The wrist action occurred in less than the time of one frame, and the time of the action was calculated to be 0.008 second. In the measurements given in Table 7-3 the range is expressed in degrees, the angular velocity in degrees per second, the moment arm length in feet, and the linear velocity in feet per second.

The sum of the velocities is 70.59 feet per second; the ball velocity in the film was measured at 70.26 feet per second. Using the sum of the linear velocities as

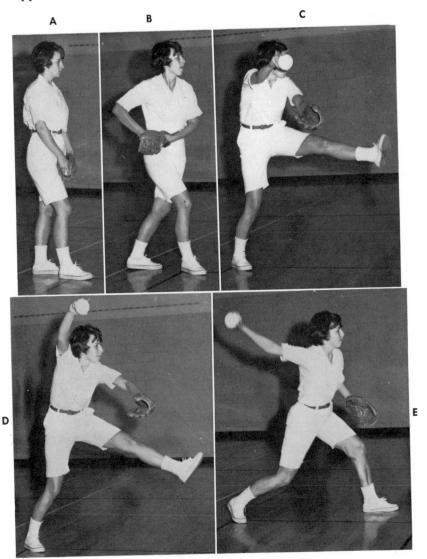

Fig. 7-1. Underarm throw.

the total, one finds the contributions of the joint actions expressed in percentages to be as follows: hip, 14.3; spine, 7.9; shoulder, 45.3; wrists, 32.4. Shoulder joint action is the major contributor, as it was in the previously reported bowling performance; wrist action in the throw with the lighter ball is more forceful.

Velocity measures of ball projections are not commonly made; however, they are a more valid measure of the force imparted by body levers than is a measure of distance. In measures made under the supervision of one of us (R. B. G.) two men, both pitchers on softball teams, had velocities of 108 and 109 feet per sec-

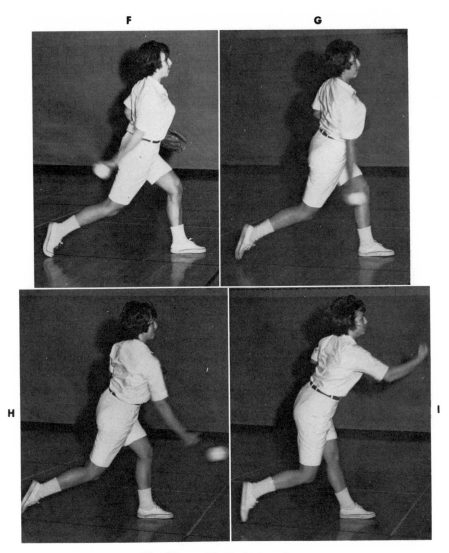

Fig. 7-1, cont'd. Underarm throw.

Table 7-3. Lever contributions to ball velocity in underarm throw

	Range	Angular velocity	Moment arm length	Linear velocity
Hip rotation	12	400	1.45	10.12
Spinal rotation	6	200	1.6	5.59
Shoulder flexion	22	733	2.5	31.98
Wrist flexion	30	3750	0.35	22.90

ond; two women majors in physical education threw balls at 65 and 64 feet per second; and a teenage girl, an outstanding pitcher in a city softball league, delivered a ball at 81 feet per second.

GOLF STROKE

The golf stroke is an underarm pattern with modifications in the shoulder action. It might be called a *reversed underarm pattern,* since for the right-handed performer, the left arm contributes the primary force, and in the downward swing the left shoulder action is abduction, rather than adduction. The skill also differs from the usual underarm pattern in that both arms are active. Although the right arm does contribute to the force, it is used mainly to support the club except for the wrist action. Broer and Houtz have classified this skill as a sidearm pattern. However, this text justifies its classification on the basis of the movement of the left arm from a horizontal position above or at shoulder level at the height of the backswing (Fig. 7-2, *C*) downward to a position parallel with the trunk axis at impact (Fig. 7-2, *E*). The observations of Broer and Houtz show greater activity in the muscles of the left arm, supporting the statement that this arm action contributes more force than the right. The sequence of joint action is the usual hip rotation, spinal rotation, and shoulder action with the wrist coming into action last. No step is taken, since the feet do not move from the starting position, but the weight shifts to the right foot on the backswing and back to the left foot on the forward swing. This shifting of weight increases the range of hip rotation (Fig. 7-2). At the height of the backswing, hip action is seen to have rotated the pelvis almost 90 degrees and spinal rotation to have turned the upper torso more. As the weight is transferred to the left foot, medial rotation in the left hip turns the pelvis toward the line of ball flight. In the skilled performer, forward hip rotation will begin before the shoulder and wrist have completed the backward movements. As the pelvis rotates forward, it will carry the arms downward. Shoulder action begins approximately at the time that the arm has reached the horizontal; wrist action will be delayed until the arm approaches the vertical (Fig. 7-2, *D*).

The moment arm lengths of hip and spinal levers must be measured from pictures taken with a camera placed in line with the flight of the ball. The moment arms are illustrated in Fig. 7-3. Depending on the length of the club and of the performer's arms and on the amount of spinal flexion, the moment arm length for hip action will be 3 to 4 feet. These factors will also affect the length of the moment arm for spinal action, which will be greater than that for the hip. The angular velocity of the hip and spine will be considerably less than that of the shoulder. A rough approximation of the linear contributions of the acting joints would be wrist, 70%, shoulder, 20%, and hip and spine, 5% each.

Because extreme accuracy is necessary in golf, Cochran and Stobbs recommend that the movement pattern be made as simple as possible; they believe that the important levers are those acting at the shoulder and wrist joints. They say that the difference between good and poor golfers may lie in the simplicity of action and the ability to generate power in the acting muscles.

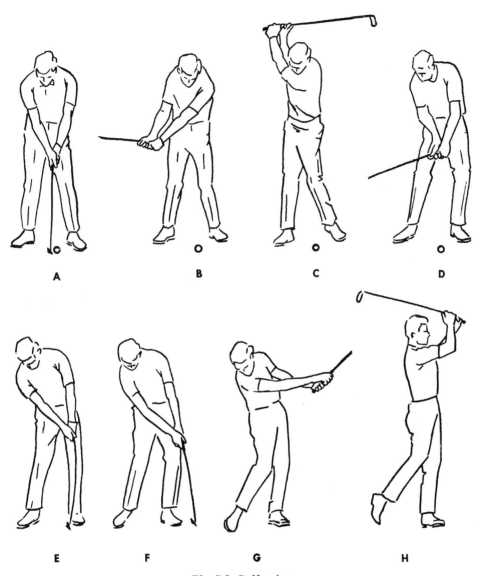

A   B   C   D

E   F   G   H

Fig. 7-2. Golf swing.

Full swings of the various clubs will have the same lever actions and the same proportion of linear contribution to the speed of the club head at the time of impact. In comparing full swings with the driver and the No. 7 iron as made by five women golfers (handicaps 4, 5, 7, 9, and 12), Brennan found that the same joint actions were used in the two swings. In the degree of joint action in the forward swing and backswing she found only one significant difference in the mean measures. Although the degree of pelvic rotation in the backswing did not differ, with the driver the pelvis had rotated 7.2 degrees farther at contact

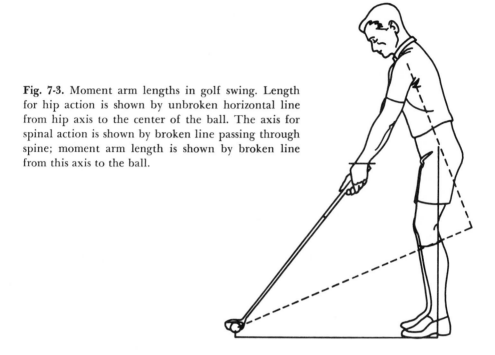

Fig. 7-3. Moment arm lengths in golf swing. Length for hip action is shown by unbroken horizontal line from hip axis to the center of the ball. The axis for spinal action is shown by broken line passing through spine; moment arm length is shown by broken line from this axis to the ball.

than with the iron. The length of the club will affect the length of all moment arms and also the path of the club head; as the club is shortened, the path will become shallower and shorter. Photographs of a No. 2 iron and a wood swung by Bobby Jones show velocities of 132 and 142 feet per second, respectively, at the time of impact. The shorter distances obtained with shorter clubs result from the lower linear velocities of the levers as well as from the higher angles of projection.

Lever action in striking activities cannot be evaluated by comparing the summed linear velocities of acting levers to the velocity of the projectile. In throwing, the distal end of each lever is the center of gravity of the object to be projected. As each lever moves, this center of gravity is moved, and at release its velocity equals that of the contribution of the levers. In striking, the projectile is moved by body levers only during the brief period of contact.

The velocity of the golf ball can be greater than that of the club head at impact. Cochran and Stobbs report that a top golfer can have a club velocity of 8800 feet per second (100 mile per hour) and that the ball velocity will be 11,880 feet per second. The difference is due to the smaller mass of the ball and also to the fact that the ball is flattened on impact and that during the 0.0005 second of contact the elastic ball pushes away from the club. These authors state that contact time is the same for almost all shots, even that of a putt—less than 1 msec.

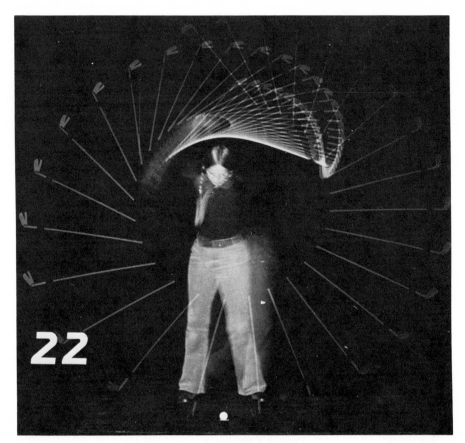

Fig. 7-4. Strobe picture of woman's golf swing, showing the use of the 5 iron. This action was photographed in frontal plane from the top of the downswing through the follow-through. As the downswing commenced, images of the club were close together and then farther apart, indicating an increase in velocity. (Courtesy Jan Sanner Merriman.)

The swing of a good golfer is so fast that detailed movement analysis can be made only with some device to aid vision. In the film of a professional golfer Cochran and Stobbs found the time from the start of the swing to impact to be 0.82 second and that from the start of the downswing to impact to be 0.23 second. The downswing was more than two and one-half times as fast as the backswing. (See Fig. 7-4.)

A study of the kinematic and kinetic aspects of the golf swing* revealed the following:

1. The line of gravity was midway between the two feet at the beginning of the downswing. This means that the force for each foot was the same.

*Cooper, J. M.: Kinematic and kinetic analysis of the golf swing. In Nelson, R. C., and Morehouse, C. A., editors: Biomechanics IV, Baltimore, 1974, University Park Press.

2. The weight shift was such that 75% occurred on the front foot and 25% on the rear at impact (mean shift).

3. After impact there was a continued shift of some weight toward the front foot with most clubs, the greatest being with the high-lofted club and the least with the driver.

4. After the impact position was reached, the performers using the highest-numbered club had a force distribution between the feet of a little more than 75% on the front and nearly 50% front and rear for the driver.

5. There was some change in the force distribution at the end of the follow-through, in that the shift was almost up to 80% on the front foot for the high-lofted club and nearly 70% with the driver.

6. The total vertical force exerted from the downswing to just at or prior to impact was from 133% of body weight for the high weight for the high-lofted club and 150% for the driver.

7. The total vertical force decreased for all clubs as impact occurred.

8. The total force exerted in the vertical direction was reduced to 80% of the total body weight, indicating that the centrifugal force of the club had pulled the body upward (Fig. 7-5).

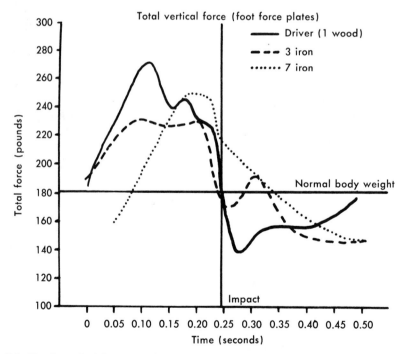

Fig. 7-5. Total vertical force during golf swing, measured by foot force plates. Note that the body weight varies from approximately 275 pounds (drives) during the downswing to 140 pounds just after impact. During the follow-through the golfer shifts body weight forward unusually far while using 7 iron.

Film measures of the swings of an average golfer, a college woman, found the average swing time with a No. 5 iron to be 1.41 seconds and with a No. 9 iron to be 1.34 seconds. The downswings were three times as fast as the backswings. Drives from the tee made by two highly skilled women golfers as they participated in a tournament were measured with a stopwatch and were found to average 0.64 (Berg) and 0.85 (Suggs) second. The swing of a highly skilled college man, measured on film, took 0.77 second; the downswing was twice as fast as the backswing. Films of Bobby Jones showed that the backswing was completed in 70 frames and the downswing in 30 frames. His downswing was two and one-third times faster than his backswing.

FIELD HOCKEY

Two members of the 1968 touring women's hockey team from the Netherlands were filmed as they executed a pass in several directions: straight ahead, diagonally right and left, and squarely to the right and to the left. The ball was sent in each direction from a standstill and also after a short dribble. Both women moved into almost the same position for each pass, and a similar joint action sequence occurred for all passes. Immediately before impact, wrist action accounted for 67% to 85% of the change in the angle of the stick. Other actions involved were pelvic and spinal rotation, shoulder flexion and adduction, and slight elbow extension.

ADDITIONAL UNDERARM PATTERNS

Detailed information on the many other underarm patterns is not available at present, but the analyses that have been presented combined with logical deductions provide insight into the contributions of levers. The underarm volleyball serve is much like the underarm throw. Instead of the player's stepping forward with the left foot, there is likely to be only a long stride in the stance, with a transfer of weight from the right to the left foot. This will limit the range and most likely the speed of hip rotation. Wrist flexion will be eliminated, since the ball is struck with the heel of the hand.

In the underarm badminton serve the long moment arm for the wrist and the speed with which the light racket can be moved make wrist action the greatest contributor to speed. In double underarm throws no hip or spinal rotation occurs, and the shoulder and wrist joints are the sole contributors. The hips are likely to be flexed, inclining the trunk to provide space for the backswing of the arms. If the hips extend during the forward arm swing, the trunk will move backward. This backward movement will decrease the speed with which the arms and wrists are moving the ball. In the double-arm throw, wrist action will necessarily be lateral (ulnar) flexion, rather than the usual type.

SUGGESTED READINGS
Bowling

Hellebrandt, F. A., Waterland, J. C., and Walters, C. E.: The influence of athetoid cerebral palsy on the execution of sport skills: bowling, Phys. Ther. Rev. **41:**106, 1961.

Reuschlein, P.: Analysis of levers contributing to the force in the delivery of a bowling ball, seminar paper, University of Wisconsin, 1962.

Widule, C. J.: A study of anthropometric, strength, and performance characteristics of men and women league bowlers, dissertation, University of Wisconsin, 1966.

Golf

Brennan, L. J.: A comparative analysis of the golf drive and seven iron shot with emphasis on pelvic and spinal rotation, thesis, University of Wisconsin, 1968.

Cochran, A., and Stobbs, J.: The search for the perfect swing, Philadelphia, 1968, J. B. Lippincott Co.

Hellebrandt, F. A., and Waterland, J. C.: The influence of athetoid cerebral palsy on the execution of sport skills: tennis and golf, Phys. Ther. Rev. 41:257, 1961.

Price, J.: Time as a measure of swinging ability in golf, thesis, University of Wisconsin, 1955.

See Bibliography for additional references.

CHAPTER 8 Overarm patterns

MECHANICS OF OVERARM PATTERN

The overarm, like the underarm, pattern is commonly used in throws and strikes. Its distinguishing feature is shoulder joint action that rotates the humerus laterally during the preparatory phase and medially during the force-producing phase. Persons who cannot readily visualize these actions may be helped by going through the following movements: Hold the upper arm at the side in such a position that, when the elbow is flexed 90 degrees, the forearm will be horizontal and pointing directly forward. Keeping the upper arm at the side, move the forearm to the right 90 degrees in the transverse plane; the forearm will now point directly to the side. The joint action that brought about this change in the position of the forearm was lateral rotation of the humerus. If the forearm is now moved back to the original position, the action involved is medial rotation of the humerus. These shoulder joint rotations can be made while the upper arm is in many positions. One position frequently used is described as follows: With elbow extended abduct the entire arm 90 degrees to the horizontal. Adjust the position of the upper arm so that, when the elbow is flexed 90 degrees, the forearm will point directly forward. Move the forearm until it points directly upward. This will be accomplished by 90 degrees of lateral rotation of the humerus. Lower the forearm until it again points forward: it has been moved to this position by 90 degrees of medial rotation at the shoulder joint. This rotation of the humerus is the outstanding characteristic of the overarm pattern; this bone is usually abducted in the force-producing phase.

Present observations suggest that next to wrist flexion medial rotation is the fastest joint action of the upper limb. Each joint action apparently has a limit to the speed with which it can be moved. Because the moment arm of shoulder medial rotation can be longer than that acting at the wrist joint, its linear velocity and therefore its contribution to the force imparted to a projectile can be greater than that contributed by wrist action.

In lateral and medial rotation of the humerus the axis passes through the shoulder joint and also the length of the humerus, whereas in the other actions at the shoulder the axis passes through the width of the humerus. The length of the moment arm in the rotating actions (lateral and medial) is the distance from the axis to the point of release or of impact. The line representing this distance must be perpendicular to the axis and also to the line of applied force. The moment arm will be longest when the forearm is perpendicular to the

135

humerus; when the forearm is flexed either more or less than 90 degrees, the moment arm will be shorter.)

With the elbow extended medial and lateral rotation can be used effectively when an implement is held in the hand. If the arm is held at the side, the elbow extended, and a tennis racket held in the hand so that it is at right angles to the arm, the racket can be moved through 180 degrees in the transverse plane. In this action pronation and supination of the forearm will add to the range and the speed as the humerus is rotated.

Other levers that are commonly combined with arm action in the overarm pattern are the same as those described for the underarm pattern; they are brought into action by pelvic and spinal rotation and wrist flexion. Their resistance arms will be those described for the underarm pattern. The lengths of the moment arms for pelvic and spinal rotation are likely to be longer in the overarm than in the underarm pattern because the humerus is usually abducted.

In the following sections the overarm pattern will be described as it is used in various skills. Again keep in mind that, until further evidence is available, no pattern can be presented as the best. However, all patterns will have fundamental characteristics of the overarm pattern.

Following are some anatomic and mechanical considerations in the overarm throw, as discussed by Tarbell:

(The variety of forms of the overarm pattern that the upper limb can perform is characteristic of the versatility of this section of the body. This limb can apply great force and also act with extreme precision. In part this is due to the structure of the connection with the trunk. The humerus is connected to the freely movable scapula. The humeral head, which is almost half a sphere, fits into a cup of cartilage that is attached to the inner surface of the fossa on the upper distal section of the scapula. This permits flexion, extension, and abduction of the humerus and the antagonistic joint actions. Variations are increased by movements of the scapula, which has no direct connection with the trunk. The scapula and clavicle are a functioning part of the upper limb and take part in practically all movements of the humerus, not adding to strength of action, but rather increasing range and versatility.

The rotational movements in throwing are accomplished by revolution of the arm around a long axis (i.e., the humerus). This action has been compared to that of a jackhammer.

The muscles acting on the scapula work like the mechanism of a revolving door. Rotating action in the opposite direction causes upward rotation. This is called a *force couple*. The longer the scapula, the farther down it the muscles attach, giving the mechanism a better chance of imparting great force to a throw.)

(The bones of the throwing arm, which includes the upper arm, forearm, wrist, and fingers, are 26 in number. In addition, this throwing mechanism is supported by a strut, composed of the clavicle and scapula. An amazing lack of stability in the shoulder girdle allows great freedom of movement. Further movement is permitted by the so-called broken hook structure, which involves the clavicle, acronium process, top of the glenoid fossa, and coracoid process (in the upward swing of the arm). The scapula moves the clavicle, and the clavicle moves on the sternum. Also the instability (or freedom) is enhanced by the gleno-humeral structure, whereby the shallow fossa permits the humerus to be relatively free. The integrity of the joint relies on a small number of muscles not considered in the great strength area.

OVERARM THROW AND PITCH

When great speed is desired in a throw, the overarm pattern is used. This uses the two joint actions that appear to have the highest speeds, wrist flexion and shoulder medial rotation. The sequence of joint actions can be seen in the football pass (Fig. 8-1) and in the baseball pitch (Fig. 8-2). Both show the step

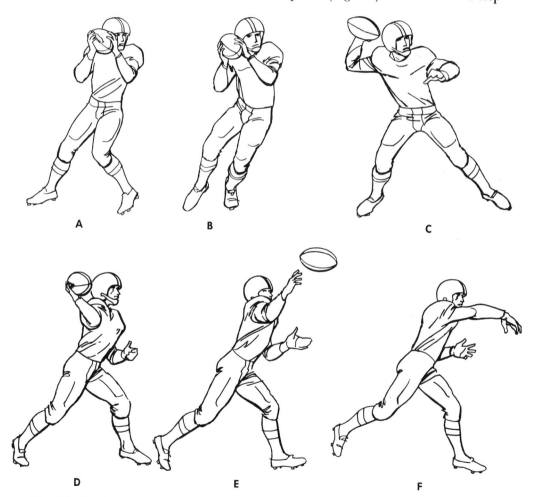

Fig. 8-1. Football pass. **C** and **D,** Lateral rotation of the humerus. **E** and **F,** Medial rotation.

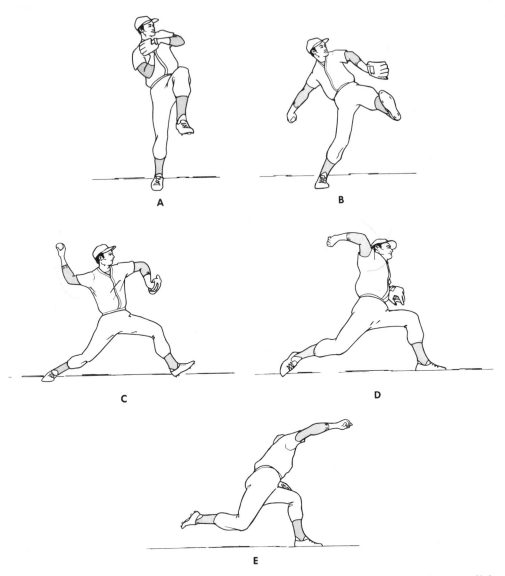

Fig. 8-2. Overarm pitch. **B** and **C**, Lateral rotation of the humerus. **D** and **E**, Medial rotation.

forward with the left foot, hip and spinal rotation, and medial rotation of the humerus. Apparently less wrist action occurs with the football throw than with the baseball pitch, which explains the greater velocity obtained with the smaller ball. Note in both series of pictures that, as the torso is rotated forward by hip and spinal actions, the humerus is rotated laterally. This timing is an important feature of complex movement patterns. The slower joints begin their forward movement as the faster more distal joints complete their backswings. No appre-

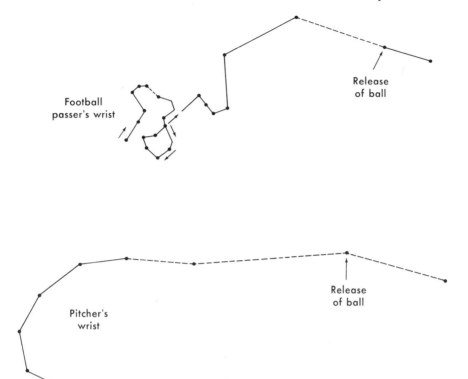

Fig. 8-3. Paths of wrists (traced from film) of two throwers, one in football and one in baseball. Note that football thrower releases the ball after the height of wrist movement has been reached and the pitcher just at the height. (Biomechanics Laboratory, Indiana University.)

ciable pause between the backswing and forward swing of these faster-moving joints is necessary. The muscles responsible for the forward swing can begin contraction to stop the backswing. The combination of backward movement and beginning contraction stretches the tendons and connective tissue in the muscles, and thus the forward movement can be more forceful.

Note that in both throws the elbow extended somewhat before the ball was released. This shortens the moment arm for shoulder medial rotation. Apparently then this action develops its greatest linear velocity before release, and this velocity must be used by the joints acting at release. However, elbow extension lengthens the moment arms for the hip and spinal levers and adds to the linear speeds of these levers at release. In both performances the right foot, as it supports the body weight during the backswing, is placed at right angles to the direction of the ball flight. This permits a greater range of pelvic rotation at the right hip.

Fig. 8-3 shows the path of the wrist in two throwing actions. The release of

Table 8-1. Lever contributions to ball velocity in overarm throw

	Range	Angular velocity	Moment arm	Linear velocity
Man				
Hip rotation	20.6	824	2.12	30.5
Spinal rotation	9.6	384	2.75	18.4
Shoulder rotation	38.5	1540	0.27	7.3
Wrist flexion	60.0	8571	0.49	73.3
Woman				
Hip rotation	20.6	735	2.32	29.8
Spinal rotation	20.9	746	2.21	28.8
Shoulder rotation	29.0	1036	0.35	6.3
Wrist flexion	42.0	5250	0.37	33.9

the ball by the pitcher is at the height of the wrist movement, but the football passer because of the spin that must be imparted to the ball releases it when the wrist is moving downward.

A physical education major, in analyzing his own football passes, measured the ball velocity as 60 feet per second immediately before release. Shoulder medial rotation contributed 62%, spinal rotation 35%, and wrist flexion 3%. He had no hip rotation during the release phase.

Film study of the overarm baseball throw of a skilled man (a major league player) and a highly skilled woman gives indications of the contributions of the four levers of the pattern and also of individual adjustments in it.

Table 8-1 gives the range of movement in degrees at the time of release, the angular velocity in degrees per second, the length of the moment arm in feet, and the linear contribution of each lever in feet per second. The time in which the joints moved through the given range was 0.025 second for the man except for the wrist, for which the time was 0.007 second. For the woman the time was 0.028 second except for the wrist, for which the time was 0.008 second. The high linear velocity for the wrist flexion shown in Table 8-1 has been questioned by later research, and the basis on which it was determined may be of interest to those who study film. Note that in the table the time for the measured range for the wrist is less than for the other joints. In the frame before release the angle at the wrist was measured; in the next frame the ball had been released, and the wrist angle had changed. The change was assumed to have occurred during the time that the camera shutter was closed, and this time, rather than the frames per second, was used to determine the velocity of the wrist joint. If this is acceptable procedure, the time cannot be longer than shutter time, and it could be less: in that case the angular velocity would be greater than reported.

The sum of the linear velocities for the man is 129.6 feet per second; the ball velocity measured on the film was 130.9 feet per second. For the woman the sum of the linear velocities is 98.8 feet per second; the measured film velocity was 95.93 feet per second.

The wrist action in both performers is the greatest contributor to the linear velocity; the hip ranks second and shoulder rotation last. Both performers extended the elbow just before release, thus shortening the length of the moment arm of the shoulder lever. The measurements for this moment arm were shorter than those for the wrist lever, showing that the ball at release is less than 6 inches from a line extending through the humerus. Shoulder action is likely to make its contribution earlier in the pattern.

In study of the moment arm lengths in the overarm throws of high school girls, the best velocities were found to be developed by the girls who had the longest moment arms for the hip rotation levers and consequently the shortest moment arms for the shoulder medial rotation levers.

The tabulation of moment arm lengths shows that for the man the moment arm for the hip is shorter than that for the spine. This is due to a leaning to the left so far that the upper spine is to the left of the hip joint at release. The lateral flexion may be the cause of the small range of movement in the spine.

Certain limitations should be remembered regarding these reported contributions of joint actions to the velocity of the projected ball. In each case the measurements are those made for one subject and were taken during the release phase, so that they do not indicate joint contributions made in earlier phases. Also cinematographic methods have improved since the reported observations were made; current work questions the accuracy of the earlier methods of measuring joint actions. The doubtful measures are included here as an illustration of a procedure that can be followed with refined techniques to determine the contributions of body levers to ball velocity.

The most detailed and extensive current study of joint actions in the overarm throw is that reported by Atwater, who observed action in three planes, using side, overhead, and rear camera views. She included fifteen subjects to provide opportunity for comparison: five skilled college men and five skilled and five average college women. Her observations include not only the release phase but also the 400 msec. preceding the release. For the skilled groups that time period encompassed almost all the overarm pattern, including the backswing; for the average women only the later stages of the backswing occurred in the selected time. Displacement of the ball was measured in three planes, and the three velocities determined were combined algebraically into one "resultant velocity." Measured joint actions were related to ball displacement on the basis of observation and logic; moment arms and linear contributions of joint actions were not studied.

In observing displacement of the ball prior to its release from the hand, Atwater found that, although the movement is primarily forward, vertical and lateral movement occur also. None of the subjects accelerated the ball continually, but all accelerated rapidly shortly before release, the men as much as 1500 to 2000 feet per second per second, skilled women, 1000 feet per second per second, and average women, 400 feet per second per second. (See Fig. 8-4.)

In comparing joint actions Atwater found that all skilled subjects used essentially the same actions but that the range and speed were generally greater for the subjects who had the fastest ball velocities at release. Some of these differences

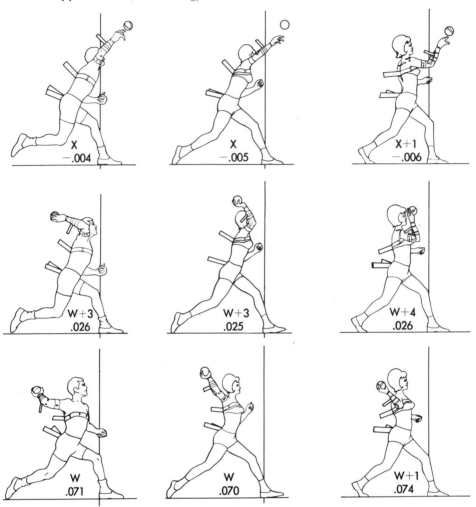

Fig. 8-4. Tracings from film study of overarm throw. Left, skilled man; middle, skilled woman; right, woman with average skill. (From Atwater, A. E.: Movement characteristics of the overarm throw, dissertation, University of Wisconsin, 1970.)

can be seen in Fig. 8-4, which represents positions at times 0.070 and 0.025 (approximately) second before release of the ball and 0.005 second after release. Note that in the lowest tracing for each subject the ball is behind the head and that this distance is greatest for the skilled man and least for the average woman. Differences in ball position at this time can be attributed largely to trunk position; the trunk of the skilled man is not yet facing the direction in which the ball is to be projected, whereas that of the average woman is facing slightly beyond that direction. To reach the positions shown in the top tracings the man's trunk moves through a greater range than do those of the women, and its rotation must therefore be at a faster angular velocity. Note also that the elbow of

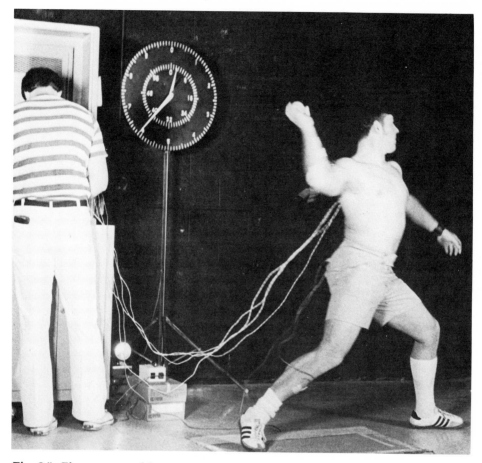

Fig. 8-5. Electromyographic apparatus used in study of overarm throwing pattern. Indwelling fine-wire electrodes were located in lateral head of triceps brachii, flexors carpi ulnaris and radialis, and pronator teres muscles. Subject as shown has started forward action of throwing arm. Also note that subject's rear foot is against force plate that could be used to obtain rear foot force during throwing action. (Calvin Fisk is the investigator, Biomechanics Laboratory, Indiana University.)

the average woman is flexed 50 to 60 degrees at release, whereas those of the skilled performers are almost completely extended.

The differences in lengths of strides are not as clearly seen in Fig. 8-4. Atwater reports considerable differences between the averages of stride lengths for the three groups; that of the skilled men was 3.87 feet; that of the skilled women was 0.52 foot shorter and that of the average women 1.57 feet shorter than that of the men. A similar finding related to stride is reported by Ekern, who studied the overarm throw of boys and girls selected as the better throwers from second, fourth, and sixth grades. Within that group she found that the better throwers, whose projected balls were fastest, have longer steps.

Fisk in a review of the data in his study "The Dynamic Function of Selected Muscles of the Forearm: an Electromyographical and Cinematographical Investigation" made the following comments:

Preliminary analysis has been made of electromyographical data obtained from 12 subjects in the study. A great deal of individual variety in the function of the four muscles [mentioned in Fig. 8-5] during the performance of the overhand straight throw and the overhand curved throw was found. Conclusions drawn from the study indicate that the electrical response generated in the muscles took place during the final movements of the "laying back of the arm," just prior to when the elbow begins its forward movement and the wrist assumes its "cocked position." Once the forward movement of the arm begins the flexors diminish electrical activity. All four muscles were more active during the throws with spin than during the straight throws; therefore, it is assumed that greater muscular effort was required to perform the throws with spin. The onset of the maximal action potential response occurred earlier and endured longer for the throws with spin and occurred earlier and endured longer among the experienced performers. The contribution of the pronator teres muscle still remains partially unsettled; however, the results do suggest that this muscle contributes to the spin imparted to the ball at release when the throws with spin were performed.*

The velocities of balls projected by the overhand throw have been measured more frequently than those of any other movement pattern. Among the reported velocities are the following:

1. Bob Feller's pitch, measured in 1946—145 feet per second
2. The throw of the winner of a city-wide contest in Philadelphia, an 18-year-old high school boy—130 feet per second
3. The mean velocity for 911 college women, reported in 1964—44.6 feet per second—and for 1072 college women, reported in 1965—42.5 feet per second
4. The mean velocity of a group of high school girls measured at the University of Wisconsin in 1959—56.4 feet per second; highest velocity in the group—90.7 feet per second
5. Mean velocities for boys and girls collected during 1956 through 1961: first-grade girls—28 feet per second—and eighth-grade girls—54 feet per second; first-grade boys—35 feet per second—and eighth-grade boys—75 feet per second (with the mean velocities for intervening grades progressively higher)
6. Individual velocities for fast balls of seven men varsity pitchers—from 86 to 122 feet per second—and for curve balls—from 75 to 108 feet per second†
7. The mean velocity for eighty high school boys, reported in 1966—68.4 feet per second
8. Standards selected after personal observation and study of available data by Atwater in 1970: for skilled women—a range of 70 to 80 feet per second, for average women—40 to 50 feet per second, and for skilled men—100 to 120 feet per second (Also see data in Fig. 8-6.)

*Prepared by Calvin Fisk after a review of data from his unpublished doctoral dissertation, Indiana University, 1976.
†Slater-Hammel, A. T., and Andres, E. H.: Velocity measurement of fast balls and curve balls, Res. Am. Assoc. Health Phys. Educ. **23**:95, 1952.

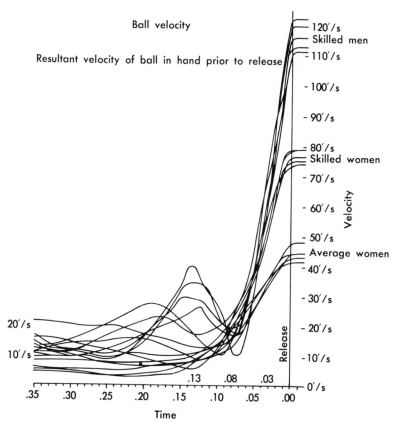

Ball velocity

Resultant velocity of ball in hand prior to release

120'/s
Skilled men
110'/s
100'/s
90'/s
80'/s
Skilled women
70'/s
60'/s
50'/s
Average women
40'/s
30'/s
20'/s
10'/s
0'/s

Velocity

Release

20'/s

10'/s

.13   .08   .03

.35   .30   .25   .20   .15   .10   .05   .00

Time

Fig. 8-6. Resultant velocities for overarm throw, calculated from measures taken from side, rear, and overhead views. At release, upper lines represent velocities of five skilled men, middle lines those of five skilled women, and lowest lines those of five average women. (From Atwater, A. E.: Movement characteristics of the overarm throw, dissertation, University of Wisconsin, 1970.)

TENNIS SERVE

The tennis serve is an overarm type of movement. At the beginning the trunk is rotated to the right (with a right-handed player) with the weight shifted to the rear foot. Note that in Fig. 8-7, *B,* as also shown in the pictures of the football pass and the overarm pitch the right foot is placed at a right angle to the intended flight of the ball. This and the flexion of the left knee and lifting of the left heel permit greater rotation of the pelvis at the right hip joint. From full extension the right shoulder (Fig. 8-7, *C*) is abducted and laterally rotated, and the elbow is flexed (*E* and *F*). At the peak of the backward movement the back is hyperextended with the wrist extended. Note the continuation of the head of the racket downward as the player's body moves forward (*E* and *F*). As the player moves the racket toward the ball, the right shoulder is medially rotated,

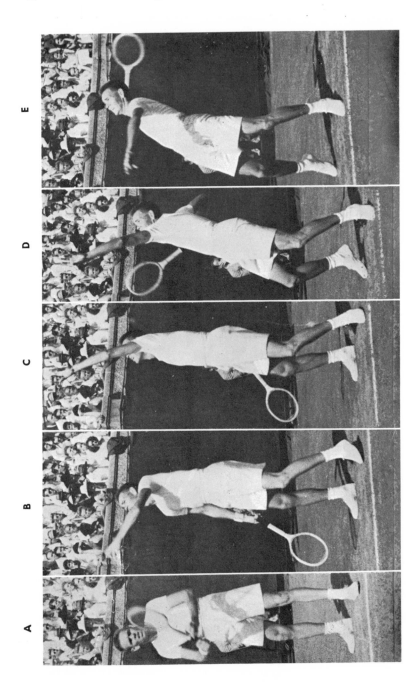

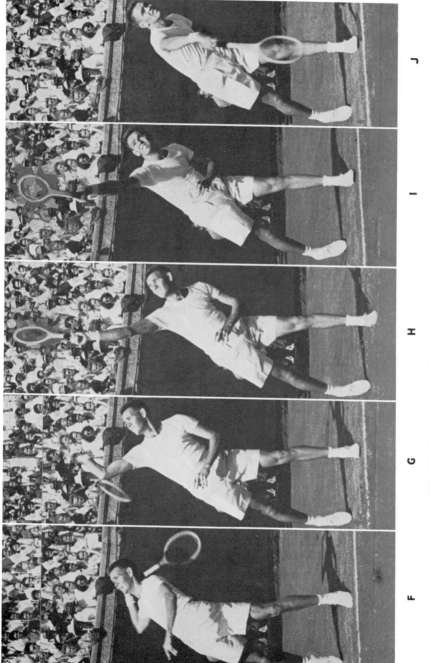

Fig. 8-7. Tennis serve. (Courtesy Scholastic Coach.)

and the elbow is extended (G and H). The trunk and pelvis are rotated to the left (H).

The tilting of the torso to the left (G and H), which here is due to abduction at the left hip, is frequently seen when height of reach is desired. This raises the right shoulder girdle and increases the length of the moment arm for spinal rotation.

In the tennis serve, medial rotation of the humerus is a major contributor to the speed of the racket. However, as in the overhand throw this action makes its major contribution before the impact phase. The humerus is laterally rotated in F; from F to G it has rotated medially close to 90 degrees. Here medial rotation imparts speed to the racket. From G to H the elbow extends to achieve height. Also during this time (G to H) the wrist makes its contribution by flexing. Except for the position of the upper arm the tennis serve and the overhand pitch are much alike. The moment arm for wrist action is lengthened by the racket, and here, as in the golf swing, wrist action will be of major importance. Plagenhoef states that racket speed is no more important than firmness of grip.

The velocity of the ball and the height of impact will determine the angle at which it should be directed to clear the net and to land in the service court. Gonzales, whose serve was measured electrically as 164 feet per second, is reported to have the fastest of measured serves. Kramer's serve was measured as 153 feet per second. These velocities will permit the ball to be directed below the horizontal. Stan Smith's serve has been reported to travel at the rate of approximately 199 feet per second.

A beginning player should develop such a velocity in the serve that the ball will clear the net and land in the service court when projected horizontally before attempting to direct the ball downward. If the impact is 8 feet above the ground and the projection is horizontal, gravitational force will bring the ball to the ground in 0.704 second ($8 = 16.1t^2$). In this time the horizontally directed ball must travel approximately 58 feet; its velocity would be $0.704x = 58$ feet, $x = 82.4$ feet per second. If the impact were 40 feet from the net, the ball would clear the net in 0.485 second, and gravity would have moved it downward 3.79 feet. This clears the net by 1.21 feet. These figures indicate that a beginning player should develop a velocity of at least 80 feet per second before attempting to direct the ball downward, unless the height of impact is considerably more than 8 feet. This is a velocity that the average college woman can develop.

A velocity of 100 feet per second has been measured in the better tennis players among college women. If impacted at a height of 8 feet and directed downward at an angle 3 degrees below the horizontal, the ball would clear the net by 4.2 inches. That angle allows little margin for error and shows the importance of the height of impact. (See Chapter 17.)

These calculations were made without consideration of air and wind resistance and ball spin. If a player is able to develop a ball velocity well over 100 feet per second, the stroke should impart spin to the ball. Plagenhoef reports that 5 men whose serves he studied had ball velocities of approximately 146 feet per second (100 miles per hour). For these projections the rackets were moving

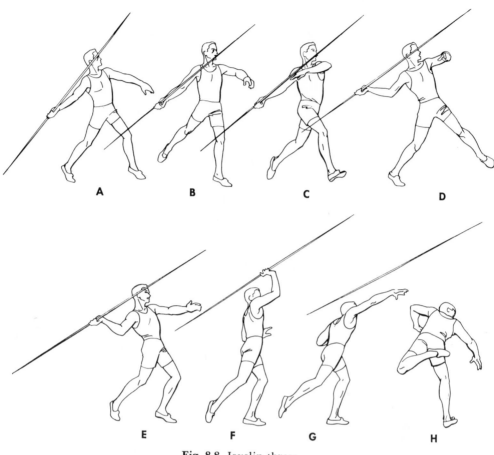

Fig. 8-8. Javelin throw.

at approximately 120 to 124 feet per second, showing that as reported for golf the ball can move with greater speed than does the striking implement.

JAVELIN THROW

The javelin throw involves a slight modification of the run coupled with an overarm throw. The run is executed at a controlled speed and involves an acceleration in its last stages. Before the last step is taken, the body weight is on the right foot; with the final step the pelvis rotates at the right hip, adding to the length of the step. As the weight is shifted to the left foot, the humerus is rotated medially, and the elbow is flexed (Fig. 8-8, *E*). The final force, added to the forward movement of the body, is derived from pelvic and spinal rotation, medial rotation and slight adduction of the humerus, and flexion of the hand.

Note the position of the pectoralis major in Fig. 8-9. It is well suited for medial rotation of the humerus. Also the action of the latissimus dorsi should

Fig. 8-9. Javelin thrower. Note position of pectoralis major.

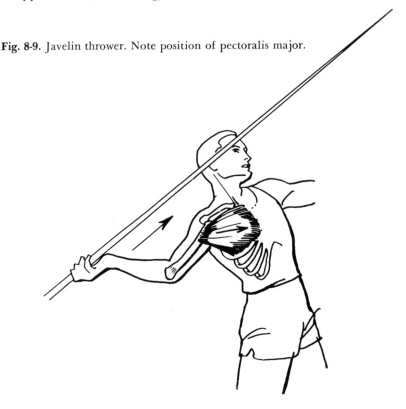

be visualized here, since it, too, is a medial rotator and its contraction would lower the humerus and pull it backward. The latter two actions are prevented from occurring by the pectoralis major. Acting together, these two muscles are excellent rotators of the arm. Note that in the javelin throw the elbow is not fully extended during the final thrust and the moment arm for medial rotation of the shoulder is almost at maximum length. In this skill medial rotation is a greater contributor than is wrist flexion.

SUGGESTED READINGS

Atwater, A. E.: Movement characteristics of the overarm throw: a kinematic analysis of men and women performers, dissertation, University of Wisconsin, 1970.

Collins, P. A.: Body mechanics of the overarm and sidearm throws, thesis, University of Wisconsin, 1960.

Ketlinski, R.: How is a curve ball thrown? Athletic J. **51:**5, 1971.

Tarbell, T.: Some mechanical aspects of the overarm throw. In Cooper, J. M., editor: Proceedings of the C.I.C. Symposium on Biomechanics, Chicago, 1971, The Athletic Institute.

Tarbell, T.: Unpublished manuscript, Biomechanics Laboratory, Indiana University, 1972.

See Bibliography for additional references.

CHAPTER 9 Sidearm patterns

MECHANICS OF SIDEARM PATTERN

The sidearm pattern, like the underarm and overarm ones, is generally used in throws and strikes. Unlike the latter two the distinguishing feature of the sidearm pattern is not the type of shoulder joint action but the lack or limitation of action at this joint. The main action in the sidearm pattern is pelvic rotation, with the arm held fairly stable in an abducted position. The lever and the resistance arm for this action include the segments described for it for the underarm pattern (Chapter 7). The moment arm for the pelvic lever can be one of the longest found in common activities. It extends from the axis passing through the left hip (for right-handed performers) to the line of applied force and includes the width of the pelvis, often the length of the whole arm, and part of the hand. The length of the moment arm is increased by the length of any implement that is used, with a tennis racket or a baseball bat the length of the moment arm could be 6 or more feet in an adult.

Other actions that are commonly combined with pelvic rotation in this pattern are spinal rotation, wrist flexion, and often a small range of shoulder adduction. (For a description of levers and resistance and moment arms, see Chapter 3.) In wrist flexion and shoulder adduction the moment arm can be greatly increased when an implement is used.

Another outstanding feature of the sidearm pattern is the plane in which the movements are made (i.e., the transverse); many movements of the underarm and overarm patterns are made in the sagittal plane.

The remainder of this chapter describes specific skills that have been observed with additions to, and modifications of, the basic pattern. As stated previously—and this point cannot be overemphasized—none is presented as the one best pattern.

SIDEARM THROW

The basic sidearm pattern, in which the shoulder and elbow joints are fixed, is rarely used in throwing light objects. Only when heavy objects are projected and in young, inexperienced children is the basic pattern likely to be observed. In a study of the sidearm and overarm throwing patterns of a highly skilled man and woman, the preliminary parts of the movements were found to be much alike. The differences were seen to be in the position of the arm and the degree and timing of elbow extension. The arm in the sidearm pattern was close

151

to the horizontal as hip rotation began, and the elbow was more fully extended at release. These arm positions would lengthen the moment arms for hip and spinal levels and shorten the moment arm for shoulder rotation. The hip action in both subjects contributed a greater proportion of the velocity in the sidearm throw than it did in the overarm pattern. The ball velocity for the man's sidearm throw was 120 and for the woman's 89 feet per second.

Continued study of the so-called sidearm throws of skilled performers has shown so much similarity to the overarm throw, especially those in which medial rotation of the humerus is followed by forearm extension, that some students have questioned classifying them as different patterns. Other observers believe that a distinguishing feature in the sidearm throw is a circular arm movement preceding release and that this is never seen in the overarm throw. Such observers say that the throw with the circular pattern should not be classified with the overarm throw. Further study of this feature is needed.

FOREHAND AND BACKHANDED TENNIS STROKES

Forehand drive. In the forehand tennis drive because of the possible length of its moment arm, the hip lever may well be the major contributor. The player faces the net as the ball is impacted, and the moment arm for hip action includes the width of the pelvis and the length of the arm and racket. This could well be more than 6 feet. However, that length must be adjusted to the height of the ball and its distance from the body. The adjustments are made by adducting the upper arm and flexing the elbow. These adjustments place the arm in an advantageous position for using medial rotation of the humerus, an action that is often observed. Since medial rotation of the humerus can be made with great speed, the force of impact with the shortened lever may more than equal that developed with the longer hip lever. Many writers advocate a firm wrist on impact, and this is often interpreted as a locked wrist. Whether a stationary wrist joint resists the force of the oncoming ball better than a wrist that is flexing is questionable. Perhaps the advantage of fixing this joint is that it eliminates the necessity for so timing its action that the racket face is brought to the desired position at impact.

In a cinematographic study of two skilled men to determine the factors influencing the direction of ball flight in the tennis forehand, Gelner found that in a drive to the right the racket had not reached a position in which the face was parallel to the net and that contact was made in line with the right shoulder. In a drive to the left the racket had passed the position in which the face was parallel to the net, and contact was made in line with the left shoulder. Neither subject pointed the forward (left) foot in the intended direction of flight, but when driving to the left both pointed that foot more toward the center of the net than they did when driving to the right.

Backhanded drive. As impact is made in the backhanded tennis stroke, the weight is on the right foot, and the fulcrum for hip action is also on the right, instead of the usual left. Thus the width of the pelvis is eliminated from the length of the moment arm. Study of the film of two skilled college women and two college men members of the varsity tennis team showed that all rotated the right humerus during the stroke. This rotation is, of course, lateral rather than the usual medial. The sequence of contributing joints was hip, shoulder, and wrist. All used wrist action, which in this stroke is extension, rather than flexion. Adjusting joint actions—shoulder abduction and elbow extension—were observed as the stroke was executed. In this study no attempt was made to observe shoulder action, and the angular and linear velocities of the acting levers were not measured. The ball velocities were measured in two situations: one in which the ball was suspended at a height chosen by each subject and one in which a tossed ball was impacted after a bounce. For the suspended balls the highest velocities obtained for the women were 92 and 101 feet per second and for the men 95 and 101 feet per second. For the tossed balls the highest velocities for the women were 95 and 96 feet per second and for the men 95 and 102 feet per second.

BATTING

The action used in batting normally is started from a position in which the performer has assumed a wide base of support (Fig. 9-1, *A*). The weight is mainly on the right foot, which is at right angles to the intended flight of the ball to permit freedom of pelvic rotation in the right hip. As the weight is transferred to the left foot, the pelvis is rotated at the left hip, turning through 90 degrees (*B* to *D*). The bat is moved forward in the transverse plane first by the turning of the torso (*B* and *C*) and finally by wrist action (*C* and *D*). The speed that the bat develops is shown by the blurring in *D*. A slight movement at the shoulder joints takes the upper arms forward and away from the trunk. The main contributing levers are those acting at the hip and wrist joints; the lengths of the moment arms for these levers have been greatly lengthened by the bat. Strong muscles acting at the wrist are important because they must hold the bat in the horizontal position, resisting gravitational pull, and move it with great speed in the final force-producing phase.

Note that the head is turned to the left in *A* and *B* to focus on the approaching ball. As the torso turns to the left, the head does not turn with it but remains facing toward the ball. Many coaches believe that if the batter's head moves to the left as the bat is swung the left shoulder will be elevated, thus changing the path of the bat and reducing the possibility of contacting the ball.

After studying the film, Breen concluded the following:

(1) The center of gravity of the body follows a relatively level plane, thus indicating a level swinging of the bat. (2) Each hitter is able to adjust his head to a position from which he can get a better look at the flight of the ball for any given pitch. (3) The leading forearm tends to straighten immediately as the bat is swung toward the ball, immediately moving the end of the bat and resulting in faster bat speed. (4) The length of the stride is the same for all pitches for any single good hitter. (5) The body is bent in the direction of the flight of the ball after contact has been made, thus putting the weight on the front foot.*

*Breen, J. L.: What makes a good hitter? JOHPER **38**:36, April, 1967.

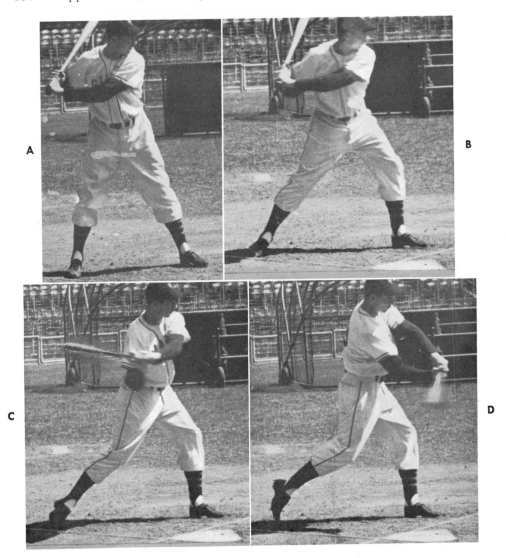

Fig. 9-1. Batting. (Courtesy Scholastic Coach.)

Another factor to consider in batting is the center of percussion. By way of explanation, if one bat is suspended and struck by another at its center of oscillation, it will swing as smoothly as a pendulum without being jarred. If the suspended bat is struck at any other point, it will shake or shiver and not vibrate smoothly. The center of oscillation is coincident with the center of percussion. This center is that point at which the blow produces the least effect on the center of suspension. Thus a baseball batter can hit a ball with more veloc-

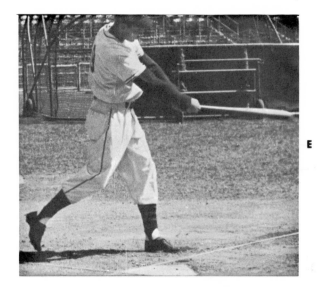

E

Fig. 9-1, cont'd. Batting.

ity if the ball strikes the bat at the center of percussion. Otherwise it will "sting" the hands.

DISCUS THROWING

The discus throw is an excellent example of the basic sidearm pattern, to which has been added a preparatory movement of the entire body. In the area (a ring with a diameter of 8 feet 2½ inches) within which the body is permitted to move, the progression includes total rotation of the body one and one-half times as well as movement from the back to the front of the space. Some of the world's best performers use all the ring starting well to the back and ending with the final step at the front of the ring.

The first step is taken with the left foot, which is moved toward the front of the ring and placed in line with the right foot. As the steps continue, they resemble those of a sprinter more than do those shown in Fig. 9-2. As the turns are made, the knees are flexed, and the right arm is held fairly close to the side; both positions lower the center of gravity and aid in balance. The arm position also moves the center of gravity of the rotating body closer to its axis and enables it to turn with greater speed. The speed of rotation during the stepping should accelerate and be as fast as is possible and still maintain balance.

On the final step the right arm is abducted, lengthening the moment arm of the pelvic lever, which can also be increased if the discus is held as close to the end of the fingers as can be controlled. Adduction of the arm at release will start the flight well beyond the front of the ring. Wrist action in the final phase can be added to impart more velocity.

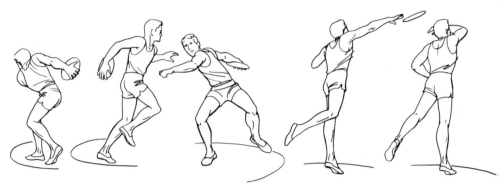

Fig. 9-2. Discus throw.

Because the discus in flight is affected by air resistance, the angle at which it is projected should be less than 45 degrees. The angle that will achieve the greatest distance will depend on the imparted velocity and the speed of the on-coming wind.

SUGGESTED READINGS

Breen, J. L.: What makes a good hitter? JOHPER **38**:36, April, 1967.

Cochran, A., and Stobbs, J.: The search for the perfect swing, Philadelphia, 1968, J. B. Lippincott Co.

Collins, P. A.: Body mechanics of the overarm and sidearm throws, thesis, University of Wisconsin, 1960.

Gelner, J.: Accuracy in the tennis forehand drive—a cinematographic analysis, thesis, University of Wisconsin, 1965.

See Bibliography for additional references.

CHAPTER 10 Pushing and pulling patterns

MECHANICS OF PUSHING AND PULLING PATTERN

The pushing pattern is commonly used to project and to move objects while one keeps contact with them and the pulling pattern to move objects while one keeps contact with them. In the push and pull both hands are often used, and in some cases no joint action may occur in the upper limbs; in such cases these limbs serve as a connection between the body and the object, or they may not be used at all. For example, in a push the shoulder girdle may contact the object, and the force will/ be derived from the action of the lower limbs. In general, one may say that in the preparatory phase of pushing the acting body segments are moved toward and in the force-producing phase away from each other. In the pull the direction of the movements will be reversed in the two phases. For efficient action in both patterns the force developed by the body should be applied in a plane that is parallel to the desired direction of movement and that passes through the center of gravity of the object to be moved. This means that contact with the object will be as close to that plane as is possible.

Of the many patterns possible, only the push used to project an object will be described. This pattern is illustrated in Fig. 10-1; in which A represents the shoulder joint and AB the upper arm, B represents the elbow joint and BC the forearm; the hand is not shown. In the preparatory position, ABC, the forearm has been drawn close to the upper arm; the shoulder is flexed 10 and the elbow 170 degrees, bringing the distal end of the forearm to the point C. To understand better the result of combined shoulder flexion and elbow extension, which will be used to develop projecting force, picture what would be the position of the distal end of the forearm if either shoulder or elbow joint acted alone. If the shoulder were flexed 80 degrees and no elbow action took place, C would move along the small arc shown by the broken line and reach a position directly above A. The distal end of the forearm has moved a slight distance upward, which is the desired direction, but it has also moved a slight distance backward, which is an undesired direction. Next, picture the position that C would reach if the elbow extended 80 degrees and no shoulder action occurred. The distal end of the forearm would be opposite the point B_1, and the forearm would be perpendicular to the line AB. Elbow extension moved C forward, a desired direction, but also downward, an undesired direction. When these joints act at the same time, the action in the undesired direction will be

157

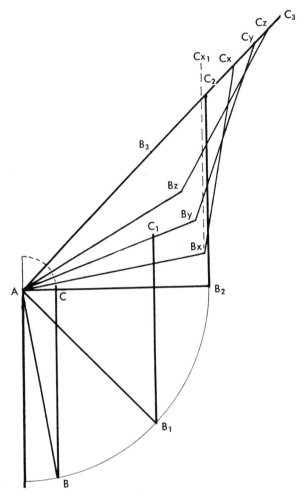

Fig. 10-1. Pushing pattern. **AB,** Upper arm; **BC,** forearm. As upper arm moves from **B** to **B₂**, equal angular velocity of the forearm will move the wrist through an arc parallel to **B-B₁-B₂**. As upper arm moves from **B₂** to **B₃**, angular movement of the forearm must be twice as fast to move the wrist along the line **C₂-C₃**.

counterbalanced by the action of the other joint. After 80 degrees of movement in both joints, C will be at C_2, which is on the desired line of projection shown by the upper diagonal line AC_3.

After these first 80 degrees of movement, the upper arm has reached the horizontal (AB_2), and the forearm is perpendicular to the upper arm (B_2C_2). From this position, as both actions continue, the elbow must extend twice as fast as the shoulder flexes if C is to move along the desired line of flight (AC_3). This is shown in the illustration; from B_2 to Bx the shoulder has flexed 10 degrees, another 10 to By, another 10 to Bz, and 15 degrees from Bz to B_3. If the distal end of the forearm is to move along the line AC_3 during this time, the elbow must extend 20, 20, 20, and 30 degrees; the result of the combined actions is shown by Cx, Cy, and Cz. If the elbow had extended only 10 degrees from B_2 to Bx, the distal end of the forearm would be at point Cx_1. Surely one must marvel at the ability of the human mechanism to make the joint adjustments necessary to keep on the line of flight. One can be confident that the speed of joint action is not voluntarily controlled; only a mental picture of the line of flight is necessary, and the nervous system somehow produces the needed actions. This suggests the importance of developing in the performer a picture of the line of flight for a projection rather than a concentration on the target, which is the final goal of a projection.

The lever and its resistance arm, which is moved by shoulder joint action, will include the entire arm and hand to the center of gravity of the projectile; the lever moved by elbow joint action will be the same except for the upper arm. In projections the hand, which is not shown here, will be moved by wrist action; its lever and resistance arm will be the same as those for elbow action except for the forearm.

Determination of the contributions of shoulder and elbow action will be more complex in this action than in the underarm, overarm, and sidearm patterns. This is because of the undesired actions. At Cz each lever, moving diagonally, will have a vertical component—up for shoulder action and down for elbow action—and a horizontal component—backward for shoulder action and forward for elbow action. The moment arm for shoulder action will be almost twice the length of that for elbow action. Part of the force of each moment arm will be used in counteracting the force in the undesired direction of the other.

If the action is made with one arm, pelvic and spinal rotation can be added to the pattern; although the contributions of the pelvis and the spine will be similar to those described in Chapter 7, in the push the range of these actions are likely to be smaller than in other projection skills. In a two-arm push the trunk is often an additional lever, moving from a flexed position by extension at the hip. In both the one-arm and the two-arm push, extension of the lower limbs may add to the force developed.

In the following sections, specific patterns will be described. Obviously if opposing directions of movement, such as those described in the preceding paragraphs, occur, the force developed cannot equal that developed in other projection skills. Again these specific patterns are not presented as best types of a general pattern; they are given to promote understanding of mechanics.

FENCING LUNGE

In fencing, upper limb action is accompanied by stepping, which is used to approach the opponent (the lunge) or to withdraw. Instead of facing in the direction of the step the trunk is turned at right angles to that direction to present a smaller target area to the opponent. To make the approach step the right thigh is rotated outward and abducted. The head, of course, faces the opponent.

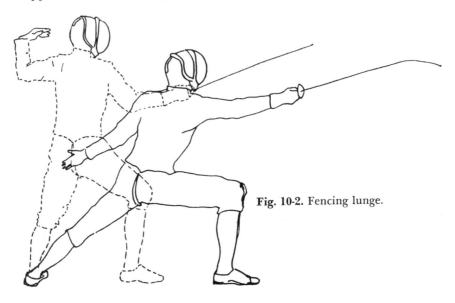

Fig. 10-2. Fencing lunge.

The pushing action of the thrust is seen in Fig. 10-2, in which the forearm extends as the upper arm, in lateral rotation, abducts. The mechanics of these actions are those described in the first section of this chapter.

The length of the reach is augmented by the step and by abduction at the hip of the supporting limb, resulting in tilting of the trunk in the direction of the thrust.

LIFTING

Lifting actions are shown in Figs. 10-3 to 10-5. When the object to be lifted is on the floor, the hands are lowered to make the contact usually by joint flexion of the lower limbs, and the possibility for extension thus achieved can then provide the needed force. Thus the work is done by the large muscles crossing the hips, knees, and ankles. In all heavy lifting the back is kept straight and acts as a single lever, with the fulcrum at the hips. In Fig. 10-5 the performer is lifting a heavy weight and attempts to apply force directly upward. Note in *A* that the arms are perpendicular to the weight. From *A* to *B* by flexion at ankle and knee the trunk has been lowered; note that in *A* the buttock is higher than the knee and in *B* it is close to the ankle. From *A* to *B* the trunk has been raised from a 45-degree inclination to a vertical position by extension at the hips (reversed muscle action). As the trunk is moved backward and upward, it undoubtedly overcomes the initial inertia of the weights, lifting them from the floor; the movement would be started by the strong hip extensors. While the weights are moving, the forearms flex, adding to the upward movement and also keeping the path of the weights in a vertical line, an important factor. Note that in *A* and *B* the weights are in the same vertical relationship to the feet.

From *B* with a widespread stance for stability, extension at ankles, knees, and

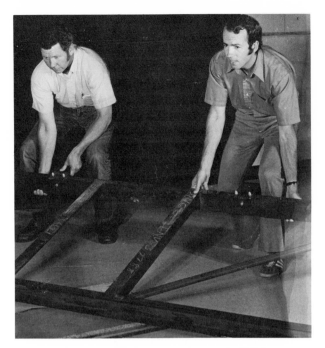

Fig. 10-3. Proper principles of lifting are illustrated by this two-man group. To assure safety, knees are bent, and the back is kept as straight as possible.

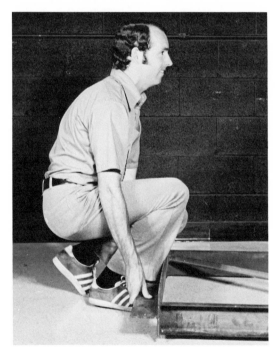

Fig. 10-4. Proper principles of lifting are illustrated here. Note that one foot is planted on the floor and is in line with the head.

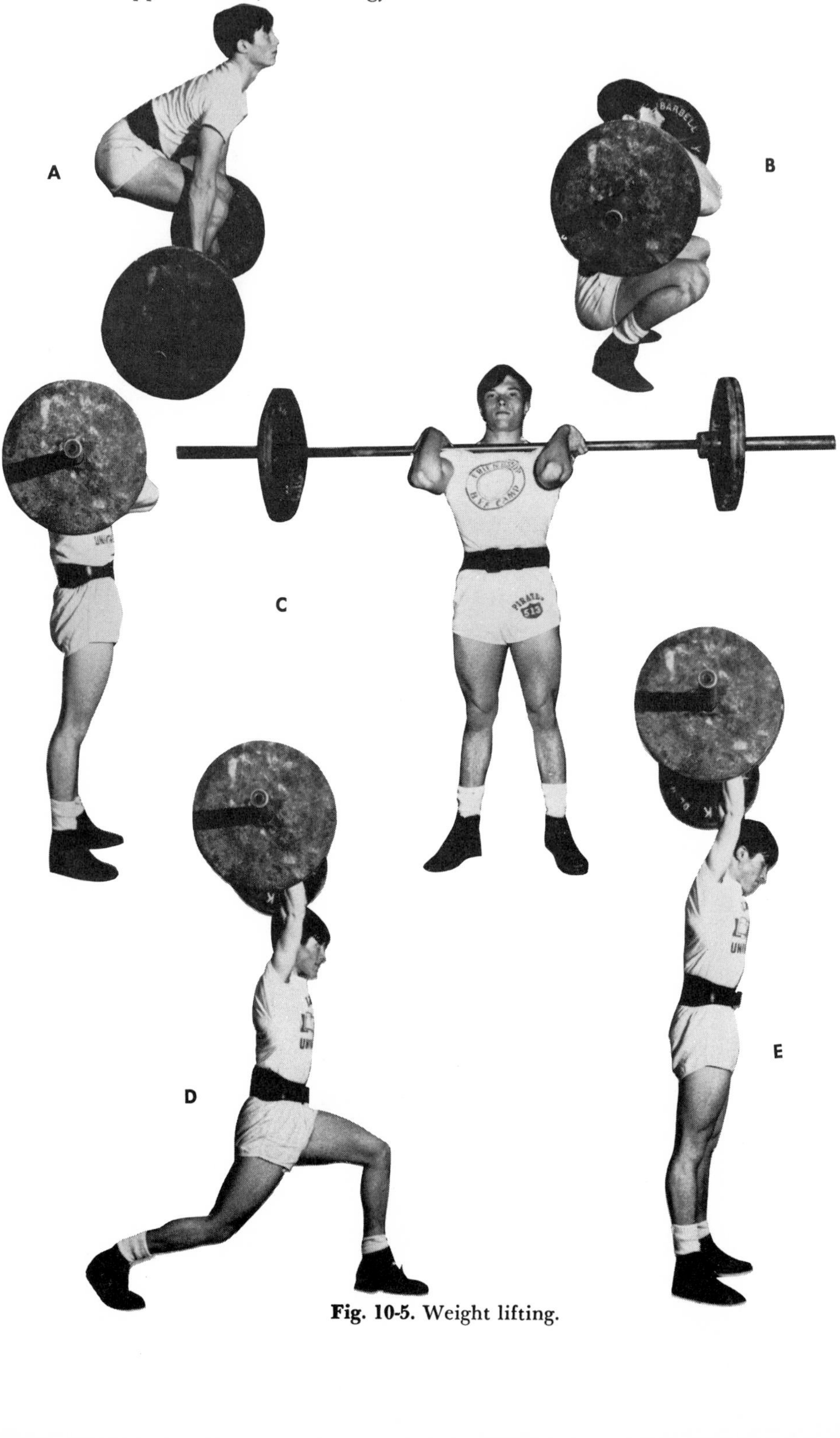

Fig. 10-5. Weight lifting.

hips raise the weights from knee to shoulder height (compare position of weights with feet [side view] in *B* and *C*). During this time, as the weight was moving, the forearms extended slightly and were responsible for the small amount of lift above the shoulders. From *C* to *D* the upper arms flexed from horizontal to vertical; the forearms extended, counteracting the backward movement of the upper arms. These combined actions added to the lift; the timing of these actions should be such that advantage is taken of the motion developed by the lower limbs. Note that the actual distance that the arms have lifted the weights is rela-

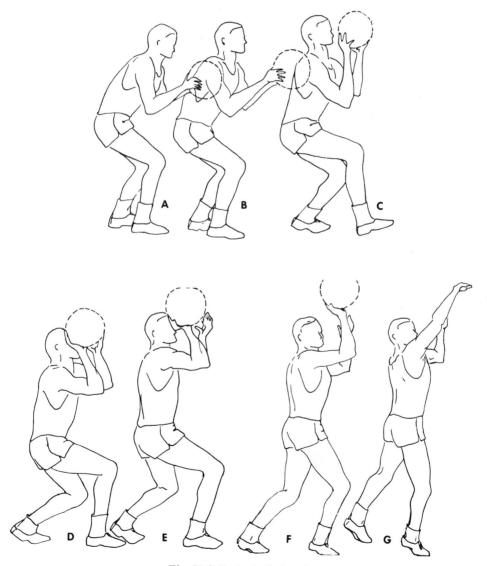

Fig. 10-6. Basketball shooting.

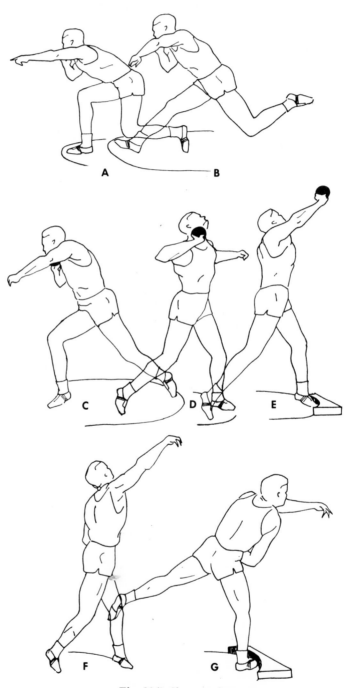

Fig. 10-7. Shot-putting.

tive to the head only, not to the feet. As the arm push is made, the body, including the arms, is lowered by the step and by knee and hip flexion. The final lift was again made with action of the lower limbs (*D* to *E*).

Mechanics of the upper limb are similar to those described in the first section of this chapter. Action in the lower limb is also a pushing pattern in which segments are moved by reversed muscle action. As the ankle extends, the proximal end of the leg is moved upward and backward; as the knee extends, the thigh is moved forward and upward. If no action occurred in the hip, the trunk would be moved forward and downward from the vertical; to prevent this movement the hip extension was adjusted to the inclination of the thigh to keep the trunk vertical from *B* to *E*. In the pattern of the lower limb, joint actions develop force in undesired directions as well as in desired ones, thus necessitating counteraction in other participating joints.

The main force throughout the lift was that developed by the lower limbs; whenever they are acting, the distance of lift is greater than when the upper limbs are acting. The muscles of the upper limbs, though not as strong as those of the lower, contribute to the lift by acting at the times when the weights are in motion.

BASKETBALL SHOOTING

The one-handed set shot in basketball is a pushing pattern in which the actions of the upper limb are almost identical to those described for the upper arm and forearm as an example of the pushing pattern in the section on mechanics in this chapter. As the performer shown in Fig. 10-6 receives the ball, the upper limbs move into a preparatory position mainly by elbow flexion (*A* to *C*). From *C* to *G* in the propulsive phase the upper arm flexes as the forearm extends.

Additional force is developed by wrist flexion (*E* to *G*) and by ankle flexion and knee extension. The ankle and knee, by moving the leg and the thigh, move the trunk forward and upward. Note that the trunk is held in a vertical position by extension at the hip. Because the supporting foot is on the same side as the pushing arm, pelvic rotation will not be a contributing factor.

The left hand is used (*C* to *E*) to balance the ball. Some players gently wag the wrist before the propulsive phase; this is believed to activate the proprioceptors.

The degree of knee flexion and corresponding hip flexion will be adjusted to the distance from the basket. Also the pattern can be carried out from a running approach rather than from the standing position shown in Fig. 10-6.

SHOT-PUTTING

The shot-putter faces to the rear, as seen in Fig. 10-7, *A,* in preparation for moving across the ring. The weight is on the right foot. From position *A* the performer hops on the right foot to place it in the position shown in *C*. This action gives a forward movement to the shot, which should be used by adding to it the final lever actions (*C* to *E*). Knee flexion (*C*) is important for development of force. As the left foot makes ground contact (*D* to *E*), the torso can be moved rapidly upward by extension of the rear (right) thigh; and, as the left foot takes the weight, the pelvis can rotate on the left limb. These two actions can accelerate the movement of the shot. Note that the upper arm is abducted to the horizontal in *D*; this position lengthens the moment arm for the lever moving at the left hip.

In the last phase of trunk rotation, shoulder adduction and flexion move the upper arm forward and upward. At the same time the elbow extends, moving the forearm forward and counteracting the upward movement of the upper arm. Final impetus is given by wrist flexion. Although these levers contribute to the force developed, as does the initial hop, the major contributor is the pelvic lever. The actions occurring from *E* to *G* are made to maintain balance.

Because the velocity of the shot is much slower than that of many objects which people project and because its release point is higher than the landing point, the projection angle should be less than 45 degrees above the horizontal. For a method of determining the best angle to gain distance see Chapter 17.

SUGGESTED READINGS

Cooper, J. M., and Siedentop, D.: The theory and science of basketball, ed. 2, Philadelphia, 1975, Lea & Febiger.

Massey, B., et al.: The kinesiology of weight-lifting, Dubuque, Iowa, 1959, William C. Brown Co., Publishers.

Mastropaolo, J. A.: Analysis of fundamentals of fencing, Res. Q. Am. Assoc. Health Phys. Educ. **30:**285, 1959.

See Bibliography for additional references.

CHAPTER 11 Kicking patterns

MECHANICS OF KICKING PATTERN

The kicking pattern, used to apply force with the foot, is a variation of running and thus is a modification of the walking pattern. The kick differs from the walk and the run in that force is applied with the swinging limb rather than with the supporting one. In the final force-producing phase the primary action is knee extension. The lever and the resistance arm include the leg and the part of the foot between the ankle and the point of impact. The length of the moment arm is approximately the distance from the knee to the point of impact.

Although little or no hip action occurs in the final phase, this joint makes an important contribution in the earlier force-producing phase. As the thigh is swung forward by hip flexion, it carries the leg and foot with it. During this time the knee flexes—an action that moves the foot backward. Film tracings show that in spite of the knee action the foot moves forward during this phase. Thigh action in this pattern contributes to the forward movement; in bowling, this is similar to the contribution of the approach steps, which move the ball forward as the arm is swinging back. The leg, then, will have not only the velocity developed by knee extension but also that developed by hip flexion, even though the latter action does not occur at impact. Immediately after impact the hip again flexes and moves the entire limb speedily upward in the follow-through. Unless one has studied slow motion action on film, the pause in hip action is not likely to be observed; hip action is often thought to be continuous.

Another valuable lever can be added to the kick by pelvic rotation, which can be acting at the time of impact. This lever is used most frequently by performers who have had training in soccer and is effective when the ball is approached diagonally. The lever and the resistance arm of this action include the pelvis, the thigh, the leg, and the part of the foot between the ankle and the point of impact. The length of the moment arm, which is perpendicular to the axis passing through the left hip (if the kick is made with the right foot) and to the line of force, will be approximately equal to the width of the pelvis.

Ankle action is used mainly to position the foot for the impact.

KICKING AND PUNTING

Studies of kicking and punting skills used in both soccer and football have shown that the major contributor at the time of impact is the lever acting at the knee joint; the hip joint makes its major contribution before impact. With

167

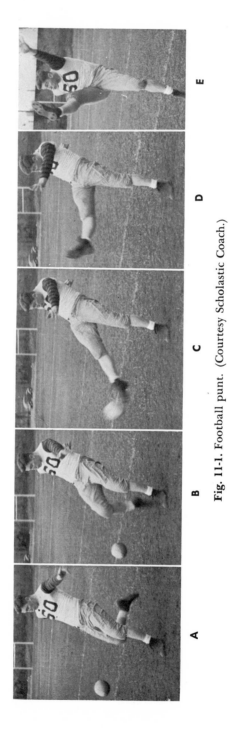

Fig. 11-1. Football punt. (Courtesy Scholastic Coach.)

any situation and performer the joint actions are so much alike that these acts (kicking and punting) can be considered the same skill. The pattern is illustrated in Fig. 11-1, where from *A* to *B* the thigh can be seen to have flexed; from *B* to *C* the inclination of the thigh has changed little if any. After *C* the thigh flexes rapidly, carrying the entire limb forward and upward.

From 90 degrees of flexion in *A* the knee extends; it has contacted the ball before *C*. Film studies show that impact is likely to be made before the knee is fully extended; this and the rapid flexion at the hip after contact protect the knee joint. Rotation of the pelvis can be seen from *A* to *C*.

Observations have shown differences in hip action at the time of impact. Some performers have no hip action; some have slight flexion, and others have slight extension. These facts suggest that, at impact, hip action is an adjustment to the position of the ball relative to the supporting foot. If this is true, studies should be made to determine whether one exact position of the supporting foot relative to a stationary ball will result in greater velocity and accuracy. The drop of the ball with reference to the foot should also be studied. Whether the foot is contacting a stationary or a moving ball, the eyes should be focused on it. Therefore the performer approaching the ball should flex the head and upper spine (Fig. 11-1, *A* to *D*).

When a step or a run precedes the kick, forward movement of the body can contribute to the force of impact. The placement of the final step differs from that of the running step. In the latter the knee flexes just before the foot makes contact with the ground, so that the foot is brought more directly under the body's center of gravity; in the kick the foot is placed well ahead of the body's center of gravity (Fig. 11-1, *A*), so that the body can be carried forward by ankle flexion, thus adding its forward movement to the force. More important is the greater range of pelvic rotation that this foot placement permits.

Similarities in thigh and knee actions are reported by Glassow and Mortimer, who studied film of an untrained 9-year-old boy punting a soccer ball and of a man, an experienced soccer player, executing a place-kick. The greatest degree of knee flexion was the same for the two performers, slightly more than 90 degrees; the rate of knee extension at impact was also the same, approximately 1280 degrees per second. The man, whose leg is longer, will have a longer moment arm for the lever acting at the knee and therefore greater linear velocity for this lever. Hip flexion, moving the thigh forward and slightly upward, occurred in both man and boy while the knee was flexing and continued as the knee extended until just before impact. Both performers extended the thigh a few degrees just before impact. This lowering has been observed in several studies; it does not add to the force of impact but is probably an adjustment to the ball position.

Much greater knee velocity for the kicks of three highly skilled Australian men is reported by Macmillian.* The average velocity for each man was 1521.3,

---

*Macmillian, M. B.: Unpublished material, Monash University, Victoria, Australia, 1970.

1788.6, and 2008.7 degrees per second immediately prior to contact. During the same time the average foot velocity was 76.5, 76.7, and 77.9 feet per second. The maximum ball velocities were faster than those of the impacting foot; they were 89.0, 89.2, and 82.0 feet per second. This phenomenon was mentioned in the discussion of golf and tennis.

Differences have been observed in the part of the foot that contacts the ball, including the toe of the shoe, the front of the foot between the toe and the ankle, and the side of the foot. Study is needed to determine the effect of each variation on velocity and accuracy.

SUGGESTED READINGS

Glassow, R. B., and Mortimer, E. M.: Soccer-speedball guide, ed. 11, Washington, D.C., 1966, American Association of Health, Physical Education, and Recreation.

Glassow, R. B., and Mortimer, E. M.: Selected soccer and speedball articles, ed. 3, Washington, D.C., 1971, American Association of Health, Physical Education, and Recreation.

Marshall, S.: Factors affecting place-kicking in football, Res. Q. Am. Assoc. Health Phys. Educ. **29:**302, 1958.

Roberts, E. M., and Metcalfe, A.: Mechanical analysis of kicking. In Wartenweiler, J., Jokl, E., and Hebbelinck, M., editors: Proceedings of the First International Seminar on Biomechanics, Basel, Switzerland, 1968, S. Karger, AG.

See Bibliography for additional references.

THE BODY
SUPPORTING
AND MOVING
ITSELF

CHAPTER 12 The center of gravity in
the human body

Man uses his levers not only to move external objects but also to move the entire body or its parts and to maintain any desired position. Movement of the whole body occurs when the base of support is changed, as it is in walking, running, and jumping and in traveling on the horizontal bar or rings when the hand provides the support. To maintain position the base is not changed—a situation seen in standing on the feet, hands, or head and in sitting.

In these activities the supporting surface is an important factor. It must be strong enough to resist the force exerted against it by the stationary body and the greater force of the moving body. The supporting surface, as it resists the force of the body, pushes back, and the force of this push moves the body and resists the downward pull of gravity. One cannot stand on quicksand because one's entire weight pushes against a small surface, but lying on the sand distributes the weight, and the downward push by each body section can be within the limits that the sand can resist.

The nature of the contacting surfaces also influences the resisting push. If the point of contact of the body slides along the supporting surface, its force against that surface is decreased, and consequently the resisting push is decreased. To prevent slide on contact, track shoes have spikes. To increase slide the underside of the skis is waxed.

Whether one attempts to maintain balance or to move the entire body, the skeletal levers move to shift the center of weight, that is, the center of gravity.

LOCATION OF THE CENTER OF GRAVITY
IN THE HUMAN BODY

The position of the human center of gravity is important for maintaining balance and for the many forms of locomotion.

Definition of the center of gravity. All masses that are within the gravitational field of the earth are constantly subjected to a pull toward the earth's center; the greater the mass, the stronger will be the force of that pull. The force of gravitational attraction that the earth exerts on a body is called its *weight.* Gravitational force pulls downward on each point of a given body. The distribution of these points determines the position of the center of gravity of the body. If a board is suspended on a support as in playground teeterboards, a downward pull is exerted on each side of the support. If the board mass on each side is equal in size and in distance from the support, the board will balance. If a child sits on one side of the balanced board, that side will be pushed downward, and the opposite side will move upward. In such unbalanced situations note that gravitational force, interestingly, is responsible for the upward as well as the downward movement. This upward movement caused by gravitational force will be shown later to be used by the body in many forms of locomotion. On the teeterboard a second child can take a position on the opposite side of the board, and, if the distance from the board is adjusted, the board and the two children can be balanced. Within every mass is a point about which the gravitational forces on one side will equal those on the other. This balance point, determined in three planes of the mass, is the center of gravity.

Center of gravity in the transverse body plane. The point of balance in the human body has long interested investigators. The earliest of these employed the teeterboard to locate the transverse plane of that point. An Italian physicist, Borelli (1608-1679), placed a nude subject on a board in the prone position and then moved the board back and forth as it rested on a knife-edged support until the total mass balanced. He reported the balance plane to be one which cut the body "between the genitals and the pubis." Somewhere within this plane would lie the subject's center of gravity. Two German brothers, the Webers, in 1836 improved Borelli's method by first balancing the board and then sliding the subject back and forth until balance was obtained. They found the transverse plane of the center of gravity to be 56.8% of the height above the heel.

Half a century later (1889) the two Germans Braune and Fischer reported that the center-of-gravity plane was 54.8% of the height measured from the soles. Their conclusion was based on finding the point of balance in four fresh "normally built" cadavers that were frozen solid. The cadavers were first balanced on a knife-edge, and then a steel rod was driven into the cadaver at the determined plane. Each cadaver was suspended by the steel rod, and gravitational force moved the mass into a balanced position. When the body attained equilibrium, a plumb line was dropped from the point of suspension to locate the transverse plane of the center of gravity.

The most convenient method of locating the plane of the center of gravity is that proposed by the two Americans Reynolds and Lovett (1909). A board of a known length is supported at either end by a knife-edge. The knife-edges are placed on scales that can be adjusted to eliminate the weight of the board. The subject lies on the board, and the plane of the center of gravity can be determined mathematically. It will be at a point on the board that can be determined by multiplying the weight on one scale by the distance from that knife-edge to the plane of the center of gravity. This product will equal that obtained by multiplying the weight on the second scale by the distance between the second knife-edge and the plane of the center of gravity. The distances are not known, but if the distance for the first scale is represented by X, the second distance will be that between the knife-edges minus X. If W_1 represents the weight on the first scale and W_2 the weight on the second scale, the question for determining the distance X will be as follows:

$W_1X = W_2$ (distance between the knife-edges $-$ X)

A subject weighing 150 pounds lies on a board with the top of the head in line with the knife-edge on scale 1. The distance between the knife-edges is 60 inches. The scale reading on the head scale is 73.5 pounds; the other scale reads 76.5 pounds. Then:

$$73.5X = 76.5 \ (60 - X)$$
$$73.5X = 4590 - 76.5X$$
$$150X = 4590$$
$$X = 30.6$$

Since the head was even with the knife-edge, the distance from the top of the head to the transverse plane of the center of gravity is 30.6 inches. If the subject is 68 inches in height, the plane is 45% of the height measured from the top of the head and 55% of the height measured from the soles of the feet.

This procedure can be used when only one scale is available, since the reading on the second scale will always be the total weight minus the reading on the single scale (Fig. 12-1). Had one scale been used in the illustration, the first step in solving for X would be the following:

$$73.5X = \ (150 - 73.5) \ (60 - X)$$
$$73.5X = 76.5 \ (60 - X)$$
$$73.5X + 76.5X = 76.5 \times 60$$

Also the equation can be written without the preliminary steps:

Total weight $\times$ X $=$ (Total weight $-$ Scale reading) $\times$ (Distance between knife-edges)

Using the scale method, other investigators have reported findings on the

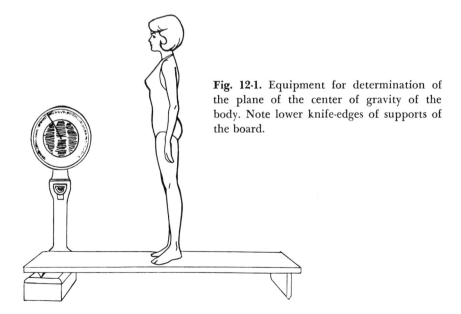

Fig. 12-1. Equipment for determination of the plane of the center of gravity of the body. Note lower knife-edges of supports of the board.

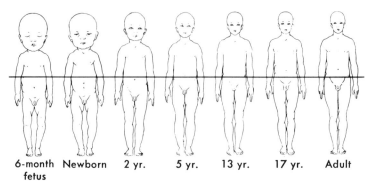

Fig. 12-2. Outline drawings of ventral aspects of the body. Body lengths are scaled to reduce all figures to same height. Transverse plane of the center of gravity is represented by transverse line. (From Palmer, C. E.: Child Dev. **15**:99, 1944.)

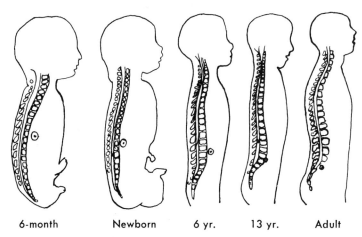

Fig. 12-3. Position of the center of gravity with reference to the spine at five different ages. (Modified from Palmer, C. E.: Child Dev. **15**:99, 1944.)

location of the transverse plane of the human center of gravity. Croskey and associates reported in 1922 that this plane is slightly higher in men than in women. The average height of the plane in men was 56.18% measured from the soles; the range of percentages was 55 to 58. For women, the average was 55.44%; the range was 54 to 58. Additional observations were made by Hellebrandt and co-workers, who found in 357 college women that the transverse plane averaged 55.17% of the height; the lowest observed was 53%; the highest was 59%.

The most extensive study is that reported by Palmer, who located the transverse plane of the center of gravity in 1172 subjects, 596 boys and 576 girls from birth to 20 years of age, and in 18 fetal cadavers. Palmer concluded that, regardless of age or sex, the plane can be estimated as follows:

0.557 height + 1.4 cm. from soles of feet (or 0.551 inch)

Since body segments differ in proportion to total height from birth to maturity, the plane of the center of gravity will lie in a different section of the body as age increases, but the proportion of height will be constant (Figs. 12-2 and 12-3).

Obviously a change in position of the limbs with reference to the prone torso will change the position of the center of gravity. If the arms are raised overhead or the hips flexed, the plane will move toward the head. Loss of body parts will also alter the position. Amputation of any part of the lower limb will raise the plane, and the height of the center of gravity will increase with the amount of body mass lost. The addition of prosthetic appliances to replace the amputated limb will lower the center of gravity toward the normal position (Fig. 12-4).

Center of gravity in the frontal and sagittal body planes. In the preceding discussion the transverse plane of the center of gravity was located at a distance from the top of the head or from the soles of the feet. In balance and locomotor activities, it is important to locate the gravity plane in the frontal and sagittal planes. To do so using the Reynolds-Lovett method, the body must be stationary

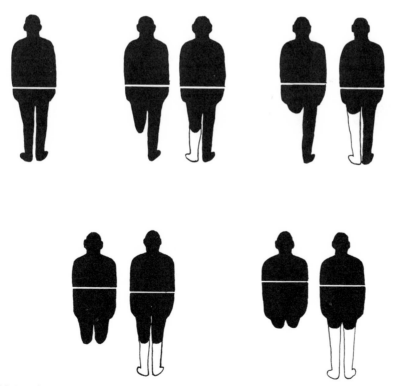

Fig. 12-4. Diagrammatic representation of the influence of amputation of lower extremities on the height of the center of gravity and compensatory effect of prosthetic appliance. (From Hellebrandt, F. A.: J.A.M.A. **142:**1353, 1950.)

on the board, and some body point must be located with reference to the knife-edges. To determine the transverse plane the top of the head was placed in line with one of the knife-edges; if the frontal gravity plane is to be located while the subject is standing, some part of the foot will be taken as the reference point, and the distance of this part from one of the knife-edges must be known. Since it is more convenient to stand near the middle of the board rather than near one end of it, a line on the board halfway between the knife-edges is convenient to take for measuring distance.

To illustrate determination of the frontal gravity plane, assume that an individual weighing 160 pounds stands on the board with the foremost tip of the toes at the halfway line. The facing scale registers 66 pounds. If one uses the equation

Total weight $\times$ X $=$ (Total weight $-$ Scale reading) $\times$ (Distance between knife-edges)

the figures will be as follows:

$$160X = 94 \times 60$$
$$X = 35.25$$

Since the distance from the knife-edge to the gravity plane is 35.25 inches and the tip of the toes is 30 inches from the knife-edge, the plane is 5.25 inches back of the tip of the toes. Often it is desirable to locate the frontal plane with reference to the ankle joint. In this case if the ankle joint is 7 inches from the tip of the toes, the frontal plane is 1.75 inches in front of that joint. A perpendicular line passing through the foot at this point is often called the gravity line; in postural measures, certain body landmarks are described in terms of deviation from this line.

When a person stands erect, the frontal gravity plane lies in front of the ankle joint and in back of the metatarsophalangeal joints. The location between these points differs with individuals and may differ from time to time in the same individual. This location between the ankles and the proximal end of the toes has been so frequently observed that it can be accepted as a human characteristic. Among the published reports are those of Cureton and Wickens, Hellebrandt, Fox and Young, and Brown. Over the years hundreds of students in our kinesiology classes have observed this phenomenon in themselves and in their classmates. Not only have they observed the location, but they have also seen that this plane is rarely stationary; it usually fluctuates, and the degree of fluctuation varies with the individual.

As the subject stands on the board for gravity-plane determination, the observer finds it difficult to make an exact scale reading because the dial needle fluctuates rapidly. The range of the needle varies with individuals but rarely exceeds 5 pounds. If one reading is desired, the best one to take is that about which the needle hovers; however, the extremes will also provide interesting information. The reason for the changes in scale readings is understood when one remembers that the body must balance on the small base provided by the upper surface of the talus at the ankle joint. Since the center of gravity of the body is ahead of the ankle joint, the body is unbalanced on this small surface. Gravitational force would tilt the body forward if no counterforce were present.

The ankle extensors provide this force; the tension in these muscles must be sufficient to withstand gravitational pull if the erect position is to be maintained. Any slight change in any body part (solid, liquid, or gas) will change the distribution of weight; this will change the force of gravitational pull and consequently change the demand on the ankle extensors. The tension in the muscles may change also. Whatever the cause the frontal plane is constantly shifting; yet it remains within the limits described. Class observations in which students are asked to lean forward as far as possible without raising the heels and then backward as far as possible without lifting the toes (and without falling) rarely find that the gravity plane has moved back of the ankle or ahead of the proximal end of the toes. It does move beyond the normal limits for the individual.

Segmental alignment above the ankle is not a universal characteristic. Individuals differ in degree of pelvic tilt, in depth of lumbar, dorsal, and cervical curves, and in shoulder girdle and head position. All these factors will affect the distribution of weight. Yet when an individual stands in a habitual position, the frontal plane of the center of gravity will fall between the ankle and the metatarsophalangeal joints.

To locate the sagittal gravity plane the subject stands on the board, with the right side toward one knife-edge and the left side toward the other. This plane has frequently been located to determine whether the subject is likely to carry more of the weight on one foot than on the other.

An arrangement for simultaneously determining the frontal and sagittal planes of the center of gravity has been presented by Waterland and Shambes. The subject takes a position on a base supported by three dial scales. Two photographs, a side and a front view, are taken by a synchronized shutter arrangement. The three scale readings shown in the photographs will equal the total weight of the subject. With these the positions of gravity lines in the frontal and sagittal planes can be calculated. These investigators have shown fluctuations of the gravity line in a "static" standing position. By placing on the supported board a paper on which the footprints of the subject were traced, they located the gravity line with reference to the feet (Fig. 12-5).

The triangular platform shown in Fig. 12-5 was used by Hasselkus to compare the postural sway of 10 women 21 to 30 with 10 others 73 to 80 years of age. Greater sway was thought to be a possible indication of aging of the neuromuscular system. Each subject stood on the platform for three 18-second periods, during which cameras recorded the scale readings every second. The area enclosed in the outer borders of the 54 calculated positions of gravity lines (such as + in Fig. 12-5) was expressed as a percentage of the functional base of support, a quadrilateral area enclosed in lines drawn along the lateral borders of the feet and across the back of the heels and connecting the heads of the first metatarsals. The older women's sway area covered an average of 43% and the younger women an average of 23%. For all subjects the position of the gravity line tended to be to the left and to the posterior of the geometric center of the functional base.

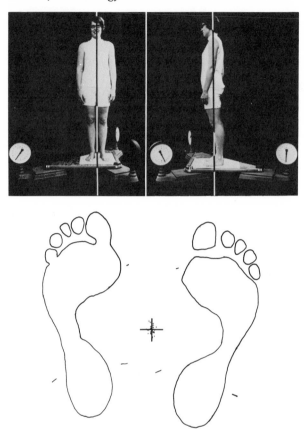

Fig. 12-5. Equipment used to determine gravity line in sagittal and frontal planes. Front and side view photographs are taken simultaneously; each view presents two of three dial scales. Gravity lines added to photographs after calculations represent the mean of thirty determinations; each dot between feet represents one determination; center point of crossed lines represents the mean of thirty determinations. (From Waterland, J. C., and Shambes, G. M.: Biplane center of gravity procedures, Percept. Mot. Skills **30:**511, 1970. Reprinted with permission of author and publisher.)

Davis devised a center-of-gravity board with accompanying three weight scales. The positions that his subjects assumed are shown in Fig. 12-6.

LOCATION OF THE CENTER OF GRAVITY IN THE MOVING BODY

Two methods, the scale and the segmental, have been used to determine the center of gravity in the moving body.

Scale method. The scale method of determining the location of the center of gravity can be used only when the body is in a stationary position. If body parts are moving, the pressure on the scale will be affected by the force of

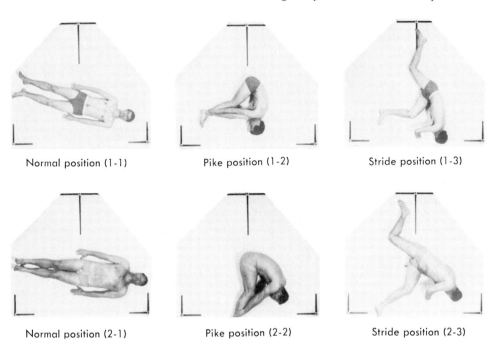

Normal position (1-1)   Pike position (1-2)   Stride position (1-3)

Normal position (2-1)   Pike position (2-2)   Stride position (2-3)

Fig. 12-6. Performer-position combinations assumed by two performers on center-of-gravity board. (From Davis, M.: Quality of data collected by the segmental analysis technique, unpublished doctoral dissertation, Indiana University, Sept., 1973.)

these movements as well as by the weight. The observer does not know how much of each scale reading is due to weight and how much to force. The plane of the center of gravity can be determined in any static position, that can be taken on the platform supported by a scale or scales. Groves has used assumed positions to determine the location of the center of gravity in various dives. Instead of one or two scales this investigator used four, each of which was attached to the corner of a rectangular plywood board. On the board subjects then assumed positions that were selected from a film of an expert diver. As presented in the published report six positions were taken for the jackknife dive and an equal number for the back dive and for the front one and one-half somersault. The positions included takeoff, high point, and entry, as well as intervening positions. As the subjects assumed the selected positions, a photograph was taken with a camera placed directly overhead. The sum of the scale readings at the right would then be equivalent to the W_1 in the previous description, and the sum of the scale readings to the left would be equivalent to W_2. If the width of the board were known, the center of gravity could be located in the frontal plane. The scale readings at the top and bottom could be used to determine the position of the center of gravity in the transverse plane. This location, measured in inches from the hip joint, could now be placed on tracings taken from the film, and the line of projection of the center of gravity could be traced. These tracings show that the center of gravity of the body when projected in flight follows a parabolic curve, the shape of which is determined by the angle and the velocity of projection.

Segmental method. Another method of determining the location of the center of gravity in the moving body is the segmental method suggested by Dawson in 1935. This method is used when the center of gravity of a performer needs to be located on a projected image, such as a motion-picture film. Locating the center of gravity in several frames of a film helps to define the path of the center of gravity for the entire movement.

This method can be illustrated by imagining three children seated on a teeterboard. One child weighs 60 pounds and is seated on the board 10 feet from the fulcrum. Another seated on the same side weighs 50 pounds and is 6 feet from the fulcrum. The third child is seated on the opposite side, weighs 90 pounds, and is 8 feet from the fulcrum. Since these body weights act as rotating forces, the effect of each force multiplied by the distance from the fulcrum is known as *torque*. On the side where the heaviest child is seated the torque will equal 90×8, or 720; on the side where the two lighter children are seated it will be $(60 \times 10) + (50 \times 6)$ or 900.

The board will not be balanced with this arrangement. To balance the board two methods are possible. First, the positions of the children may be changed. The 90-pound child might be moved 10 feet from the fulcrum, and the torque on that side of the board would then equal the 900 pounds of the opposite side. The second possibility would be to move the fulcrum. To determine the distance that the fulcrum should be moved, the percentage weight of each child in relation to the total weight of the three children (200 pounds) will be used to determine the force of each side:

$$60 \text{ pounds: } 0.30 \times 10 = 3.00$$
$$50 \text{ pounds: } 0.25 \times 6 = 1.50$$
$$\text{Total: } 4.50$$
$$90 \text{ pounds: } 0.45 \times 8 = 3.60$$

The difference between 4.50 and 3.60, 0.9, shows the number of feet that the fulcrum should be moved. To balance the board the distance between the heaviest child and the fulcrum should be increased 0.9 feet; that between the fulcrum and each of the lighter children should be decreased 0.9 feet. With these distances and the percentage weights the torque values will be as follows:

$$0.30 \times 9.1 = 2.73$$
$$0.25 \times 5.1 = 1.275$$
$$\text{Total: } = 4.005$$
$$0.45 \times 8.9 = 4.005$$

In relating this example to determination of the center of gravity in the moving body, keep in mind that the combined weight of the three children is equivalent to the entire body weight, and the percentage weight of each child is equivalent to the percentage of each body segment to the total body weight. To find the position of the center of gravity of the total body, any line (which may or may not pass through some part of the body) can be arbitrarily chosen

Table 12-1. Weights of body segments relative to total body weight for women

Segment	Bernstein	Plagenhoef	Kyeldsen
Trunk		27.0	30.1
Upper arm	2.63	2.90	2.74
Forearm	1.82	1.55	1.61
Hand	0.64	0.50	0.51
Thigh	12.48	11.50	8.26
Calf (lower leg)	4.73	5.25	5.49
Foot	1.31	1.20	1.24

Table 12-2. Weights of body segments relative to total body weight for men

Segment	Braune and Fischer	Cleaveland	Williams and Lissner	Dempster
Head and neck	0.0706	0.0703	0.079	
Trunk	0.4270	0.0703	0.511	0.494
Upper arm	0.0672	0.0625	0.054	0.035
Forearm	0.0624	0.0433	0.044	0.016
Hand	(With forearm)	(With forearm)	(With forearm)	0.005
Thigh	0.2316	0.2252	0.194	0.137
Calf (lower leg)	0.1412	0.1152	0.120	0.047
Foot	(With calf)	(With calf)	(With calf)	0.013

Table 12-3. Locations of centers of gravity of body segments for women, expressed as percentage of total segment length as measured from proximal end

Segment	Matsui	Bernstein
Head and neck	63	
Trunk	52	
Upper arm	46	48.40
Forearm	42	41.74
Hand	50	
Thigh	42	38.88
Calf	42	42.26
Foot	50	

as the line from which the position of the segmental centers of gravity will be measured. Torque values for each segment can be calculated (by the use of percentage weights). The difference between the sums of the values on each side of the line will show the distance that the line should be moved to pass through the total body's center of gravity.

In using this method the investigator must have the following information:

1. The percentage of total body weight of each segment (Tables 12-1 and 12-2)

Table 12-4. Locations of centers of gravity of body segments for men, expressed as percentage of total segment length as measured from proximal end

Segment	Cleaveland	Dempster	Matsui
Head and neck		(With trunk)	63
Trunk	53	60.4	52
Upper arm	42	43.6	46
Forearm	28	43.0	41
Hand	(With forearm)	50.6	50
Thigh	36	43.3	42
Calf	42	43.3	41
Foot	(With calf)	42.9	50

   2. The location of the center of gravity in each segment, usually reported as a percentage of the total segment length as measured from the proximal end of the segment (Tables 12-3 and 12-4)

   3. The horizontal and vertical distance of each body segment center of gravity from a vertical and horizontal axis in the form of an X- and Y-coordinate system as depicted in Fig. 12-7

The steps to follow in calculating the total-body center of gravity from a projected film image are as follows:

A. Project the image onto a piece of graph paper and trace the performer. The standard Recordak viewer is ideal for this purpose.

B. Establish a coordinate system on the graph paper in such a way that the origin is in the lower left-hand corner (Fig. 12-7). This confines all the data to the upper right quadrant, where all X and Y values will be positive.

C. From the picture select two reference points that can be viewed in all the frames to be analyzed for a given performance and that are stationary objects—for example, the center of the dial on a wall clock or an electric wall socket.

D. Record the X- and Y-coordinate values of the two reference points from the graph paper. In analysis of future frames of this same performance, these reference coordinate values must be exactly the same.

E. Record the X- and Y-coordinate values for each of the following segmental end points:

   1. Tragus of the ear

   2. Sternal notch

   3. Crotch

   4. Right shoulder

   5. Right elbow

   6. Right fingertips (distal point of right fingertips)

   7. Left shoulder

   8. Left elbow

   9. Left wrist

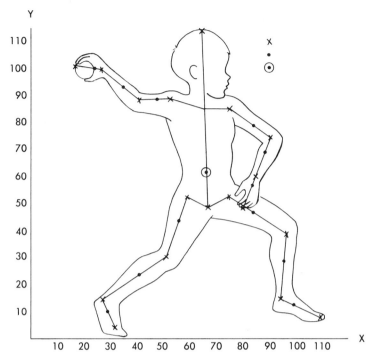

Fig. 12-7. A tracing from film of young child throwing a ball to illustrate points required to determine position of body center of gravity. **X** represents segmental end points; • marks segmental midpoints; ⊙ indicates determined body center of gravity.

10. Left fingertips (distal point of left fingertips)
11. Right hip
12. Right knee
13. Right ankle
14. Right toe
15. Left hip
16. Left knee
17. Left ankle
18. Left toe (distal point of left toes)
   These points are marked on Fig. 12-7.
F. Connect the segmental end points to form a stick figure.
G. Locate the center of gravity for each segment by the following procedures:
   1. Measure the segment lengths.
   2. Multiply this value times the appropriate percentage value from Table 12-3 or 12-4.
   3. Measure this amount from the proximal end of the segment. Mark this spot as the center of gravity for the segment; that is, if the trunk and head measure 10 cm. then the center of gravity for this segment would

Table 12-5. Segmental center of gravity locations, based on Fig. 12-7 and the coordinate values once segmental weight factors are considered

Segment	X coordinate	X value weighted	Y coordinate	Y value weighted
Head and neck	(With trunk)		(With trunk)	
Trunk	65.0	33.41	76.0	39.01
Upper arm (left)	81.5	2.45	81.0	2.43
Forearm (left)	88.0	1.41	69.5	1.11
Hand (left)	83.5	0.50	57.0	0.34
Thigh (left)	83.5	10.77	48.0	6.19
Calf (left)	95.5	4.58	30.0	1.44
Foot (left)	99.0	1.49	13.0	0.20
Upper arm (right)	48.0	1.44	89.0	2.67
Forearm (right)	35.0	0.56	93.0	1.49
Hand (right)	23.5	0.14	101.0	0.61
Thigh (right)	55.5	7.16	44.5	5.74
Calf (right)	41.0	1.97	24.0	1.15
Foot (right)	29.0	0.44	10.0	0.15
Total body		66.32		62.53

be 0.604 × 10 = 6.04 or 6.04 cm. from the crotch (using Dempster data on men).

4. Repeat the procedure for all segments.

H. Record all the X- and Y-coordinate values for each segment's center of gravity.

I. Multiply the X values for each segment's center of gravity times the percentage of the total body weight contributed by that segment (Table 12-5). Sum these values. This sum represents the location of the center of gravity of the total body in the X, or horizontal, plane.

J. Repeat step I using the Y values for each segment's center of gravity.

K. The X- and Y-coordinate total-body center of gravity can be located on the graph paper.

Table 12-5 contains sample coordinate values based on the image in Fig. 12-7.

Care must be taken when using the segmental method. A study by Davis on the validity, reliability, and objectivity of the segmental method revealed some of its limitations.

The precision of the estimation of the center of gravity is significantly affected by the type of segmental data applied. Segmental data collected on men should not be used when analyzing the movements of women and children.

Davis also found the validity of the segmental method acceptable for use in kinematic analyses; however, he states that at the present the method is not refined enough to be used for kinetic analyses.

When kinetic information is needed, it must come from equipment designed specifically for the purpose of measuring forces, such as force plates, accelerometers, and strain gauges.

In Davis's study the reliability of the segmental method was high with intraclass correlations of $R_x = 0.9682$ and $R_y = 0.9443$ when the same center of gravity was identified from three repeated measurements.

In contrast, the objectivity of the segmental method was low. The reason for the inconsistency in measurements taken by several observers appeared to be related to individual interpretations of the locations of segmental end points. This was not a problem when testing the reliability.

No further investigation after Braune and Fisher's experiments mentioned in Chapter 2, was made until 1955, when Cleaveland, using eleven college men, determined the weight of body segments and located the center of gravity of each. Marks on the body indicated the limits of each segment, and the body was lowered into a tank of water to each mark in succession. The weight of each segment was calculated by the weight lost and the amount of water displaced at each stage of submersion. The center of gravity of each segment was located at the point at which half the amount of weight was lost. Also in 1955, Dempster published a report on the dissecting and weighing of segments of eight men cadavers. Using these findings as a basis, Williams and Lissner presented percentage weights and locations of the center of gravity for body segments.

The segmental limits used in the observations of these various investigators were not identical, and consequently the percentages differ, as do the locations of the centers of gravity.

These measures and calculations illustrate a method by which the path of the body's center of gravity can be depicted in any skill. Such a procedure was used by Sparks, as seen in Fig. 12-8. To do so there must be a vertical and a horizontal reference line, neither of which has to pass through some part of the body, as did the lines in the illustration. The number of film frames necessary to determine the path will depend on whether the body is in flight or whether segments are changing position while the body is supported on a stationary base.

When the body is in flight, once the contact with the supporting surface has been broken, the path of the center of gravity is determined by the velocity and direction imparted to it at takeoff and by gravitational pull. It is now a projectile and can be treated as such. The line of flight can be found by the method described in Chapter 17. Once the body is in flight, no segmental movement will affect the path of the center of gravity. Therefore, it is necessary to locate the position of the center of gravity at only two points (and the corresponding times). One must always be the first frame in which contact has been broken—in which the body has just begun its flight. The second can be any frame before landing, but it is well to select a frame that is as far as possible from the first. The frame selected will depend on the number of frames included in the film. The choice of the second frame is as far as possible from the first because there are always likely to be measurement errors; the longer the time and the distance that are measured, the smaller the percentage of error. Since the in-flight path of the center of gravity will be a parabolic curve, the equation for that curve can be calculated from any two points on the curve. In this text

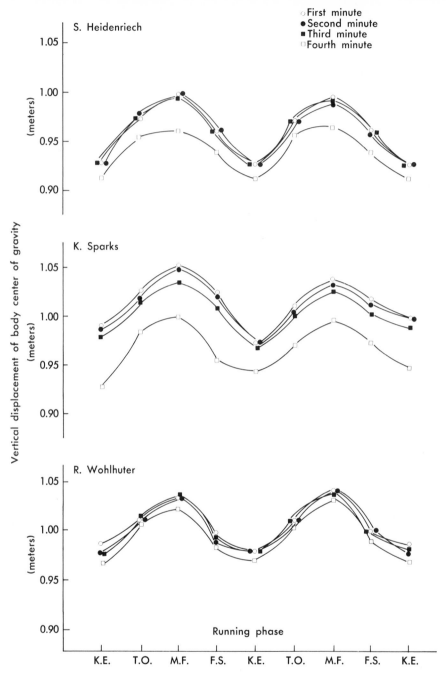

Fig. 12-8. Vertical displacement of body center of gravity of runners for each minute in 4-minute–mile run. All three runners show the effect of fatigue during fourth minute. This was due to greater flexion of knees and general alteration of running style. **K.E.,** knees even; **T.O.,** toe off; **M.F.,** midflight; **F.S.,** foot strike. Stride for two phases is shown. (From Sparks, K. E.: Physiological and mechanical alterations due to fatigue while running a four-minute mile on treadmill, unpublished doctoral dissertation, Indiana University, May, 1975.)

when direction and velocity of body projections are reported, they have been determined by this method.

When the path of the center of gravity is depicted while the base is stationary and segments are moving, its position should be found in every film frame. In such situations the center of gravity is not a projectile, and movement of a segment will affect its path. To determine the path of the center of gravity in the takeoff phase of a standing broad jump, Johnson drew the vertical references line through the metatarsophalangeal joints and the horizontal line along the bottom of the toes. At the time the heels left the floor she found the center of gravity to be 28.6 inches above the floor and 3 inches ahead of the metatarsal joints. As the knees and hips flexed and the arms moved downward from the height of the backswing, the center of gravity moved downward and forward to a position 21.9 inches above the floor and 10.4 inches ahead of the metatarsophalangeal joints. (See Fig. 15-9.) At takeoff the center of gravity was 29.3 inches above the floor and 22.8 inches ahead of the metatarsophalangeal joints. Note that interestingly the center of gravity was ahead of the toes at the time that the heels were raised—a further indication that gravitational pull, not muscle action, tilts the body (raising the heels). As the muscles act and move body segments, the position of the center of gravity is changed, so that it is outside the base of support, and the body falls forward, a fall that is controlled by the ankle extensors.

Calculations to determine the position of the center of gravity by this method involve a relatively long and involved process; yet understanding of the effect of segmental positions will be furthered by a limited number of determinations. If films are not available, various positions can be taken on the gravity board: for example, the subject may stand on the board in a stride position with feet separated at a measured distance and trunk flexed at a measured angle or may lie on the board with upper and lower limbs held at measured angles to the trunk. Segmental calculations can then be compared with scale determinations.

For more extensive studies, work can be reduced by means of recently developed techniques. Motion analyzers and digitizers used in conjunction with computers (on-line or separate) can greatly increase the number of frames that may be feasibly analyzed in a given time.

(See *Kinesiology Review*, 1968, for article by Garrett, Widule, and Garrett. Also see Scheuchenzuber's center-of-gravity computer program found in Appendix D and Bates' program. The latter is more detailed with several subroutines. Several graduate students have used it for analyzing their data in their doctoral dissertations.)

SUGGESTED READINGS

Bates, B. T.: The development of a computer program with application to a film analysis: the mechanics of female runners, unpublished doctoral dissertation, Indiana University, Aug., 1973.

Bernstein, N.: The co-ordination and regulation of movements, Oxford, England, 1967, Pergamon Press, Ltd.

Clauser, C. E., McConville, J. T., and Young, J. W.: Weight, volume, and center of mass of segments of the human body, AMRL-TR-69-70, Aug., 1969, Wright-Patterson Air Force Base, Ohio.

Cleaveland, H. G.: The determination of the center of gravity in segments of the human body, thesis, University of California, 1955.

Dempster, W. T.: Space requirements of the seated operator, WADC Tech. Rep., July, 1955, U.S. Department of Commerce.

O'Connell, A. L., and Gardner, E. B.: Understanding the scientific bases of human movement, Baltimore, 1972, The Williams & Wilkins Co.

Palmer, C. E.: Studies of the center of gravity in the human body, Child Dev. 15:99, 1944.

Scheuchenzuber, H. J., Jr.: Kinetic and kinematic characteristics in the performance of tethered and non-tethered swimming of the front crawl arm stroke, unpublished doctoral dissertation, Indiana University, Aug., 1974.

Steindler, A.: Kinesiology of the human body under normal and pathological conditions, Springfield, Ill., 1955, Charles C Thomas, Publisher.

Williams, M., and Lissner, H. R.: Biomechanics of human motion, Philadelphia, 1962, W. B. Saunders Co.

See Bibliography for additional references.

CHAPTER 13 Balance activities

MECHANICS OF BALANCE

To maintain balance, humans, like all animals and inanimate objects, must keep the center of gravity in an area within and directly above the supporting base. The larger the base, the greater the range in which the center of gravity can be moved without the body's falling. The closer to the base the center of gravity is, the greater will be the angle of tilt necessary to move the center of gravity outside the base area. Thus the stability of the body is often said to be increased as the center of gravity is lowered. The human being can use many body segments as a base—the feet, one foot, the hands, one finger (in the case of some acrobats), the head, the thighs, or the entire body. The segments above the base can be adjusted to bring them into various positions. No general balance pattern exists, but whatever the base and the positions of the segments above it the center of gravity must be kept over the base area if balance is to be maintained.

STANDING UPRIGHT

Human beings are bipeds whose upright posture makes them distinct from all other animals. Morton and Fuller say that "in his body form, in his completely erect bipedism and mental development, Man possesses characteristics that separate him undeniably from all other living creatures."* They are of the opinion that the physical differences that distinguish the human from other closely related animal forms developed as a result of reaction to the force of gravity. To maintain an erect position humans had to evolve certain skeletal and muscular changes. The human foot became the sole weight-bearing organ. Concerning the human foot arrangement, Morton and Fuller state, " (1) It permits the body center to occupy its central position over the area of ground contact so that the margin of postural security is equal forward and backward; (2) it places the direction of structural unbalance toward the front so that the muscular tension needed to maintain our erect posture is imposed

*Morton, D. J., and Fuller, D. D.: Human locomotion and body form, Baltimore, 1952, The Williams & Wilkins Co.

entirely upon the large and powerful calf muscles; (3) the weaker anterior group of muscles is released from any active counterbalancing tension."* In addition, they stress the value of the anteriorly unbalanced position of the body center in aiding the initiation of forward movement. They also state that the only contact with the ground that a human being has is the bony architecture of two feet, and consequently the balance is on this small contact area.

Human lower limbs are much straighter than are those of partially bipedal animals and are extended in line with the body. The human gluteus maximus as an extensor of the hip is unusually large and is counter-balanced by the large quadriceps femoris in front. The latter arrangement helps prevent the knee from flexing, which would cause a person to fall in moving forward as the foot strikes the ground.

The use of the arms and hands to support the body weight in the hanging position while the body was moved by a change in the position of the hands (called brachiation) enabled man's ancestors to develop changes in the arms and hands that produce free mobility in the shoulder girdle and wide movement in all directions in the shoulder joint. The upper limbs were lengthened and strengthened, and the movements of supination and pronation were developed in the forearms. The hand, including the digits and thumb, is common to certain related animal forms, but the human hand is the most flexible and dexterous. These skeletal changes in the upper limb began when the arms were given a weight-bearing function.

When descendants of these arboreal ancestors returned to terrestrial living, some found that the lower limbs could be used efficiently for locomotion, and thus the hands and arms were freed for manipulation. This form of bipedism and gravitational pull again developed structural changes. To provide better balance, man developed his one unique skeletal part, the human foot. Bony segments above the foot were altered, and among these was the pelvis, which gradually took a vertical, rather than a horizontal, position to support the weight of the torso better. To meet this function the pelvic bones shortened, thickened, and broadened. (For a detailed description of this evolutionary change, see Napier.) Howell says, "Man is a biped with a unique pelvis, and although neither cursorial (running) nor saltatorial (jumping) in a strict sense, his adaptations should receive some attention. His pelvis has been shortened (craniocaudally) and broadened. The ilium has expanded not only ventrally but dorsally (thereby accentuating the greater sciatic notch). The chief muscular stimuli concerned with the shortening of the ilium seem undoubtedly to be the proper anchorage in the erect posture of the abdominal muscles and the broadening and shortening of the gluteus medius complex; the iliacus is probably but little responsible. The position of the thigh in the upright posture has tended to reduce to zero the angle of the leverage of the hamstring muscles—a quandary that the ischium has met by migrating dorsally, thus helping, but to a rather

*Morton, D. J., and Fuller, D. D.: Human locomotion and body form, Baltimore, 1952, The Williams & Wilkins Co.

poor degree, the functioning of the hamstring muscles. As a result the ilioischiatic angle (of the axes of these two elements) apparently is less than in any other mammal. The pubis tends to follow the ischium dorsally."*

Since human lower limbs perform the functions of both weight bearing and locomotion, structural differences exist between the human and the lower animals. Essentially the human being is less equipped to run, jump, or even stand than are other animals. However, the upper limbs are free for manipulation. Structural differences from the feet to the pelvis provide for the weight-bearing and locomotor functions. Similar differences, especially the lumbar curve, are present in the spinal column and torso to adjust to the upright position. The C-shaped curve of the spine in an infant develops into the anterior, posterior, or lateral S curve of the adult. During the period of creeping and progress into walking the spine undergoes changes especially in the lumbar region to enable the child to become an upright creature. Keith states that the lumbar curve is seen only in the human species.

Medawar states, "The 'vertebral column' is not a column at all but is more like a cantilever having the four legs as piers. The vertebral column of a human being is no longer a simple uninflected arc; it bends slightly forwards in the neck, slightly backwards in the thoracic cage, forwards again in the lumbar region, the small of the back, and backwards in the fused vertebrae that form the sacrum. That is the mature pattern; in development, the neck flexure appears somewhat before birth, and the lumbar flexure between the ninth and eighteenth months of age."† The center of gravity of the human body is elevated to a position high above and to the outer borders of the feet, the supporting parts. This unstable and potentially mobile structure must be held in a standing position by continuous muscular action because of the fact that it is a high vertical structure with a small base.

Above the midline any body portion that is moved to the rear or front to any great extent makes the maintenance of balance more difficult. Also a person whose body design is unusual, such as large or tall, or who has a specific body part that is unusually large or long may find that these conditions have an effect on the ability to maintain an upright position. For example, a person with a heavy, tall body and small feet will experience some difficulty in standing and walking comfortably. His base is not large enough to allow him to withstand as great a displacement of force as he should. However, Morton believes that this instability is an aid in the initiation of forward movement. Joseph has said, "One may therefore conclude that in the posture of standing at ease (military position) in most subjects, stability at the ankle joints is maintained by the calf muscles, mainly soleus, at the knee and hip joints by the appropriate ligaments and at the vertebral joints by only some parts of the sacrospinales muscles. There are no apparent differences between the sexes with regard to the leg and thigh

*Howell, A. B.: Speed in animals, Chicago, 1944, University of Chicago Press.
†Medawar, P. W.: The uniqueness of the individual, New York, 1958, Basic Books, Inc., Publishers.

muscles. Movements such as swaying at the ankle joints or flexion at the knee or hip joints or flexion of the vertebral column result in activity in the appropriate muscles, usually the extensors, which resist the force of gravity."* In other words, not all muscles are used to maintain the standing position as would be more likely in a vigorous movement, such as running. The specific muscles used are rightly called *postural muscles.*

Hellebrandt has said that standing is really movement on a stationary base and that swaying is inseparable from the upright stance. Hellebrandt and others have shown that considerable sway occurs in forward, backward, and sideward directions. One of us (J.M.C.) has had his students measure the amount of sway that occurs during 5- and 10-minute periods of standing erect without moving (other than swaying) and with the feet placed close together. The longer the individual stands, the greater is the amplitude of sway. Usually after 15 minutes the individual will tend to faint and fall to the floor. One individual in a special experiment was able to stand erect for 25 minutes with his feet in a bucket of ice water. At the end of 25 minutes he fell to the floor and had to be revived. In speaking of a study of standing. Hellebrandt and Franseen state: "Weiner (1938) in South Africa combined the factors of exercise and a hot, humid environment in studying the ability to stand. He found that most of his adult male Bantu subjects could tolerate an hour of quiet standing after shoveling gravel for an equal period of time. When, in controlled experiment, the standing was undertaken in a cool room, no cases of collapse occurred."†

The muscles act as "little hearts" in helping push the blood back through the veins to the heart. When this action is lacking, the blood pools in the feet, and the individual faints from lack of blood in the brain. Feet have increased in size as much as one and one-half shoe sizes after prolonged standing. A walk of one-half mile reduced the feet to normal size.

Concerning sway, Hellebrandt and Franseen have said: "There is general agreement that stance is steadied when the eyes are open and focused on a fixed point and least stable with the eyes closed. Distraction reduces sway. When the feet are together, the stance is unsettled. Turning the toes out to an angle of 45 degrees or separating the feet so as to equalize the coronal and sagittal diameters of support steadies the stance. Sway is much greater in the anteroposterior vertical orientation plane than in the transverse. Height and weight correlate poorly with stability. Thus the body may compensate in other ways for mechanically disadvantageous factors in physical build. Though kaleidoscopic at first sight, when carefully made, postural sway patterns are characteristic for each person and highly reproducible. There is lack of agreement chiefly as to whether stance training reduces postural instability or not, and whether fatigue

---

*Joseph, J.: Man's posture—electromyographic studies, Springfield, Ill., 1960, Charles C Thomas, Publisher.
†Hellebrandt, F. A., and Franseen, E. B.: Physiological study of the vertical stance of man, Physiol. Rev. 23:220, 1943.

is reflected as readily, as often implied, in an augmentation of sway."* Joseph has listed several studies on sway. For example, one study showed that activity in the muscles of the calves of the legs was greater when subjects wore high-heeled shoes (2½ inches) than when they were barefoot. The increased muscular activity resulted from the unstable position created by the high-heeled shoes. Activity in the gastrocnemius muscle was increased the most.

The term *posture* has many meanings, depending on the person who is defining the term, as illustrated in the following discussion.

In 1889 Braune and Fischer described a posture in which a vertical line erected from the ankle intersected the axis of the knee joint, the axis of the hip joint, the axis of the shoulder joint, and the ear (Chapter 12). This linear alignment of the body in an erect position presented a convenient posture from which to measure deviations, since all reference points fall along the same line. This posture, in which no part deviates from the vertical line, was named the *Normal-stellung,* or *normal standing posture.* Other postures, such as the relaxed and military, were also described, and deviations from normal posture were discussed. Normal posture does not correspond with the usual position of the body and can be maintained only momentarily. The usual position of the body is a more relaxed posture. Although no attempt was made by Braune and Fischer to depict the normal standing as the ideal posture, such an interpretation became widespread. Many logical reasons have been given to support the contention that the normal posture of Braune and Fischer is the ideal one. Most of the reasons were based on the relationship of this posture to the healthy function of the internal organs. Posters showing this normal posture are displayed today on many schoolroom walls to depict a perfect standing position. Modifications are also seen in posture charts showing a similar "normal" sitting position —an unnatural but "ideal" position.

The statistical interpretation of normality is in terms of the frequency distribution of a population. In a healthy population the normal posture would be that assumed by the majority. Observations of people standing in line before ticket windows or on street corners reveal that practically no one is using the *Normal-stellung.* Instead people shift from one position to another while standing or sitting. An investigator attempting to measure the usual postures of a population would be confronted with the task of erecting a frequency distribution of postures assumed by each person from day to day in various conditions of heat and cold, sickness and health, and sadness and joy. For women as well as for men a researcher would face the additional problem of fashion changes. After the model posture of each person has been determined, the frequency distribution for this population could then be erected. This statistical expression of normality of posture derived by the frequency of occurrence of one posture among others would necessarily include the range of differences and the amounts

*Hellebrandt, F. A., and Franseen, E. B.: Physiological study of the vertical stance of man, Physiol. Rev. 23:220, 1943.

of deviations from the normal that could be expected from time to time. Thus the statistical normal posture cannot be a fixed value.

The physiologic concept of normality is that condition in which the organs and systems of the body function efficiently. Body postures affect physiologic functions. For one thing the energy requirements of different postures vary considerably. The rigid military posture requires about 20% more energy than the easy standing position. An extremely relaxed standing position requires about 10% less energy than an easy standing position. If one stands so as to be practically hanging on the ligaments (completely relaxed as much as possible), little more energy is used than in sitting or reclining. Hellebrandt and co-workers determined that the energy cost of standing is relatively small and that oxygen consumption during graded degrees of gravitational stress deviates insignificantly from the normal variations characteristic of recumbency.

Blood pressure rises when a person assumes a rigid, erect posture because of the muscular effort involved. The respiratory efficiency is difficult to assess in the resting state, since only a small part of the available lung tissues would provide ample area for the small requirement of gaseous exchange. Because of this excessive respiratory tissue the small gain in maximal diaphragmatic excursion and vital capacity because of changes in posture is inconsequential. Thus from the point of view of physiologic efficiency the rigid, erect posture is not the normal, since the efficiency of metabolic and circulatory systems is reduced.

Extreme curvature and poor alignment produce physiologic changes and are considered to be pathologic. Just how much deviation is possible without causing impairment of health and inefficient function of vital organs is a subject of discussion by several authors with some disagreement. Minor deviations do not appear to greatly affect the health and efficient function of the internal organs.

Erect posture is commonly associated with attitudes of readiness, self-confidence, and assurance. A relaxed or slouched posture may generally connote laziness and incompetence. For this reason the erect posture is the one most often aspired to and considered normal. Wells has stated that relatively little is known about the upright posture, so that one should be careful of what one says about it. Hellebrandt and others have stated that one should not think of a standing posture as involving a rigid set of anatomic landmarks—lobe of ear, tip of acromion process, middle of trochanter, and head of fibula—in alignment. Certainly the erect posture gives a better appearance, since clothes fit better, the physique is shown to better advantage, and the face is held up so that attentiveness is indicated. Fashion models, stage and screen actresses, and beauty contest winners assume erect and stately postures to appear to the best advantage before an audience. However, exceptions have occurred in successful individuals. Superior intelligence and tremendous energy are sometimes housed in a body that is habitually slouched. Some great athletes assume a habitual posture of extreme relaxation.

Normal posture, then, is that which best suits one's own condition and the conditions of the environment. During attention to a stimulating situation the normal posture will be erect. In a condition of distress because of sad circumstances normal posture will be characterized by a general sagging of all body parts. In extreme fatigue the normal posture will be that which conserves energy. The normal posture of physical attractiveness is one that displays the special qualities of the physique to the best advantage.

Metheny states her concept of posture as follows: "There is no single best posture for all individuals. Each person must take the body he has and make the best of it. For each person the best posture is that in which the body segments are balanced in the position of least strain and maximum support. This is an individual matter."* Goldthwaite and associates have stated, "There is not and cannot be one posture which is normal for all individuals and to which all individuals should conform."† Joseph points out that there is no single correct posture and that it is difficult to place anyone in an arbitrary grouping. Hellebrandt and associates drew the following conclusions from one of their studies: "(1) Gravitational stress patterns are highly individual. (2) Body alignment measured repeatedly during uninterrupted standing is variable. (3) There is no relation between the Wellesley posture score and the anteroposterior eccentricity of the center of gravity. (4) The evidence is contrary to theoretical expectation. It is suggested that the lack of association between the variables studied may be due to reliance on a posture criterion more related to esthetic than physiological concepts."‡

To sustain oneself in the upright position, one must maintain the skeletal structure in an elongated position against the force of gravity by a continuous interaction of the postural muscles. The extensor muscles carry the major load. Morton and Fuller state, "When body weight is transmitted by the legs upon the feet, it is received at the ankle joints, which are back of the midpoint of anteroposterior length. Consequently, as viewed laterally, the columns of support represented by the leg bones are inclined slightly forward to form an angle of about two to three degrees in relation to the perpendicular dropped from the body center. This means that in order to hold the body center over the central point of ground support, a constant state of forward unbalance must be maintained by continuous tension on the large calf muscles."§

The sustained contraction of the muscles supporting the upright position is termed *postural tonus*. The stimuli that produce the volley of nerve impulses that continually excite the postural muscles can arise from every sensory organ of the body. Loud noises, bright lights, strong odors, and jarring shocks all increase the postural tonus. In the absence of such stimuli the postural tonus is diminished.

---

*Metheny, E.: Body dynamics, New York, 1952, McGraw-Hill Book Co.
†Goldthwaite, J. E., et al.: Essentials of body mechanics in health and disease, ed. 5, Philadelphia, 1952, J. B. Lippincott Co.
‡Hellebrandt, F. A., Riddle, K. S., Larsen, E. M., and Fries, E. C.: Gravitational influences on postural alignment, Physiotherapy Rev. 22:149, 1942.
§Morton, D. J., and Fuller, D. D.: Human locomotion and body form, Baltimore, 1952, The Williams & Wilkins Co.

The major stimuli of postural tonus arise from several sources. These so-called righting reflexes are often classified as follows: (1) labyrinthine sense, concerned mainly with the inner ear and otolithic chamber, (2) tonic neck-righting reflexes, (3) visual, or optical, reflexes, (4) proprioceptor, or kinesthetic, sense, (5) extensor or antigravity reflexes, (6) spinal stretch reflex, and (7) plantar reflexes. The portion of the brain controlling most of these reflexes lies in the ventral part of the midbrain just behind a section located immediately in front of the third cranial nerves. The facilitory mechanism of the spinal muscles has its source in the spinal cord, the brain stem, and the cerebellum and cortex (Chapter 4). These reflexes and actions have been ably studied by Magnus and Sherrington.

The movement of the head from side to side affects labyrinthine and tonic neck reflexes. The tonus of the muscles in the neck is most affected when the head is thrown backward, and the muscles in the neck are most relaxed when the head is allowed to come forward in complete relaxation. Many performers need to relax the neck muscles just before competing in sports, so as not to have these muscles in contraction during the movement.

In the antigravity muscles the so-called stretch reflex is well developed. The extensor muscles of the joints involved in weight bearing, the abdominal muscles, and even the adductors of the scapula are all a part of this arrangement. As the body starts to sag from the pull of gravity, this reflex takes over and causes contraction in the extensor muscles to hold the body upright. (See Chapter 4.)

The spinal stretch reflex augments the work of the antigravity muscles in keeping a person in standing position. Pressure against the sole of the foot by the ground elicits a reflexive contraction of the extensor muscles of the lower extremity of the legs and again aids in maintaining an upright position.

The sensory organs of the inner ear contribute stimuli to postural tonus through the impulses that arise when the head is moved. Tiny particles of calcium, called *otoliths,* are suspended like silt in the fluid of the semicircular canal of the ear. When the head is tilted, the otoliths drift from one part of the wall of the canal to another. As the otoliths touch the sides of the walls, they press against a few of the many hairlike sensory nerve endings that line the semicircular canal. This pressure of the otoliths on the sensory nerve receptors causes the rise of impulses that ultimately produce sensations that are perceived as position. Only slight stimuli are necessary to evoke the reflexes that keep the body erect. The importance of this postural reflex is demonstrated by the reaction of a person whose semicircular function is lost and who must rely on muscle and tendon proprioceptors, visual stimuli, and other sensations to maintain an erect position. Such a person has extreme difficulty in standing erect with eyes closed unless he can touch some stable object with his hand to establish the sense of position. Even when semicircular canal function is intact, the body, as stated previously, is continually swaying forward and backward and from side to side while standing. The body sways until sufficient stimuli are produced to evoke the righting reflex. The response to this reflex is to make the muscular adjustments necessary to return the body to the erect position. The body again starts to sway after this response and would fall if the reflexive adjustments did not once again take place.

The frequent contraction and relaxation of the postural muscles during this continual falling and catching of oneself has a beneficial influence on moving the blood and lymph through the muscles. In this way, circulation is maintained, and working fibers are supplied with food and prevented from becoming choked by their own excreta.

Visual impressions are important in the maintenance of erect posture. These sensations establish relationships to objects about the individual. The effect of training on the effectiveness of visual impressions is brought out by experience in a "fun house" in which one enters a room whose walls, floor, and ceiling are constructed at unusual angles. Standing quietly erect in this room is difficult. In fact, if the eyes are closed, stability is improved because the sensations from the deep proprioceptors, the inner ear organs, and the touch receptors in the soles of the feet provide more customary information.

These reflex actions keep the center of gravity within the base of support. Normally the center of gravity is located between the ankle and the metatarsophalangeal joints, thus providing a margin of safety to the rear and front of the foot.

Other sensations that act to change the tonus of the muscles that are active in holding the unstable framework erect in standing may make marked modifications in the standing position. A view of a horrifying scene (unless one is conditioned to it) may elicit such intense responses that the chemistry of the blood will be changed and the irritability of the muscles altered. Depending on the degree of stimulation the resulting tension may be increased or decreased. A loud noise causes the body to become rigid. Music can be either exciting or soothing. A slap on the back causes stiffening, whereas a gentle back massage is relaxing. A whiff of spirits of ammonia is stimulating, whereas odors associated with comfort, such as that of fresh bed linens, have an opposite effect. Other sensations, such as thirst, nausea, fatigue, heat, cold, love, hatred, tickling, and itching, also vary postural reactions.

Military postures. The military posture of attention is an unnaturally immobile position in that the chest is elevated, the head is erect, the chin is drawn inward, and the feet are together with the weight distributed on them evenly (Fig. 13-1). In this position, stress is placed on the long back muscles, the extensors of the hip, and the muscles in the calf regions. The knee extensors are more relaxed because the center of gravity falls in front of the axis of the knee joint. The position of attention cannot be maintained for long periods because of fatigue resulting from poor circulation and constant muscular tension. A formal but less strenuous posture, called *parade rest,* is ordered when a military formation is prolonged. Parade rest is assumed with the feet apart, increasing the base of support and thus diminishing muscular tension. If either attention or parade rest is held too long, leg circulation is hindered, and a loss of sensation occurs in the legs. In some individuals, quiet standing for 20 minutes causes so

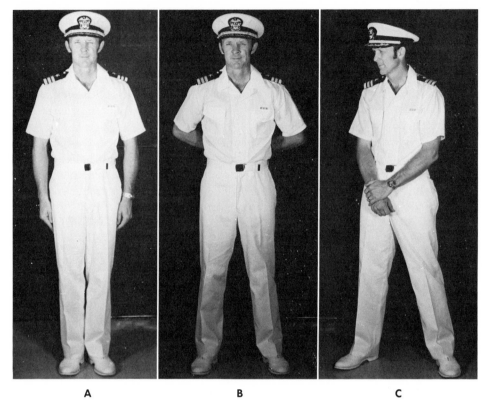

Fig. 13-1. Military postures. **A,** Attention. **B,** Parade rest. **C,** At ease.

much pooling of the blood in the legs that cerebral anemia results. Such pooling is prevented by slight movement of the legs. In the military postures of at ease or parade rest a certain amount of shifting of the legs is permitted, which favors circulation and relieves muscular tension, as Joseph has stated.

Individual differences in stance. Differences in standing posture are often linked with differences in nutrition, climate, and training. Certain races are commonly observed to have a characteristically rigid posture; others tend to be kyphotic or lordotic. These different postures can often be traced to differences in nutrition, climate, or training.

Among the various body types obese persons are likely to have the most erect posture as a result of the effort required to support excessive fatty tissue. Fat persons twist as they walk, and to reduce the amount of this turning they stiffen and take short steps. Persons with large abdomens often lean slightly backward to balance the weight in front. Some short, stocky people stand erect to make themselves appear taller and slimmer. Extremely thin individuals often lack the muscular strength needed to hold themselves erect. Many tall girls voluntarily slouch to appear more nearly the size of their shorter men companions. Attractiveness is spoiled by following this procedure. Specialization in certain forms of hard work or strenuous athletic activity results in adaptations of posture. A coal miner carries the head and shoulders forward and the arms slightly bent in the position of work. The side horse specialist in gymnastics tends to become overly round shouldered and kyphotic if this activity is not balanced with others that exercise contralateral musculature. Postural adaptations to specialized events may also be counteracted by a conscious effort to improve the carriage at all times when the person is not bent to the task.

Structural deformities cause postural compensations. A short leg produces scoliosis. This may be corrected by elevating the heel to lengthen the short leg. Pronated feet result in an anteriorly tilted pelvis and lordosis, which are corrected when the pronation is remedied.

Effect of pregnancy. The later weeks of pregnancy are marked by a large forward displacement of the center of gravity because of the combined weight of the embryo, its surrounding amniotic fluid, and the massive uterus. The resulting postural compensation is a slight backward lean and a backward shift of weight in the lumbar region. More weight is borne by the heels. The backward lean (although the center of gravity stays over the base) becomes more exaggerated as the pregnancy progresses. This adaptation occasionally corrects a customary slouch.

Effect of shoe heel height. Julius Caesar is thought to have been the first to discover the advantage of elevating the heels. He observed that when heels were added to the sandals of his legions the soldiers were able to march farther with less fatigue. When the calcaneus is elevated about ½ inch above the level of the base of the ball of the foot, its shaft is brought to a tangent with the Achilles tendon, and thus the gastrocnemius and soleus muscles are able to exert a greater force in plantar flexion. If shoes without heels or with higher heels are worn after an individual has become accustomed to wearing heels of a certain height, the legs and feet become fatigued more quickly. The effect of the height of the heel on body position in standing is shown in Fig. 13-2. Note that the sagittal length of the supporting base is shorter in *B* and *C* because of outward rotation at the hips as well as raising the heels. The head height is greater in *B* and *C*. Because in *B* and *C* the inclination of the foot is greater than it is in *A,* the leg has been moved back with reference to the foot by ankle extension. If segments above the knee were to move with the leg, the body's center of gravity would move toward the ankle. To prevent this, upper segments have moved forward; note in reference to the background lines that the buttocks and the tip of the nose are farther forward in *B* than in *A* and farther forward in *C* than in *B.* Thus the center of gravity is kept in the customary position between the ankle and the outer end of the metatarsals. These joint adjustments illustrate reflex actions that occur in standing.

Standing at work. Continued standing may result in a pooling of blood and other fluids in the feet and lowering of the arches to such an extent that the foot may increase in size as much as one to two shoe sizes. This may explain why clerks, dentists, ticket takers, and barbers commonly wear shoes at work that

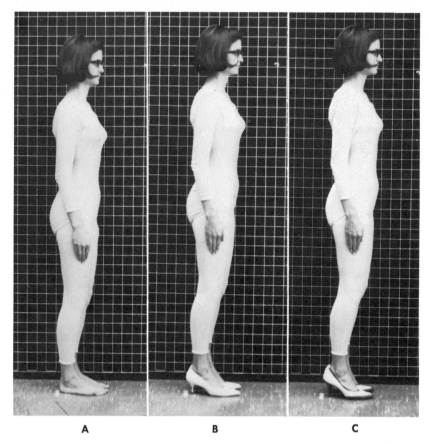

A　　　　　　　　　B　　　　　　　　　C

Fig. 13-2. Effect of shoe heel height on body position in standing.

are lacerated at the toe, ball, and top to allow for the expansion to take place. Probably in such work two pairs of shoes should be worn, one pair in the morning and a larger one in the afternoon. A compromise in the form of loose-fitting shoes is sometimes made. However, this is a poor solution because, when no support is given, pronation occurs. A good shoe for standing is constructed so that most of the weight is borne on the outside of the foot, since this part of the foot is supported by strong ligaments, whereas the inside of the foot is supported by long, thin muscles that are easily fatigued.

Posture of readiness. The standing posture is affected by a person's anticipation of forthcoming action. If no action is anticipated and the conditions of the external environment are unexciting, the response will be a relaxed posture. This is so well known that athletes can simulate a relaxed posture to deceive their opponents. In a game of basketball a forward about to receive a pass can often deceive the guard by assuming a relaxed posture and passive countenance.

The posture of readiness when a rapid or strong movement is about to be

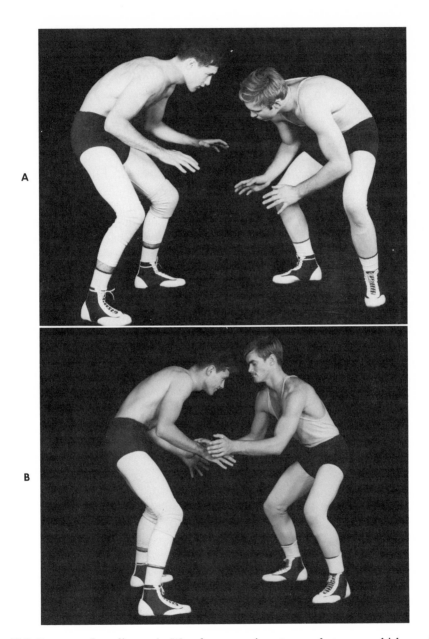

Fig. 13-3. Postures of readiness. **A,** Wrestlers are using staggered stances, which are best for moving rapidly forward or backard. **B,** Wrestlers are using parallel stances, which are best for moving right or left. (From Boring, W. J.: Science and skills of wrestling, St. Louis, 1975, The C. V. Mosby Co.)

performed is an alert one. The peak of attention is reached between 1 and 2 seconds after concentration is directed to the situation. The posture adapts to the condition; after the peak of attention is past, the posture either is relaxed or becomes unstable because of extreme tremor, resulting possibly from accommodation of the coordinating centers in the nervous system.

The position assumed during a state of readiness is in accord with the immediate tasks to be accomplished (Fig. 13-3). If the direction of movement is not known, the weight should be distributed over the surface of both feet. When the direction is known, the center of gravity should be shifted toward the anticipated direction. A slight flexion may occur at the ankle, causing the equilibrium of the body to be unstable and thus facilitating movement. The head, arm, and leg positions are also adjusted to the action to follow. The infielder in baseball leans forward and rises on the toes as the ball is pitched. The base runner taking a one-stride lead off the base will lean toward the next base and rise on the toes as the ball is pitched. In each instance the mechanical equilibrium of the body is disturbed, and movement is commenced. The football quarterback in T formation crouches with the arms forward and the heels of the hands close together in a position of readiness to catch the ball. Such postures of readiness should not be held motionless for an extended length of time, since proprioceptor sensations, which govern the senses of position and relationship of the body parts to objects in view, will be diminished and have to be reestablished before accurate movement can be accomplished. For this reason, the golfer waggles the club near the ball while adjusting position in readiness for the swing. The batter in baseball does the same thing while poised for the pitch to heighten the sensation of the position of the bat in relation to himself and to the path of the ball.

The causes of poor posture and the defects that are associated with pathologic handicaps should be the topic of discussion in books on adapted and corrective physical education. The discussion here has been centered only on the standing position of man.

BALANCING ON HANDS

To keep the base of support wide when the handstand is being executed the fingers are spread as widely as possible. The hands are turned slightly outward, so that the fingers will be able to help counteract movements to the outside, and the thumbs are turned inward to maintain balance. A plumb line dropped through the center of gravity should fall at the base of the fingers to provide a supporting area from the heel of the hand to the tips of the fingers and thumb, through which the gravity plane can move without the performer losing balance. This is especially true in the execution of the *one-armed handstand*. Also important in the performance of this move is to hold the parts of the body (arms, torso, and legs) in a relatively stationary position, so that control is centered at the shoulder area, where the large muscles (deltoideus, triceps, pectoralis major, and latissimus dorsi) are able to exert their force (Fig. 13-4). If the elbow and knee joints are flexed, loss of balance is often the result.

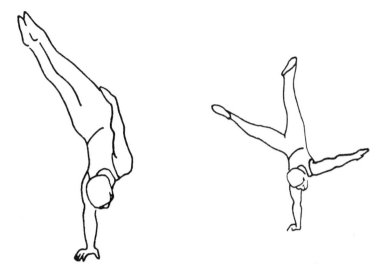

Fig. 13-4. One-armed handstand.

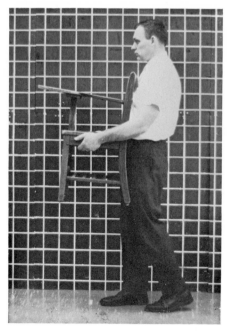

Fig. 13-5. Body position with load resting against abdomen.

CARRYING OBJECTS

Carrying an object increases the weight that must be supported by the feet and affects the positions of the gravity planes with reference to the body. If the carrier is to remain upright, these planes must be kept within the area of the supporting foot; segmental adjustments must be made. This is usually done by altering the trunk position. If the object is held in front of the body, the trunk will be inclined backward (Fig. 13-5); if held in back the trunk will be inclined forward (Fig. 13-6); and if to the side the trunk will be inclined to the opposite side (Fig. 13-7). When loads are carried on the head, there is no inclination. Visitors to regions in which carrying objects on the head, especially among women, is common frequently comment on the excellent carriage of these people. Undoubtedly the additional weight high above the feet requires careful alignment of body segments.

Walking with a heavy load alters the stepping pattern. The center of gravity is not allowed to fall as far forward as it does in normal walking. With the load the step will be shortened, and the center of gravity will be held over the supporting foot for a longer time. It is interesting to note that when bulky packs of produce are loaded onto the backs of Mexican Indians by fellow workers the

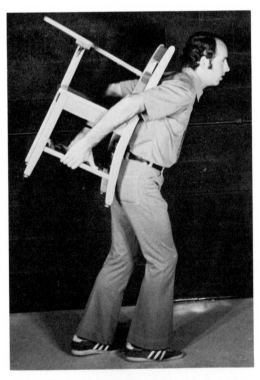

Fig. 13-6. Body position with load on back.

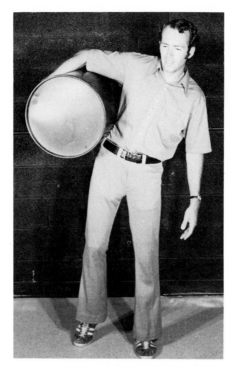

Fig. 13-7. Body position with load resting on side.

carrier cannot sit down during the 10-mile trip from the fields to market because once the load is lowered he cannot lift it without assistance.

SUGGESTED READINGS

Cureton, T. K., Jr., and Wickens, J. S.: The center of gravity in the human body in the antero-posterior plane and its relation to posture, physical fitness, and athletic ability, Res. Q. Am. Assoc. Health Phys. Educ. 6(2) (supp.):93, 1935.

Hellebrandt, F. A., and Franseen, E. B.: Physiological study of the vertical stance of man, Physiol. Rev. 23:220, 1943.

Joseph, J.: Man's posture—electromyographic studies, Springfield, Ill., 1960, Charles C Thomas, Publisher.

Loken, N. C., and Willoughby, R. J.: Complete book of gymnastics, Englewood Cliffs, N.J., 1959, Prentice-Hall, Inc.

See Bibliography for additional references.

CHAPTER 14 Arm-supported skills*

MECHANICS OF ARM-SUPPORTED SKILLS

In many gymnastic skills the body is supported by the hands as it is rotated in a vertical or horizontal plane around the support. In the vertical plane as the body rotates downward, gravitational force aids; as the body rotates upward, gravity resists the movement. Therefore on the downswing the skilled performer will move the body center of gravity as far as possible from the center of rotation; this is done by full hip extension and shoulder girdle depression. On the upswing the center of gravity will be moved toward the center of rotation by hip flexion and shoulder girdle elevation. In skills in which the body is rotated in the horizontal plane, the joint actions will be those that tend to keep the center of gravity directly over the supporting base.

SIMPLE UNDERSWING

The simple underswing (swinging back and forth) is a preliminary movement that is used in preparation for the execution of more advanced moves. The hands provide the point of support and the center of rotation. To develop a simple underswing the hips should flex on the upswing (forward or backward), thereby shortening the radius of rotation (with the result that the center of rotation moves closer to the center of support). The performer, by elevating the shoulder girdle when directly under the point of support, may also help increase the angular velocity. In gymnastic terms this is known as *hollowing* the chest. At the end of the swing as the body starts downward, the angular velocity can be increased by hip extension and shoulder girdle elevation.

GIANT SWING

This exercise may be done both backward and forward. On the upward swing the radius of rotation is shortened by flexion of hips and also by shoulder girdle elevation. Actually the hollowing of the chest has the effect of causing a slight flexion as well as depression of the shoulders to take place. (If the arms were flexed, the radius of movement would be shortened much more; however, in topflight gymnastic competition the flexing of the arms is considered poor form.) This brings the center of gravity closer to the center of support (shorten-

*This chapter was revised in consultation with James Brown, gymnastics coach, Indiana University.

206

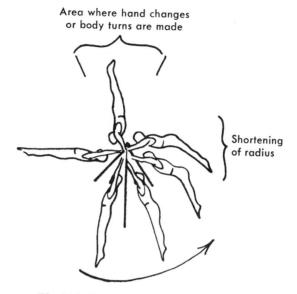

Fig. 14-1. Reverse grip giant swing on high bar.

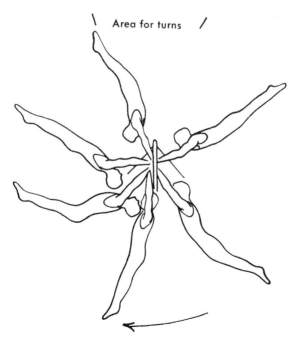

Fig. 14-2. Back giant swing on high bar.

ing the radius) and in turn accelerates the upward angular velocity. As the center of gravity moves over the center of support (the hands), the grip has been moved upward, and the performer momentarily pushes the body up to a handstand balanced position. On the downswing the body is fully extended. The extension is made just before the body reaches the high vertical position to gain the full effect of gravity and to develop the greatest possible velocity in preparation for the next upward swing. (See Figs. 14-1 and 14-2.)

Following are kinetic findings reported by Vallière* on performers executing the backward giant swing:

1. A decline in force was exerted during the descent phase.

2. A sudden increase of force coincided with the greatest shoulder joint velocity.

3. A drop in force coincided with the whiplike action of the legs occurring at the bottom of the swing.

*Vallière, A.: Kinetic and kinematic analysis of the backward giant swing on the still rings in gymnastics, doctoral dissertation, Indiana University, Aug., 1973.

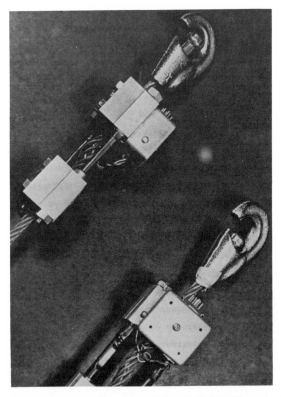

Fig. 14-3. Special strain gauge transducers used by André Vallière in his study of backward giant swing. (See also Figs. 14-4 and 14-5.)

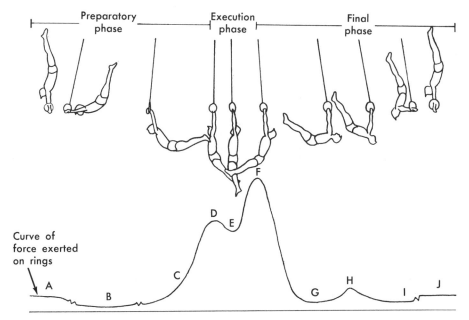

Fig. 14-4. Kinetic and kinematic diagram of backward giant swing executed on still rings. Selected points on strain gauge recording were synchronized with corresponding body positions taken from film sequence. (From Vallière, A.: Kinetic and kinematic analysis of the backward giant swing on the still rings in gymnastics, unpublished doctoral dissertation, Indiana University, Aug., 1973.)

4. A sharp increase in force moving to a maximum coincided with the upward lift of the body in the ascent phase. (See Fig. 14-3 for a view of his special apparatus; also see Figs. 14-4 and 14-5.)

STUNTS ON PARALLEL BARS

In the swing from the supine position (Fig. 14-6) on the parallel bars, much of the skill depends on adjustments made to keep the body's center of gravity over (or near) the supporting hands. Note that in the supine position the arms are tilted to the left and the hips are flexed; both adjustments move body mass toward the vertical plane of the hands. In the prone position the elbows are flexed; this is a reversed muscle action moving the upper arm and with it the upper portion of the trunk to the right to balance the lower limbs. In the final position, extension of the spine and backward rotation of the pelvis have moved the lower limbs close to the support to balance the head and shoulder girdle. As the arms moved to the right on the downswing, the effect of gravitational force was increased by increasing the distance between the hands and the center of gravity; on the first part of the upward swing as the elbows flexed, that distance was shortened to make better use of the momentum developed on the downswing.

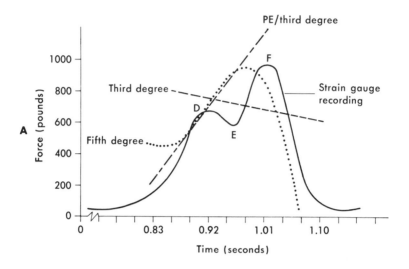

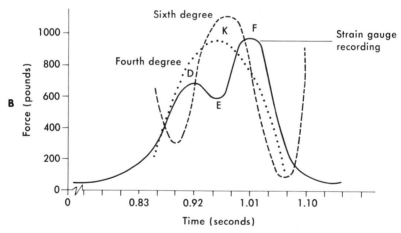

Fig. 14-5. A, Comparison of vertical forces obtained from the film when using third and fifth degree of polynomial equation with vertical forces obtained with the use of strain gauge transducers for tenth subject. **B,** Comparison of vertical forces obtained from the film when using fourth and sixth degree of polynominal equation with vertical forces obtained with the use of strain gauge transducers for tenth subject. (From Vallière, A.: Kinetic and kinematic analysis of the backward giant swing on the still rings in gymnastics, unpublished doctoral dissertation, Indiana University, Aug., 1973.)

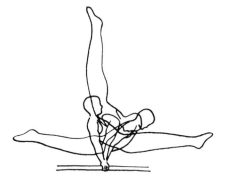

Fig. 14-6. Swing in support position on parallel bars. A deduction would be made for bent arms shown in prone position; thus this competitor would lose points.

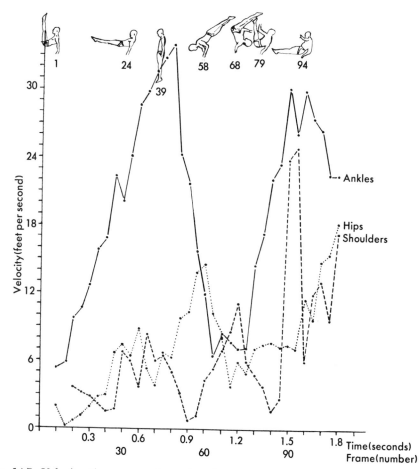

Fig. 14-7. Velocity time curves for selected points on the body in the somersault on parallel bars (front dismount).

Movements made during the somersault on parallel bars are shown in the traced positions of a skilled gymnast (top of Fig. 14-7). The plotted lines show the velocity in feet per second of three body points—ankle, hip, and shoulder. As one would expect, the fastest is the ankle, which is the greatest distance from the center of rotation, the hands.

FLYAWAY

The flyaway is a type of dismount that usually follows a giant swing. The performer first does a giant swing and then prepares for the flyaway by speeding it up. The radius of rotation is shortened as the body passes over the bar. This is done by flexing the hips and depressing the shoulder girdle. (The arms could be flexed, but this is considered poor form.) The back is then arched (by extension) just before coming directly under the bar on the downswing. This

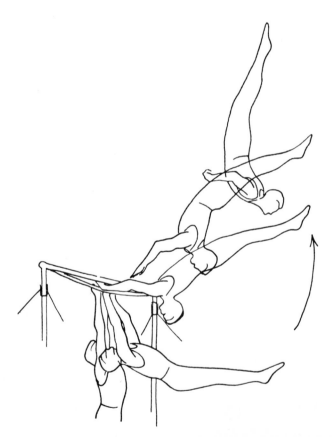

Fig. 14-8. Flyaway (layout) from back giant swing on high bar. The head appears to extend too early. Although some gymnasts still do extend the head in this manner, it would generally be considered too early to obtain maximum lift. In the last drawing, arms should be extended to lift the center of mass of the body upward.

arching helps shorten the radius as the body rises in the upswing and aids in accelerating the angular velocity. As the body rises above the horizontal, the arch is continued with the head held well backward (upper back and head extension) and the hips and arms (slightly) flexed (Fig. 14-8). The reaction from the bent bar gives added upward velocity to the performer. Centrifugal force pulls the body away from the bar.

KIP SWING

In executing the kip swing (Fig. 14-9) the performer flexes the hips and depresses the shoulder girdle. Note how close the body is to the bar before mounting it.

ACTION ON STILL (STATIONARY) RINGS

The performer on the still rings demonstrates the principles of good balance by shortening the lever arm (radius) and also shows the value of continuous movement throughout the exercise.

Back uprise to a handstand on rings. In this exercise (Fig. 14-10) the performer swings the body to and fro by alternate trunk flexion and extension to gain momentum, and on the downswing the radius (the distance from the hands to the toes) is lengthened. The center of gravity is kept under the point of suspension of the cables. On the upswing the radius is shortened by arching the back and in-locating (internal rotation of the humeral head in the glenoid fossa) the shoulders. (This helps overcome the force of gravity and gives the performer accelerated upward angular velocity.) The body is moved forward, placing the center of rotation nearer to the point of support (hands), which is kept behind an extended line from the shoulders. The center of gravity is still kept under the point of suspension of the cables and rings. As the point of support moves under the point of suspension of the rings, the center of gravity moves upward and inward at the same rate. The performer pulls the body up by forceful scapular abduction and shoulder extension and then pushes upward

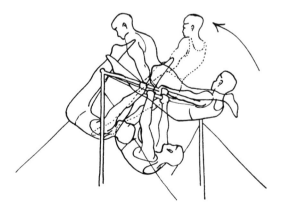

Fig. 14-9. Kip onto high bar.

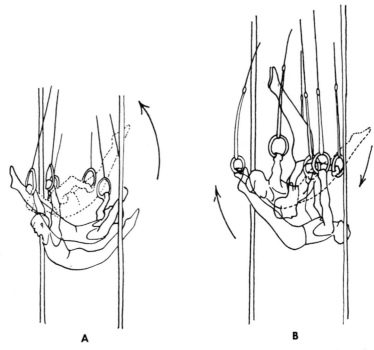

Fig. 14-10. A, Back uprise to a handstand on rings. **B,** Shoot to a handstand on rings.

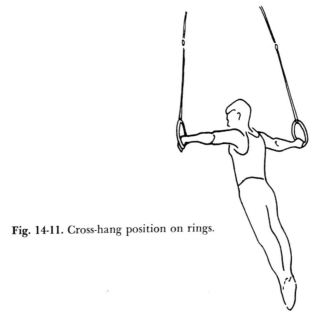

Fig. 14-11. Cross-hang position on rings.

to a handstand in continuous motion as the rotary swing diminishes. This is accomplished by flexing the hips and abducting the scapulae. (See Fig. 14-10, *B*, and 14-4.)

Since the rings should be as stationary as possible while the exercises are being performed, the performer should attempt to stop or prevent movement of the cables. Usually swing occurs when the performer fails to keep the center of gravity under the point of support and along the rope suspension line. When, the swinging begins, it is difficult to stop, and thereafter all movements on the rings are difficult to execute. Developing a certain amount of swing is inevitable during the course of a competitive routine, and the accomplished gymnast learns to "kill," or stop, the swing in some movements and use it to advantage in others. Usually one of two things happens: the swing continues to increase (most commonly) or may be controlled or partially dissipated. Movement of the center of gravity of the body against the direction of the swing may help control or stop it.

Cross-hang position on the rings. The cross-hang position is an exercise of simple joint action requiring tremendous strength because the supports (the hands) are not directly above the body's center of gravity but rather at arm's distance from it horizontally. To maintain the arm position the shoulder adductors must contract forcefully. The elbow and wrist joints must be stabilized; however, the muscular effort for maintaining the positions of these joints is not great if the shoulder position is held. From this position upper trunk rotation takes place to either the right or the left (Fig. 14-11).

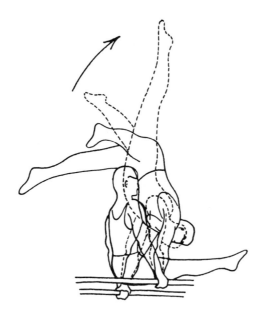

Fig. 14-12. Straight arm and leg press to a handstand on parallel bars.

STRAIGHT ARM AND STRAIGHT LEG PRESS TO A HANDSTAND

This move is executed on the parallel bars in free calisthenics and on the rings. Proper execution again involves keeping the center of gravity over the base of support. The hips and shoulders are flexed during part of the move, keeping the body mass closer to the base of support and enabling the joint action to be in a good position for the stronger muscles to act. This exercise may also be done with the legs placed in a straddle (hip abduction) position. This position causes the center of gravity to be lower, and the move is easier to accomplish (Fig. 14-12). Scapular abduction and elevation enable the performer to maintain this position.

After a cinematographic study of his own actions in the felge handstand Lascari found that with the adoption of an early drop in the execution after 6 months of practice he was able to attain an immediate straight arm position in the regrasp, which he had rarely achieved in years of previous work. The felge is considered a difficult exercise, and the straight arm position is achieved by only a few of the most skilled gymnasts.

SIDE HORSE ACTIVITIES

The moves on the side horse are normally those of pendulum-like swinging, rotary movements, and variations of these two.

A type of *pendulum-like swinging* is observed in the execution of simple leg cuts and scissor actions (Fig. 14-13). The points of suspension of the pendulum are the shoulder joints. The radius is shortened as the performer moves the center of gravity nearer to the base of support on the upswing and is lengthened on the downswing to increase angular velocity. This is accomplished by flexing the hip, accompanied by flexion and lateral rotation of the trunk. On the up-

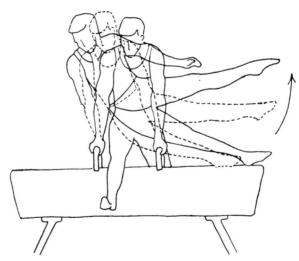

Fig. 14-13. Pendulum swing in scissors action on side horse.

swing the top thigh is abducted. The resistance arm of the level (distance from the point of support to the center of gravity of the combined mass of the trunk and lower limbs) is also shortened on the upswing and lengthened on the downswing. As the upswing diminishes until the velocity is zero (with the upward velocity and the pull of gravity nullifying one another), the performer flexes the hip and flexes and laterally rotates the trunk and executes leg crosses and scissorlike actions.

When high double leg circles are executed, the center of gravity must be kept over the center of rotation and base of support during most of the move. The body rotates about the center of support by means of lateral trunk flexion with the shoulders held more or less at the same elevation (Fig. 14-14). The shortening of the radius and raising of the center of gravity during the movement allow the return swing to be made more easily. Takemoto and Hamaido liken this action to the spinning of a top. No pause (or slowing down) may occur while the action takes place, or the performer will fall off the apparatus.

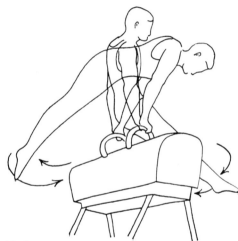

Fig. 14-14. High double leg circle on side horse.

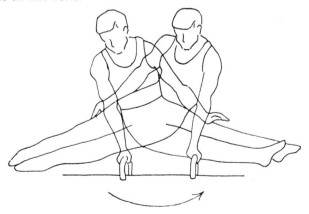

SUGGESTED READINGS

Gowitzke, B. A.: Kinesiological principles applied to gymnastics, Kinesiology Review, p. 22, 1968.

Lascari, A. T.: The felge handstand—a comparative kinetic analysis of a gymnastic skill, dissertation, University of Wisconsin, 1970.

Monpetit, R., and Boulonne, G.: Biomechanical analysis of the backward swing on the parallel bars (French), Movement 4:135, 1969.

Vallière, A.: Kinetic and kinematic analysis of the backward giant swing on the still rings in gymnastics, doctoral dissertation, Indiana University, Aug., 1973.

See Bibliography for additional references.

CHAPTER 15 Locomotion on land and in water

GENERAL ASPECTS

Types of locomotion. Locomotion includes all activities in which the entire body is moved by the action of its own levers often with the aid of gravitational force. The most common forms of body displacement are running and walking, in which the center of gravity is transferred from one foot (base) to the other. This successive alternation of supporting bases occurs also in walking on the hands and, when the weight is suspended from a hand support, in traveling on the horizontal ladder, the boom, and the traveling rings. In some forms of locomotion the hands and feet may alternate as the supporting base, as they do in cartwheels and handsprings. Crutches are extensions of the arms; in walking, their distal ends are the equivalent of hands, and this is similar to walking on the hands and feet. Pole vaulting is crutch jumping.

Dives that end in the inverted position are a transfer of weight to a new base. If a dive ends in the upright position, the takeoff and landing bases are the same. This manipulation of the takeoff base to receive the projected center of gravity is seen in hopping, in standing jumps for distance and height, and in many trampoline skills.

The essential feature in all locomotion is the movement of the entire body from the point of contact between a body segment and the supporting surface. To achieve this movement some part of the body must apply force to a surface, and the surface must resist, not give way to, the force. The resisting surface pushes back, and this reaction moves the body in accordance with Newton's third law of motion, which states that, whenever one body exerts a force on another, the second always exerts on the first a force that is equal in magnitude but oppositely directed.

Swimming differs from the previously mentioned forms of locomotion in that the body rests in a layout position on the supporting surface. Yet here too the entire body is moved, and the portion of water that supports the body changes. This type of contact is seen also when the body, while lying on a surface, moves itself by rolling.

MECHANICS OF STEPPING PATTERN

Walks, runs, and jumps are modifications of stepping, which is a human reflex pattern. This pattern can be, and often is, elicited in an infant held upright with the feet in contact with a surface. It can be seen months before the infant is able to stand, and adults, not knowing that stepping is a reflex act, often assume that the child is advanced in motor skills. When the child is able to stand, though hand contact with some support may be necessary to maintain the upright position, intent will inhibit the reflex or permit it to function. If he wishes to remain in one place, foot contact does not fire the stepping; if he wishes to move toward an object beyond his reach, the built-in joint actions occur. He is not aware of the joint actions; he knows only that he has moved. Intent, a cortical activity, set off the pattern that resulted in lifting one foot and then transferring the weight to it. After the child has learned to stand and walk, the joint actions of the early stepping are modified with continued use. The early wide stride is narrowed; hip flexion of the swinging limb is decreased, and therefore the foot is not lifted as high; and the step is lengthened.

Once walking is well established, progression to running is easily made, since the nervous system no longer needs the assurance that the forward foot has made contact before the rear foot is lifted. Then the rear foot can give its final push before front foot contact, and since both feet are in the air at the same time a running pattern has been achieved. With practice, additional modifications can be made, and a number of other patterns can be developed, such as the hop, skip, jump, and leap. All are achieved without conscious direction of joint action; the child has a general idea of the desired pattern, and somehow the nervous system provides the necessary joint actions. The general idea of the new pattern may have come from observation of other performers, or perhaps the child may have produced the pattern and made efforts to repeat it.

Although desirable changes in the stepping pattern are unconsciously made by the young child, it is possible after a certain age to make them voluntarily. If they are consciously made, the teacher, at least, should have an understanding of the mechanics. For the instructor it is not enough to know that extension of hip, knee, and ankle are necessary when the body (i.e., its center of gravity) is to be moved; there should be understanding of the contributions that each moving segment makes to the desired action—the contributions that each makes to the force that will move the body.

For such understanding, three features should be kept in mind. First, whenever the toes are not free to move (as is the case when they are in contact with the supporting surface and supporting the body weight), each segment proximal to the toes is moved by reversed muscle action. Metatarsophalangeal joint action moves the foot, not the toes; ankle joint action moves the leg, not the foot; knee joint action moves the thigh, not the leg; hip joint action moves the trunk, not the thigh.

Second, gravitational force is a major contributor to segmental movements in locomotor patterns. When the body's center of gravity is not directly above the ankle joint, gravity tends to initiate movement in that joint. If the center of gravity is in front of the ankle joint, gravitational force tends to flex the ankle. If muscles at the ankle contract and prevent such movement, gravity can raise the foot; if the action is moving the center of gravity forward, the heels will be raised; if the action moves the center of gravity backward, the fore part of the foot and the toes will be raised.

Third, locomotor patterns are pushing patterns—pushing against the supporting surface. As described in Chapter 11 in the discussion on the mechanics of the pushing pattern, some segments will move in a direction other than that of the desired line of force. Counteraction to the undesired movements must occur. Also as a segment moves, it carries with it all segments proximal to it. As the leg moves (when the foot is fixed), it also moves the thigh and trunk; as the foot moves, it moves the leg, the thigh, and the trunk. Therefore the movement and position of a segment are determined not only by action at the joint at its distal end but also by the movements of the segments distal to it. To describe and explain the movements of a segment the movement of the segment immediately distal must be described (measured), and the angle at its distal end must be described (measured).

Measurement of joint angle is familiar to students of movement; measurement of segmental position has not been widely used. This position is described as the angle that the line of the segment makes with a horizontal line and is known as the *angle of inclination*. The angle can be measured from the front or the back. If the segment is perpendicular, its angle of inclination is 90 degrees, whether measured from the front or the back; if the segment is inclined forward 45 degrees, the angle of inclination is 45 degrees measured from the front and 135 degrees measured from the back. Obviously the sum of the front and back measures will always equal 180 degrees. In describing angles of inclination one must know whether measures were made from the front or the back.

With these characteristics of the locomotor pushing pattern as background understanding, contributions of moving segments in a modified stepping pattern will be described. The descriptions will be based on the line tracings in Fig. 15-1, which were made from a film showing the joint actions in a standing broad jump. The segmental contributions shown will be similar to those in any form of locomotion in which the foot contacts the supporting surface and in which force is derived from ankle, knee, and hip action and from the pull of gravity. In the illustration broken lines represent segmental positions while the toes are in contact with the supporting surface and the foot has been raised *(A)*. Unbroken lines represent the segmental positions at the time of the last toe contact just before takeoff *(E)*. In the time between *A* and *E* all segments and joints have made their contributions to the propelling force.

The other tracings *(B* through *D)* do not represent actual positions during takeoff for the jump; they are presented to show counteractions and to illustrate the interaction of inclination angles. In *B* the foot inclination is that which it has at takeoff *(E)*; this change results from metatarsophalangeal action, which is caused by gravitational pull. In *A* it can be seen that the center of gravity is in front of the metatarsophalangeal joints. If no action occurs at ankle, knee, or hip, gravity will rotate the foot, leg, thigh, and trunk as one unit around the metatarsophalangeal joints, bringing the four segments to the positions shown in *B*. The foot has reached the position desired at takeoff; the other segments are

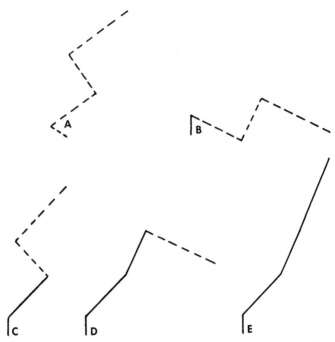

Fig. 15-1. Effect of joint actions on higher body segments in locomotion, as illustrated by joint actions in standing broad jump. All broken lines represent the angle that a segment makes with the segment below at the position shown in **A,** a phase in the crouch. All unbroken lines represent these angles as they are in **E,** the takeoff position. Note that ankle extension moves the leg, thigh, and trunk backward. Main forward and upward force is due to extension at knees and metatarsophalangeal joints.

in undesired positions, and some joint action must prevent them from reaching this position.

The logical action would be leg movement because it would raise not only the leg but also the thigh and trunk. This is shown in *C,* where the leg has been moved backward by ankle extension. If foot action is completed before leg action begins, the segments would reach the inclinations shown in *B.* The most casual observer of the takeoff knows that these positions do not occur. However, if the number of degrees of movement of the leg equals at all times the number of degrees of movement of the foot, the inclination of the leg will remain constant—always be the same as it is in *A, C, D,* and *E.* As a result of simultaneous action of two segments, the inclination of the leg can be held constant. Because the leg inclination is the same in *C* as in *A* and because no knee or hip action has occurred, the inclination of the thigh and trunk are the same in *A* and *C.* However, the position of these segments with reference to the toes is not the same in *A* and *C.* They and the foot and leg have been moved forward and upward by action at the metatarsophalangeal joints, an action caused by gravitational pull.

Tracing *D* shows the effect of knee extension if there is no hip action. As the knee extends (*C* to *D*), it moves the thigh first forward and upward until its inclination is 90 degrees; beyond that its movement is forward and downward. Up to the 90-degree position the thigh moves against gravity; beyond that, gravity adds to its speed. Thigh movement can be seen to be the greatest contributor in moving the body's center of gravity in the desired direction, since it moves the heaviest segments—the thigh and trunk and with the latter the arms and head. From the trunk position in *D* that segment will be moved backward by hip extension; this will occur simultaneously with knee extension, thus keeping the trunk inclination close to that which it has in *A*. Hip extension serves much the same purpose as ankle extension; it maintains direction, moving opposite to the direction of the segment below.

In summary, the main propelling force in the stepping pattern is derived from knee extension; to this is added the force of gravity, which rotates the entire body around the metatarsophalangeal joints. Ankle and hip extension keep the center of gravity in an advantageous position to move it in the desired direction.

The segmental lines in the illustration and the discussion of their changes in position have shown that inclination of a segment is determined not only by the joint action moving the segment but also by the inclination of the adjoining distal segment. For example, in *C* the inclination of the trunk is 45 degrees measured from the front, and in *E* it is 65 degrees. The joint action that moves the trunk is hip extension. In *C* the hip angle is 90 degrees; in *E*, 180 degrees. Hip extension of 90 degrees has occurred, which would move the trunk backward. The thigh in *C* has an inclination of 135 degrees measured from the front; in *E* it has an inclination of 65 degrees, which moves the thigh and the trunk 70 degrees closer to the front horizontal. The combined action of hip extension and thigh inclination has moved the trunk 90 degrees backward and 70 degrees forward, a change of 20 degrees backward. This accounts for the change in trunk position from 45 to 65 degrees.

Although ankle, knee, and hip do extend in skills in which the entire body is moved, the functions of the joints differ. Understanding of the function of each should aid in determining what changes should be made in a pattern to increase its efficiency.

PROGRESSION BY FOOT ALTERNATION
Walking

Walking is a form of locomotion in which the center of gravity of the body is carried alternately over the right and left foot. At all times one foot is in contact with the supporting surface, and for a brief phase both feet contact the surface. In addition to muscular force, other forces aid in the progression. These are gravity and the momentum of the body once forward movement is under way.

If walking starts from a stationary position, the first joint action to occur is ankle flexion. This is a result of decreasing the amount of tension exerted by the ankle extensors in the standing position when the center of gravity is in front of the ankle joint. When walking is initiated, the ankle extensors permit the

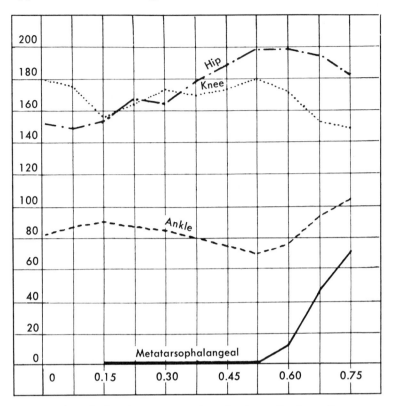

Fig. 15-2. Joint actions during foot contact phase in the walk of a college woman. Time in seconds is shown at the bottom; angles between body segments are shown in degrees at the left. Downward slope of lines indicates flexion, and upward slope indicates extension.

center of gravity to move beyond the forward limit that is habitual in standing. The nervous system permits this because one foot will be moved forward to receive the body weight. As the forward-moving foot is placed on the walking surface, the momentum of the moving body and the push from the rear foot carry the center of gravity over the new support. As each new foot contact is made, joint adjustments in that limb use and facilitate the already developed momentum.

Joint actions of lower limbs. Joint actions of the lower limbs include those of the supporting and of the swinging limb.

Joint actions of supporting limb. Movement at the hip, knee, ankle, and metatarsophalangeal joints from the time that the heel makes contact with the walking surface until the toes leave that surface is shown in Fig. 15-2. A graph such as this one presents detailed and exact information that if described verbally would require many times the space taken by the graph. Here you can see the direction of each joint action, its degree in a given time, and the relationship between actions. Students should develop ability to interpret such graphs and to visualize the joint actions and the body positions shown at each time interval. In the illustration they should see that the heel makes contact at 0 second in time; then for the first 0.15 second, the ankle joint is extending, thus bringing the entire foot in contact with the walking surface. From this point all joint actions will be reversed muscle actions: ankle flexion inclines the leg farther forward; knee action moves the thigh; and hip action moves the trunk.

Because after 0.15 second the center of gravity is in front of the ankle joint, gravitational force will flex it; this action is controlled by the ankle extensors, which lengthen. Hip and knee extension will be the result of contraction of the extensors at these joints. At 0.525 second the leg has reached the desired degree of inclination (not consciously determined), and the ankle extensors contract with force enough to resist gravity, which now acts on the metatarsophalangeal joints and raises the foot from the surface. At point 0.60 second the other (advancing) foot is making contact; then the center of gravity is moved over that foot by the forward momentum developed in the time from 0.15 to 0.60 second and by the final push with the toes and extension at the ankle of the rear foot. Note that the hip and knee are flexing in this final phase. Further explanation of the function of joint actions will be presented in the section on inclinations of the segments.

Joint actions of swinging limb. After contact the rear foot must be swung forward to establish the new contact. The swing, occupying 0.45 second, is accomplished by hip flexion. From full extension it flexes 34 degrees, bringing the thigh ahead of the trunk. Just before contact the hip extends slightly (3 degrees), lowering the limb for contact.

The knee, which was flexed 50 degrees as the foot left the ground, continues to flex for a brief period—0.075 second. This action lifts the foot from the ground and also shortens the resistance arm for the hip action, thus reducing the energy needed for moving the limb forward.

The ankle joint, which was extended 115 degrees as it left the ground, flexes immediately, lifting the forepart of the foot to clear the ground. Flexion continues until the last 0.075 second before contact. Then extension begins and continues until full foot contact is made.

Inclinations of segments of supporting limb. In all locomotor and balance activities, movement of any joint in the supporting limb changes the inclination of the segments above that joint. In standing, ankle flexion inclines the legs, thighs, and trunk toward the horizontal; extension moves these segments away from the horizontal. In most forms of locomotion simultaneous action is likely to occur in the joints of the supporting limb. These may counteract the effects of distal joints or increase them. (See the discussion on the mechanics of the stepping pattern in this chapter.)

The angle made by each segment with the horizontal in walking is shown in Fig. 15-3. The angles are those between a horizontal line drawn through the joint at the distal end of the segment and a line drawn through the segment. All angles are measured from the front except that for the foot, which is measured from the back. Foot measures shown begin at the time the foot is in full

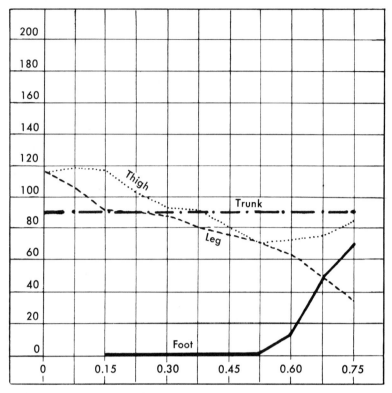

Fig. 15-3. Angles of inclination of body segments during foot contact phase in the walk; joint angles are given in Fig. 15-2. All angles are measured from front horizontal except those of the foot. Note constant inclination of the trunk, resulting from the adjustment of hip joints to thigh inclination.

contact, and its inclination is therefore 0 degree until the heel is raised. At 0.525 second the heel leaves the contacting surface, and the angle of inclination changes from 0 degree to 72 degrees as the final push is made.

Leg inclination during full foot contact is changed by ankle action only. As ankle flexion occurs, it is paralleled by the change in leg inclination. However, when foot inclination begins to change at 0.525 second, foot inclination and ankle action affect leg inclination. Fig. 15-2 shows that as foot inclination begins, the ankle starts to extend at the same rate as the foot inclines; the inclination of the leg remains constant. If ankle extension occurs at the same rate as foot inclination, the inclination of the leg remains constant. If foot inclination is greater than ankle extension, leg inclination will increase. These changes are shown in Fig. 15-3. From 0.525 to 0.75 second the ankle extends 36 degrees, and the foot inclines 72 degrees. During this time the leg is inclined forward 36 degrees.

Inclination of the thigh is determined by the inclination of the leg and by knee action. Knee extension moves the thigh toward the front horizontal; forward inclination of the leg moves the thigh in the same direction. From 0.15 to

0.525 second the knee extends 26 degrees, as shown in Fig. 15-2, as the leg inclines forward 20 degrees. The thigh during this time is moved 46 degrees toward the front horizontal. In the last phase of foot contact the knee flexes 50 degrees, moving the thigh away from the horizontal as the leg inclines 36 degrees. Thigh inclination during this period decreased fourteen degrees.

Inclination of the trunk will be determined by thigh inclination and hip action. As the thigh inclines forward, the hip extends at the same rate, keeping the trunk at a constant angle. This is efficient mechanics, eliminating the effort that would be required if the trunk inclination changed.

Additional joint actions. The joint actions just described provide the major forces in propelling the center of gravity in walking. At the same time other joints contribute to the total movement. Among these contributions are rotation of the pelvis on the supporting femur because of medial rotation in the hip joint. These actions lengthen the stride. At the same time the swinging limb is rotated laterally at the hip to keep the foot along the desired line of direction. The torso is also rotated by spinal action to keep the shoulders facing the desired line of progression. As the speed of walking increases, the rotation of the spine is aided by shoulder action with the right arm moving forward as the left foot advances.

Variations in stride. The joint actions and segmental inclinations shown in Figs. 15-2 and 15-3 are those of a college woman walking at what she considered her average speed. As the speed of walking changes, the relative duration of the support and swing phases changes also. In slow walking the stance phase may be almost twice as long as the swing phase; in fast walking, the stance and swing phases are likely to be equal. In slow walking gravitational force contributes less; the inclination of the leg decreases, and the length of the step is shortened. Whatever the speed the same joints are acting, and each will be making the same type of contribution. However, variations occur in timing, range, and speed of joint actions.

The number of steps per time unit varies with the speed of the walk and the length of the lower limbs. Morton and Fuller report that a man 5 feet 8 inches in height took 100, 112, 122, and 130 steps per minute when walking 2.5, 3, 3.5, and 4 miles per hour. A man 6 feet ½ inch in height walking at the same speeds took 92, 100, 108, and 115 steps per minute.

In studying the energy cost for nineteen college women walking on a treadmill electrically driven at 2, 2.5, and 3 miles per hour, Baird found the optimum rate (ratio of the amount of work to the oxygen consumption) to be between 2.5 and 3 miles per hour. A strobe picture enables the investigator to integrate time with body and joint positions. (See Fig. 15-4.)

Skiing

The basic element in skiing skill is the ability to control the position of the center of gravity of the body. The skis become the base of support and increase the range through which the center of gravity can be moved in the sagittal plane

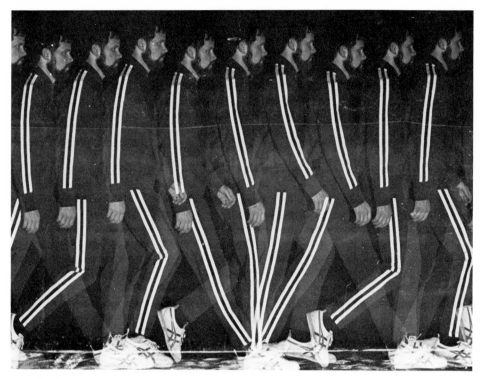

Fig. 15-4. Strobe photograph of walking, taken at 300 flashes per minute. Note the change in position of the foot from that of flat to that with the toe just touching the floor.

without losing balance. Van der Stok observed this range in an expert woman skier.

The transverse and frontal planes of the center of gravity were first located by the scale method; the intersection of these planes was marked by a point on the body to represent the center of gravity. Standing on the gravity board the skier leaned forward in ski boots as far as possible without falling; then she leaned backward as far as possible. This was repeated with attached skis. Films were taken during the leans, and on tracings showing the body during the greatest leans lines were drawn from the determined center of gravity to the ankle. The angle made by each line with the vertical was used as a measure of the degree of lean. In ski boots the forward lean was 11 degrees, and the backward lean was 1 degree. With attached skis the leans measured 30 and 10 degrees. The enlarged base made possible a forward lean almost three times as great and a backward lean ten times as great as that without the skis. With the skis the center of gravity was moved beyond the length of the boots; without the skis it remained within boot length.

In progressing on level ground the body does not lean, as it does in normal walking. In normal walking the center of gravity is allowed to fall ahead of the supporting foot. If this were done on skis because of the lack of friction between the ski and the snow, the supporting ski would slide backward. In progressing on skis the weight is transferred to the foot coming from the rear when it reaches the level of the supporting foot. As the forward moving foot slides ahead, the center of gravity is kept in a vertical line over the ski, and the rear foot can push the weight ahead. The poles aid in preventing a slide backward.

In skiing on a downslope the major propelling force is gravitational pull. In this situation if the center of gravity were vertically above the skis, the feet would be pushed ahead of the center of gravity. To prevent this the center of gravity is brought in front of the feet, slightly in front of a line perpendicular to the slope of the hill. Since gravity is the propelling force, the speed of movement can be altered by lowering the center of gravity (decreasing the speed) and by raising the center of gravity (increasing the speed). This is done by flexing the ankles and knees.

Movement of the center of gravity in the frontal plane is the means of controlling direction. If the weight is greater on the right, the skier will be turned to the left.

Running

Running is a modification of walking and differs from the latter in two aspects with reference to foot contact. First, during one phase in running neither foot is in contact with the ground; second, at no period are both feet in contact. Although these differences necessitate differences in joint action, the same joints and segments are used in running and walking; differences in degrees and timing can be expected. Also once speed in running has developed, the force of body momentum is greater and contributes more to forward movement of the body. The action of the swinging leg in running is greater in range and speed and is likely to contribute most to the movement of the body.

Again action and interrelationship of joints can be best shown on graphs.

Joint actions of lower limbs. The joint actions of concern here are those of the supporting and of the swinging limb.

Joint actions of supporting limb. In Fig. 15-5 are shown the angles of the lower limb measured on a film of Herb Elliot as he neared the finish line in the 1500-meter race in the 1960 Olympic Games. The time per frame for this film was not available, but the speed of the camera can be assumed to have been approximately 64 frames per second. The support phase was therefore approximately 0.075 second. Elliot landed with full foot contact, and the ankle flexed immediately and continued to do so for 0.03 second. This action would be due to the forward momentum of the body, causing rotation at the ankle joint. At 0.03 second ankle extension begins, preventing further rotation at the ankle joint; the forward momentum cannot now rotate the body around the ankle joint, and its force must act at the metatarsal joints. This action continues to the takeoff. Angle extension, as the foot (except for the toes) is lifted, moves the leg backward and upward from the positions to which it would be carried by the metatarsophalangeal action. The knee flexes at contact, easing the force

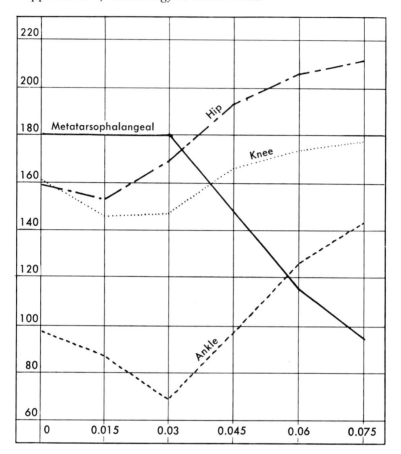

Fig. 15-5. Joint actions of supporting limb during foot contact in the run. (Taken from a film of an Olympic contestant.)

of impact as the foot touches the ground. During the final 0.045 second the knee extends, carrying forward the entire body except for the supporting leg and foot. This action is due to contraction of the knee extensors and the forward momentum of the body. The hip joint also flexes at impact and then begins extension to maintain the angle of inclination of the trunk.

It is interesting to compare the joint actions of the skilled runner with those of a college woman who had had no special training in running. In Fig. 15-6 are shown the joint actions of the woman as she ran at top speed. The pattern of action is the same for the two runners; that is, the direction of joint movement is the same. The differences are in speed of action and in range and are shown in Table 15-1.

Comparison of information in Figs. 15-5 and 15-6 shows that except for the metatarsophalangeal joints the range of movement for the man is greater especially in the knee and hip joints. Also the speed of the man's actions is greater

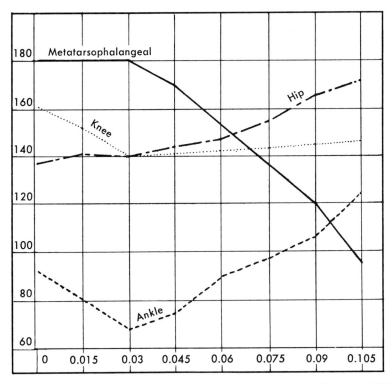

Fig. 15-6. Joint actions of supporting limb during foot contact in the run. (Taken from a film of college woman with no special training in running.)

Table 15-1. Comparison of joint actions of trained man and untrained woman in running

Joint action	Elliot			Woman		
	Range	Time	Velocity (degrees/ sec.)	Range	Time	Velocity (degrees/ sec.)
Metatarsophalangeal extension	86	0.045	1911	85	0.075	1133
Ankle extension	73	0.045	1622	56	0.075	746
Knee extension	32	0.045	711	6	0.075	80
Hip extension	59	0.06	983	32	0.075	426

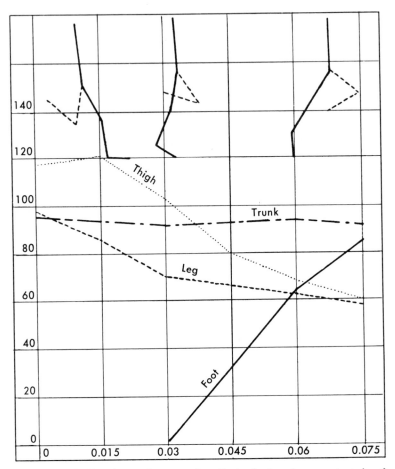

Fig. 15-7. Segmental inclinations of supporting limb during foot contact in the run. (Taken from a film of an Olympic contestant.)

in all joints; in the knee it is more than 8.8 times as great. Further comparisons can be made of the angles of inclination.

Joint actions of swinging limb. The joint actions of the swinging limb can be visualized from the line representations of positions shown in Figs. 15-7 and 15-8. Those of primary interest are the hip and the knee. In the takeoff the rear limb is about to leave the ground, and the swing will begin with the extended hip and knee. During the period of no contact, this limb will reach the position of the rear limb shown at contact. During this time, which for Elliot equals the support phase, the hip joint has not yet brought the thigh in line with the trunk, but the knee has flexed through almost 120 degrees, bringing the heel to hip level. At contact the hip flexes rapidly, bringing the thigh down in line with the trunk and then up toward the front horizontal at takeoff. During the first two thirds of support, the swinging knee flexes, bringing the leg closer to

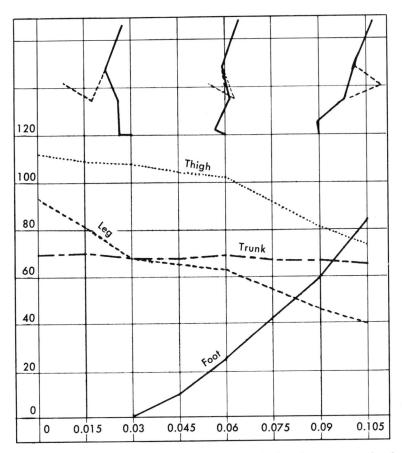

Fig. 15-8. Segmental inclinations of supporting limb during foot contact in the run. (Taken from a film of college woman with no special training in running.)

the thigh. This moves the center of gravity of the limb toward the fulcrum (the hip) and facilitates its flexion. The speed with which the thigh and leg are swung forward and upward during contact adds to the projecting force. Observation of a vigorous kick will show that the swinging limb can move the whole body forward. (One film of an expert football punter shows that the body is moved forward more than 2 feet with no observable action in the supporting limb.) According to Fenn and Fortney better runners bring the thigh closer to the horizontal at takeoff.

From the position at takeoff the leading limb during flight prepares for contact by extending the hip, thus lowering the entire limb, and the knee is extended, thus increasing the length of the stride. In other film observations, some runners have been seen to flex their knees just before contact; this moves the foot back under the body and decreases the possible backward push on contact.

In such cases the forward movement of the total body is greater than the backward movement of the foot because of knee flexion; there seems to be an advantage in this knee flexion, since it rotates the distal end of the leg backward; as foot contact is made, ankle flexion rotates the proximal end of the leg forward. Thus the direction of leg rotation before contact is continued after the foot is placed on the ground.

Angles of inclination of supporting limb. The graphs in Figs. 15-7 and 15-8 show that to understand movement in running both joint and inclination angles must be considered. The inclination of the trunk of both runners remains at an almost constant angle during foot contact, and yet the hip joint (which moves the trunk) has extended 59 degrees (in the man) and 32 degrees (in the woman). (See Table 15-1.) In both runners, thigh inclination has equaled hip action. The graphs show that foot inclination is the same for both, approximately 85 degrees; leg inclinations differ, indicating a difference in ankle action. During foot rising the man's leg inclines 12 degrees and the woman's more than twice that. If the man's action is better running mechanics, the primary cause of the woman's poor performance may be the small range of ankle extension. Do her extensor muscles lack strength, or does the reflex for ankle flexion fail to respond with sufficient strength? Leg inclination could explain the difference in thigh inclination. That of the woman is less. Greater thigh inclination combined with her leg inclination could be too much for balance. This comparison of good and poor performance illustrates the value and limitations of film in studying movement. A possible cause of poor performance has been suggested; its validity needs testing.

Additional joint actions. The pelvis rotates to a greater degree in running than it does in walking. When the thighs are separated, the pelvis is rotated on the supporting femur. As one thigh is swung forward, the pelvis rotates forward on the same side, adding length to the step. Hubbard says that improvement in running is due to an increase in the length of stride, rather than to an increase in rate of movement. The comparison of the two runners described here suggests that both factors influence speed.

The arms swing in opposition to the legs. They aid in maintaining a forward position of the upper trunk, which would otherwise tend to face in the same direction as does the pelvis. The arm swing also affects the center of gravity of the whole body. At takeoff one arm is raised to the front and the other to the back. These positions raise the center of gravity of the total body, which reaches its highest point at takeoff. Shortly after contact when the thighs are parallel, the arms are at the side of the body with the elbow joints approaching extension. The arms now tend to lower the center of gravity of the entire body, which reaches its lowest point at this time. Modern sprinters are deemphasizing the backward extended movements of the forearms for a more rapid arm movement. This seems to be associated with increased leg action.

Variations in running stride. The differences between an untrained and a trained runner have been shown. The trained one was finishing a 1500-meter race as he was filmed. His joint actions differ from those of a sprinter. Any runner, in reducing speed, increases the proportion of time of contact and decreases the number of steps per minute. The part of the foot that contacts the ground varies also; it may be the heel, ball, or entire foot. A carried object, such as a football or a hockey or lacrosse stick, affects the swing of the arms. The length of the limb and distribution of weight also results in individual differences in joint action.

It has been said that a sprinter inclines the trunk more than does the long-distance runner. Slocum and Bowerman question whether any good runner, regardless of the distance of the run, inclines the trunk forward beyond the vertical after the acceleration of the start. They also maintain that there is a backward tilting of the pelvis accompanied by flexion of the spine and that this so-called flatbacked position increases the ability to rotate the thigh laterally. (Lateral rotation of the thigh is needed to place the foot in the desired direction as the pelvis is rotated forward over the supporting hip.) The lower-limb actions of a sprinter and a distance runner are the same in general appearance, but there are differences in detail. The sprinter has greater hip flexion in the swinging limb and thus raises the flexed knee higher; he also has a longer stride and more strides per second, and less of the foot contacts the ground. Other investigators (Sparks, for example) found trunk inclination to be 2 to 4 degrees forward of the vertical.

In reviewing publications on the direction of foot movement immediately before contact, Fortney found that authors did not agree on this direction but also that in most cases they did not make clear whether they referred to movement with reference to a fixed point in space or to a fixed point in the body. In studying film of eight elementary school boys whose runs were photographed when they were in the second grade and again in each of the three following years, Fortney found that the heel moved forward with reference to a fixed point in space and that there was no apparent difference between runners classified as good and those classified as poor. However, she found that the heel moved backward with reference to a point within the body (the knee). Since the forward movement of the total body was greater than the backward movement caused by knee flexion and hip extension, the foot moved forward immediately prior to contact.

Other findings by Fortney point out differences between the good and the poor runners. At the beginning of the flight phase the good runners had greater flexion in the leading limb at the knee and the hip, the latter bringing the thigh closer to the front horizontal; at the beginning of the contact phase the good runners had greater knee flexion in the rear limb, bringing the heel closer to the buttock.

The path of the center of gravity of the body during the running stride has been studied by Beck. The subjects, twelve boys ages 6 through 12 years representing the first six grades, were selected from their classmates as those having the better time scores in a 30-yard run. Beck found that regardless of age all paths were wavelike, reaching the high point shortly after the body was airborne. After the high point the center of gravity moved downward through the next foot contact and for a short time afterward. The next rise began while the foot was in contact with the ground and continued through the takeoff, and the cycle was then repeated. With increased age there was an increase in the horizontal and vertical distances that the center of gravity traveled during each stride; also the stride became longer. With age the percentage of the total stride time represented by foot contact decreased, and of course that of flight time increased. The horizontal velocity of the center of gravity increased with age; for the flight phase, however, the percentage of the horizontal velocity decreased, and for the support phase it increased.

Track starts and initial sprinting phase. In running races it is desirable to move the body forward as rapidly as possible from the start. This is especially important in sprints, and most investigators have thought that the start is faster when executed from a crouching position. Yet some researchers (e.g., Ward) have found that from a standing position top runners negotiate the first half of a 100-meter dash faster than they do from a crouching position. The center of gravity at the start from a standing position is at the same height as it would be 15 yards from the starting line with a crouching start.

It has been found through experience that the start is faster if blocks are provided for the push; they, too, increase the amount of push that can be directed horizontally (Fig. 15-9).

Since most sprinters use the crouching start because the results from the standing start are as yet not conclusive, the discussion here is stated in terms of the crouching start.

As the runner takes the crouching position, hands, feet, and rear knee are in

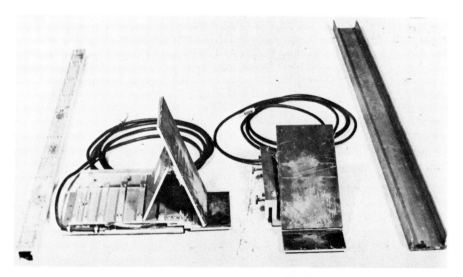

Fig. 15-9. Starting blocks and center rails used in Paul Ward's study of the stand-up start. (From Ward, P.: An analysis of kinetic and kinematic factors of the standup and the preferred crouch starting techniques with respect to sprint performance, unpublished doctoral dissertation, Indiana University, Aug., 1973.)

contact with the supporting surface with the rear foot supporting little of the body weight. The distance between the hands and the forward foot is short enough to force the spine to flex (arch); the value of this flexion will be shown later. In the "get set" position, which precedes the actual start, the rear knee is raised from the surface until the rear leg is inclined some 25 to 30 degrees as measured from the front. (However, some runners completely extend the rear leg.) Both thighs are moved upward and forward by knee extension, thereby moving the trunk and the center of gravity farther forward. At the same time the spine flexes more; the head is held at the same height that it had in the first position.

As the trunk is raised, the rear foot pushes by sudden knee extension, which moves the thigh forward. Film has shown that the feet are moved slightly backward preceding the push. This push is of short duration because the limb must be moved forward quickly for the first step. Before the rear foot has left the block, extension of the front knee begins, moving the front thigh forward. Both knee actions are examples of reversed muscle action and are the primary sources of power for putting the body into motion. The leg of the front foot keeps a fairly constant inclination, adjusting its position to the movement of the foot. The trunk, which has been inclined slightly above the horizontal during the push of the rear foot, is raised somewhat as the rear foot is moved forward for the first step. Since the center of gravity is ahead of the supporting front foot, gravity will rotate the foot about the metatarsophalangeal joints. In general, the action is that described in the discussion on mechanics of the stepping pattern in this chapter. A noted coach has increased the height of the front block to decrease the amount of backward movement of the front foot and thus decrease the time that the foot pushes against the block.

The first five or six steps after the push differ from the steps of the run. There is either no period or only a short one in which both feet are off the surface. Because the center of gravity is so far ahead of the takeoff foot, little upward projection is given to it, and the succeeding step must be taken quickly to prevent it from falling below the desired line of flight. After the first step the trunk is gradually raised, thus increasing the amount of upward direction given to the center of gravity; with this change the steps can be gradually lengthened to equal those which will be used in the sprint stride.

During the striding action of the lower limbs the arms move in opposition to them. The upper arms are moved by shoulder joint muscles, and the forearms are held in approximately 90 degrees of flexion to shorten the moment arm of the shoulder levers.

At the starting signal the contacting segments leave the surface in sequence. According to Bresnahan, who observed twenty-eight trained sprinters, all right handed, the order of breaking contact in all subjects was left hand, right hand, right foot, left foot. The average time between the signal and the left-hand break was 0.172 second and between the signal and the left-foot break 0.443 second. Bresnahan also observed one left-handed sprinter, for whom the breaking order was reversed—right hand first and right foot last.

As the hands are raised, the spine extends, counteracting the pull of gravity on the upper trunk while the lower trunk is supported by the feet. As the spine extends, it moves the head and the center of gravity forward. In looking at film of this action the viewer is reminded of Gray's statement: "By arching and extending its back, a galloping dog greatly increases the power and length of its stride."*

The forces made against the blocks by runners using the standing and crouching starts are shown in Figs. 15-10 and 15-11 for comparison. Also in the crouching start note that the front foot in most instances exerts force over a longer time but for less maximum force. (The impulse is greater for the front foot force × time.)

The effect of foot spacing on velocity in sprints was studied by Sigerseth and Grinaker. The subjects were twenty-eight men college physical education majors. In the crouching start the feet were separated 10, 19, and 28 inches, and times were checked at 10, 20, 30, 40, and 50 yards. At every distance the time for the 19-inch start was the lowest, but the records were statistically significant only when the means for the 19- and 28-inch starts were compared for the 10, 20, 30, and 50 yards.

*Gray, J.: How animals move, London, 1960, Cambridge University Press.

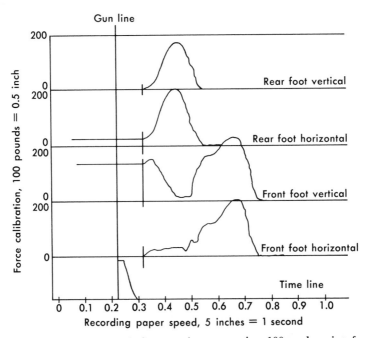

Fig. 15-10. Typical force graph for a sprinter, running 100-yard sprint from a stand-up start (subject No. 103). (From Ward, P.: An analysis of kinetic and kinematic factors of the standup and the preferred crouch starting techniques with respect to sprint performance, unpublished doctoral dissertation, Indiana University, Aug., 1973.)

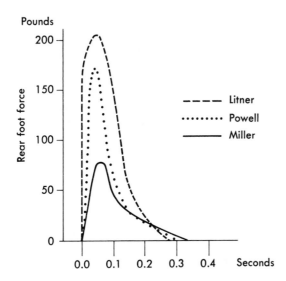

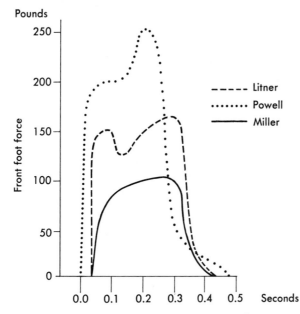

Fig. 15-11. Starting block force curves for three runners using a crouch start. (From Barlow, D. A., Bates, B. T., and Vallière, A.: Unpublished study, Indiana University, 1973.)

Speed in running may be stated as follows: speed = stride length × stride frequency. Length of stride is dependent on several factors: (1) It is positively correlated with the ratio of leg length to body height, (2) directly proportional to the amount of force exerted to propel the body into the air during pushoff, and (3) inversely proportional to the amount of braking force at touchdown. Runners with short legs have shorter strides and thus must have greater stride frequencies to run at the same speed.

Following are certain set mechanics agreed on by investigators Barlow and Cooper:

1. Block spacings vary from 11 to 15 inches partially dependent on leg length. This arrangement enables the sprinter to attain a fast start.

2. In the set position the front knee joint angle should be near 90 degrees, since the sprinter remains longest over this leg before leaving the blocks.

3. The rear leg is near extension (varying from 140 to 170 degrees) to react to the gun signal as soon as possible and to apply nearly maximum thrust.

4. The head of the sprinter is relaxed and extended downward. It is the first body part to move to impel the body in the desired direction.

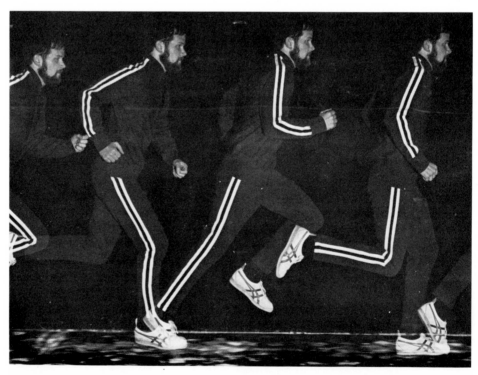

Fig. 15-12. Strobe photograph, taken at 300 flashes per minute. The foot, arm, and leg action are seen clearly in their sequential relationships. (Photograph by Phil Henson, Biomechanics Laboratory, Indiana University.)

5. A sprinter usually takes about 0.11 second to react to the gun.

6. The time of exit of the rear foot from the rear block (mean time, 0.270 second) was less than Morris found for untrained sprinters (mean time, .343 seconds).

7. The mean time spent in the blocks by the front foot was 0.446 second, showing a greater time spent there by this foot.

8. The greatest horizontal force against the blocks was exerted by the rear foot. However, the front foot generates slightly more force over a longer time.

9. The first step by the best sprinter off the blocks was longer and closer to the ground.

In middle-distance running, Sparks found the following:

1. The best runners depend on their ability to consume and to use oxygen efficiently. These same top runners supply more energy by the aerolic system and therefore produce less oxygen debt.

The better runners are more airborne during the race; that is, they are in the air slightly longer than they are on the ground. The reverse often happens as they become fatigued.

2. As the stress of the run becomes greater toward the end of the race, often the stride is shortened, and to keep up the pace the stride frequency increases. The center of gravity is lowered, and the knee lift (knee flexion and extension) is decreased as fatigue sets in.

In distance running the same mechanical effects from fatigue can and often do occur. Stress tolerance and ability to consume and use oxygen efficiently may delay or even prevent the occurrence of mechanical faults. A strobe picture of a runner in action (Fig. 15-12) shows the leg and arm action in one plane clearly. Also the outward rotation of the foot is depicted.

STANDING JUMPS (PUSHING OFF WITH BOTH FEET)
Standing broad jump

This type of jump is most frequently used in elementary schools as one measure of motor ability and physical or motor fitness. It is a modification of the walking step—a modification that low-level performers frequently do not achieve. These performers take off from one foot when they attempt to take off from both, a reflex or inherent reaction to maintain balance.

Joint actions in takeoff phase. The following analysis of the mechanics of the jump is based on a film of a 12-year-old girl whose score ranks above the ninety-fifth percentile in a nationwide sampling of girls 12 to 17 years of age. The discussion is based on the graphs of joint angle and segmented inclinations shown in Figs. 15-13 and 15-14. The lines in the illustrations begin at the time that the heels leave the ground and show that the propelling actions occur in the slightly more than 0.25 second from raising of the heel until the final thrust is made. For the first 0.18 second as the foot is raised from the floor, no action (or very little) occurs in the ankle joint, except for the slight flexion and immediate recovery at 0.09 second. This lack of ankle extension is noteworthy, since many authors attribute rising on the toes to ankle extension. These graphs, like many

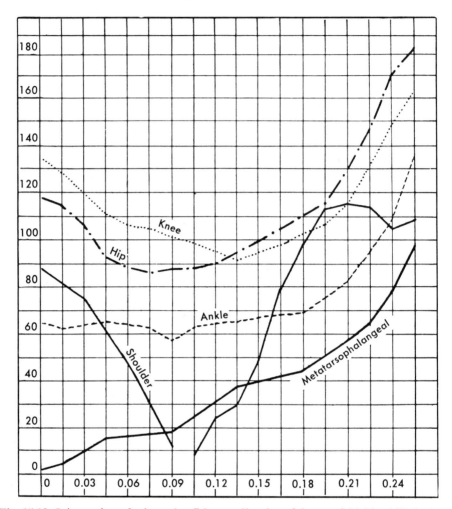

Fig. 15-13. Joint actions during takeoff in standing broad jump of highly skilled 12-year-old girl. Time in seconds is shown at the bottom; angles between body segments are shown in degrees at the left. For lower-limb joints, downward slope of lines indicates flexion and upward slope extension. Note lack of action in ankle joints until 0.18 second; also at this time all joints except those of the shoulders increase speed of extension. All shoulder joint action is flexion.

others, show that, as the center of gravity of the body is moved downward by gravitational force, the foot rotating at the metatarsophalangeal joint is moved in an upward direction. This occurs only when the ankle extensors prevent ankle flexion. This apparent paradox—movement in an upward direction because of gravitational force—was also noted in connection with teeterboard action.

Once the leg has reached the desired angle of inclination, ankle extension parallels metatarsophalangeal extension from 0.135 to 0.21 second (Fig. 15-13), and by this means the inclination of the leg is kept almost constant (Fig. 15-14).

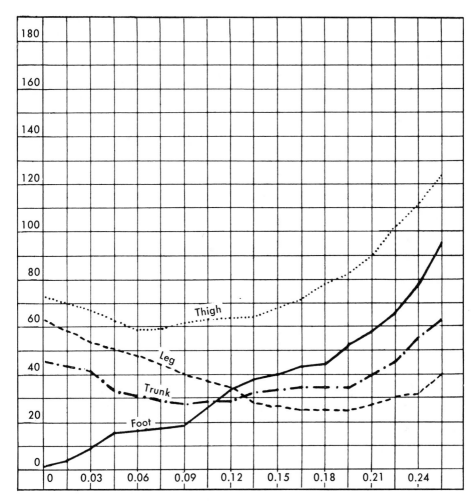

Fig. 15-14. Angles of inclination of body segments in standing broad jump of joint angles shown in Fig. 15-13. Note small range of movement in the leg and trunk and large range of movement in the foot and thigh.

In the final 0.03 second, ankle extension exceeds metatarsophalangeal action, and the leg is raised 10 degrees, adding to the upward thrust.

The knee flexes for the first 0.135 second, carrying the thigh downward and backward in reference to the knee. However, from 0.06 to 0.135 second the thigh is not inclined backward with reference to the horizontal because the forward inclination of the leg at this time exceeds knee flexion. At 0.21 second the thigh reaches the vertical, and after this point all joint actions increase in speed. Up to 0.21 second, thigh extension has lifted the thigh and the torso against gravitational pull; after that time both thigh extension and gravity are applying force in a downward direction. All joints (metatarsophalangeal, ankle, knee, and hip) react to this change in gravitational pull; all increase in speed. Here is an example of the marvelous capacity of a living organism to adjust to a situation; one can be assured that these adjustments are not voluntarily controled. The nervous system reacts to balance and to the speed of the thigh; guided by the intended action, it provides the necessary joint movements.

The shoulder measures shown in Fig. 15-13 are those of the angle formed by lines drawn through the upper arms and the trunk. As the heels leave the ground, the arms are back of the trunk at an angle of 88 degrees. They are moved downward by shoulder flexion, pass the trunk between 0.09 and 0.105 second, and reach the height of their swing just before the thighs reach the vertical.

In this swing the arm movement affects the position of the center of gravity of the entire body, tending to move it forward and downward until the arms pass the trunk and then forward and upward.

In studying the standing long jump of twenty boys (five each at ages 7, 10, 13, and 16 years) who were selected as average jumpers, Roy found that the knee, ankle, and metatarsophalangeal joints reached peak angular velocity at takeoff except for one 10-year-old whose maximal knee velocity occurred 0.07 second prior to takeoff. Using measures derived from film and a force platform, Roy concluded, "Kinematics of jumping are well established by the beginning of school age and remain essentially constant through mid-adolescence for average performers."*

Factors affecting the distance of the jump. The standing broad jump is customarily measured from the toes at takeoff to the point where the heels touch the ground in landing. This distance is determined by three factors: (1) the distance to which the center of gravity of the body is carried forward by the lean at takeoff, (2) the horizontal distance through which the center of gravity is projected during flight, and (3) the distance beyond the center of gravity that the heels reach on landing. Felton compared these factors as shown in the performances of five high-scoring college women, whose jumps averaged 86.38 inches, and of five low-scoring ones, whose jumps averaged 42.78 inches. At the time of takeoff the centers of gravity of the high-scoring group averaged 30.62 inches in front of their toes; for the low-scoring one the average distance was 18.74 inches. The heels of the high scorers landed 5.56 inches ahead of the center of gravity and the heels of the low scorers 3.60 inches ahead. The degree to which the center of gravity is in front of the toes at takeoff is affected mainly by the degree of knee extension. The 12-year-old girl whose joint actions were shown in Fig. 15-13 reached a knee extension that was 16 degrees less than 180 degrees. In Felton's comparison of high-scoring and low-scoring women the average knee extensions were 165.7 and 141 degrees. The degree of extension may be due to the balance mechanism. Also the strength of the ankle extensors could influence the amount of lean, for the tension in these muscles must move or hold all parts of the body above the ankle joint.

The position of the thigh at landing is the determining factor in the length

*Roy, B.: Kinematics and kinetics of the standing long jump in seven, ten, thirteen and sixteen year old boys, dissertation, University of Wisconsin, 1971.

of the reach. The more closely the thigh approaches the horizontal, the longer is the reach. When the thigh is nearly horizontal on landing, the legs are almost vertical. This landing position enables the body momentum to carry the center of gravity over the stationary feet. In a running broad jump the horizontal velocity during flight is greater, and the legs can reach farther without the likelihood of the body's falling back of the contact point. The horizontal position of the thighs changes the position of the center of gravity and permits that point to approach closer to the ground before the landing contact is made. This increases the time of flight, adds to the horizontal distance gained during flight, and facilitates forward rotation of the body at the ankle, thus decreasing the possibility of falling backward. Observation of hundreds of films of children by one of us (R. B. G.) has shown that the position of the thighs at landing is a distinguishing feature between high-scoring and low-scoring broad jumpers.

The flight adds the greatest proportion to the distance of the jump. The range of flight is determined by the angle and velocity of the projection. Unlike those situations in which the takeoff and landing are in the same horizontal plane, a 45-degree angle is not the best to gain distance. Whenever the center of gravity is higher at takeoff than at landing, as it is in the standing broad jump, an angle of less than 45 degrees adds to the distance that the projectile will travel. The horizontal component of velocity becomes greater as the angle is decreased. (See Chapter 17.)

Measures of velocity and distance. A measure of the velocity of the center of gravity is rarely made; yet this is the most valid evaluation of the force developed in the takeoff. Halverson found an average velocity in the jump of kindergarten children to be between 6 and 7 feet per second, and the highest (for a boy) was 8.28 feet per second. Felton calculated the mean velocity of five high-scoring college women to be 8.11 feet per second and that of five low-scoring women to be 5.66 feet per second. The highest velocity was 9.22 feet and the lowest 5.02 feet per second. With horizontal and vertical scores from Roy's study, projection velocities of the center of gravity were calculated to be 8.9 feet per second for ages 7, 10.0 for age 10, 10.5 for age 13, and 12.9 for age 16. The increase from age to age was due to greater horizontal velocity, whereas vertical velocity changed little, indicating that with age the center of gravity is lowered at takeoff.

Distance scores for various age groups are fairly common. To these are added here unpublished scores for elementary school boys obtained at the University of Wisconsin. For the first grade the average was 46 inches, and for the eighth grade it was 76 inches. The scores for intervening grades fell between these; the score for each grade was higher than that for the grade below it.

Standing jump for height

The standing jump for height is widely used as a test item and its successful performance adds to playing ability in many sports. Sargent was the one who first proposed the jump for height as a measure of motor ability. In 1921 he said, "I want to share what seems to me the simplest and most effective of all tests of physical ability with the other fools who are looking for one."* Since that time many investigators have found the Sargent jump test or the "jump and reach" a valuable item in a test battery. For games in which an attempt is made to catch or to strike a high ball the ability to jump is an asset. The receiver of a forward pass in football, the infielder and outfielder in baseball, the spiker in volleyball, and the basketball player who attempts to tip a ball toward the basket or to a teammate after a held ball will play more effectively if they can add to their reach by a jump for height.

Film comparison of joint actions in the broad jump and the jump for height of the same performer indicates minor differences in the action at the knee, hip, and shoulder. These are much like the actions in the standing broad jump (Fig. 15-13). The ankle joint action is an important key to the differences in the direction of the two projections. In one skilled performer (a college woman) in the first third of the time between raising of the heel and final thrust, the ankle flexed 10 degrees in the standing broad jump and 5 in the jump for height. Since ankle flexion carries the center of gravity of the body forward and thereby increases the effect of gravitational pull (which pulls the feet except for the toes from the floor), the difference in metatarsophalangeal action at this time (15 degrees and 5 degrees) is to be expected. Beyond this point the ankle joints extended at the same rate until the final thrust, when the action in the jump for height exceeded that in the jump for distance. The first reached an extension of 134 degrees and the second an extension of 123 degrees. The leg in the first was closer to the vertical with reference to the ankle. Since the foot in the first third of the projecting time had been lifted farther from the floor in the broad jump, gravitational action was greater, and the foot rose more rapidly. At the final thrust in the broad jump the foot was at an angle of 78 degrees with the horizontal (measured from the back) and in the high jump at an angle of 44 degrees.

Since the inclination of any segment affects the inclination of all segments above it, in spite of the similarities of proximal joint actions in the two jumps the difference in foot inclinations results in differences in inclination of the remaining segments. In the observed actions the inclinations (measured from the front and with those in the jump for height given first) were as follows: leg, 91 degrees and 44 degrees; thigh, 102 degrees and 60 degrees; and trunk, 80 and 37 degrees (Fig. 15-15).

In the broad jump gravitational force adds to the final push; in the high jump it adds little or nothing. Without the aid of gravity the velocity in the jump for height is slower.

Racing dive

The racing dive is an excellent example of the action of the lower limbs described in the discussion of mechanics of the stepping pattern in this chapter. However, in this skill the projection force is directed almost horizontally with

*Sargent, D.: The physical test of a man, Am. Phys. Educ. Rev. 26:188, 1921.

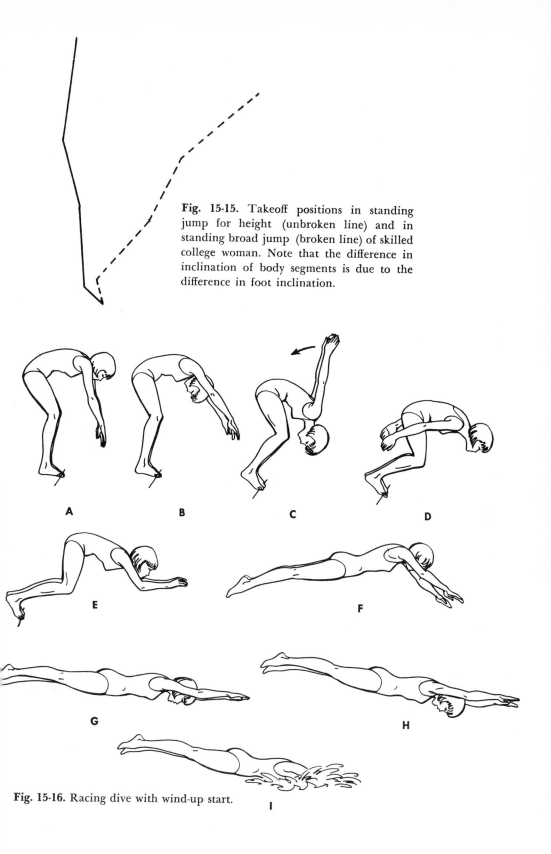

Fig. 15-15. Takeoff positions in standing jump for height (unbroken line) and in standing broad jump (broken line) of skilled college woman. Note that the difference in inclination of body segments is due to the difference in foot inclination.

A

B

C

D

E

F

G

H

I

Fig. 15-16. Racing dive with wind-up start.

little in the vertical direction. Therefore the directing segment, the leg, will be close to the horizontal in the force-producing phase. The dive is illustrated here by tracings taken from film of a woman diver, a national champion (Fig. 15-16).

In *A* the diver stands at the edge of the pool with feet separated to bring them in line with the hips for an effective push. The eyes should be looking downward and forward at approximately 45 degrees. In *B*, flexion of spine and head and forward raising of the arms with reference to the feet have moved the body's center of gravity forward resulting in ankle flexion. This flexion is possible because the ankle extensor muscles have permitted it by lengthening contraction. The importance of streamlining is evident as the body readies itself to become a projectile in the air. The path of the center of gravity is determined at takeoff. The conservation of energy law could apply here (that is, energy can be neither created nor destroyed); thus the change is from potential to kinetic energy, resulting in the transfer of momentum, which is in fact the basic mechanical principle applied to the wind-up start technique (Fig. 15-16).

The newest racing start technique is the grab start, whereby the swimmer holds onto the starting platform until the gun is fired and enters the water sooner than when using the wind-up start and at a lower angle. He gains in execution because of being into the swimming action sooner. (See Fig. 15-17.)

In *C,* ankle extensors are contracting with sufficient force to prevent flexion at that joint; now gravitational force rotates the entire body around a fulcrum that is the point of contact between the feet and the edge of the pool. Also in *C,* preparation has been made for the final application of force. The arms have moved backward; the knees have flexed; the hips have increased flexion, bringing the trunk close to the thighs; and the spine has flexed. The last action, like that described in the crouching start for running races, prepares for spinal extension, which will add to the power and distance of the body's flight.

Note that the change of inclination of the legs *(C to E)* is due to changes in foot inclination, not to changes at the ankle joint. Application of final force is delayed until the legs are at, or close to, the desired direction. From *D* to *E* the beginning of the force-producing phase is seen—forward movement of the arms, facilitated by slight elbow flexion, spinal extension, and beginning knee extension. From *E* to *F* the knees and ankles have extended vigorously. In the last-named action, since the feet no longer support the body weight, ankle extension will move the feet; however, knee extension, because the feet resist a horizontal push, will be reversed muscle action and will move the thighs. During the forward, downward movement of the thighs, trunk inclination will be maintained close to the horizontal by hip extension, a direction technique.

From *E* to *H,* head flexion can be seen; this will affect the position of the center of gravity within the body, to which gravitational force will respond by changing the inclination of the entire body. The upper part will incline downward and the lower part upward. At entry the inclination of the body is approximately 10 degrees; because this angle is small, the dive will be shallow, and forward momentum will be much greater than downward momentum will be. The diver will glide until the momentum is equal to that of swimming speed.

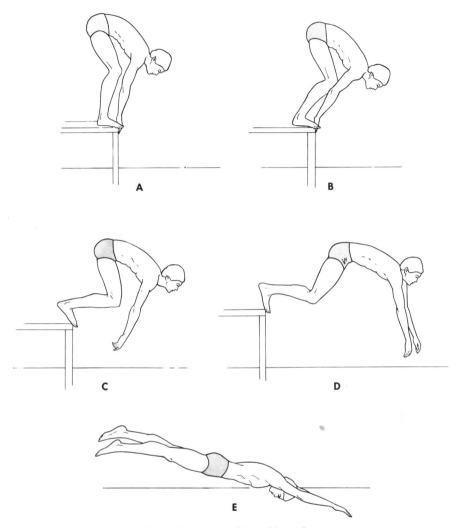

Fig. 15-17. Racing dive with grab start.

The major propelling forces are knee extension, gravitational pull, and the final thrust from the feet and toes.

RUNNING JUMPS—SINGLE-FOOT PUSH
Running long jump

The running long jump is a modification of the running stride. The differences can be seen by comparing the line representations shown in Fig. 15-7 with those in Fig. 15-18. On contact the center of gravity in the jump is seen to be farther back than it is in the run. After contact the jumper relies on the momentum of the run to carry the body mass forward by permitting the ankle joint to flex.

Adjustments to bring the center of gravity of segments closer to the fulcrum

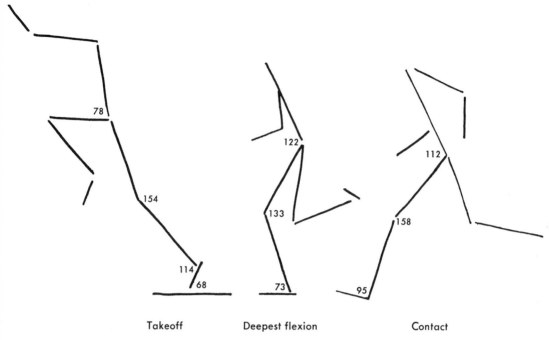

| Takeoff | Deepest flexion | Contact |

Fig. 15-18. Running long jump.

(the contact point) are made by knee and hip flexion in the supporting limb and by hip flexion in the swinging limb. As the supporting limb reaches the point of deepest knee flexion, ankle extensors prevent further flexion at that joint, and the pattern described for walking, running, and the standing broad jump follows; that is, the heel is raised from the ground. At deepest knee flexion the center of gravity is almost over the foot and will be moved forward rapidly by knee extension of the supporting leg, hip flexion of the swinging limb, and shoulder flexion of both arms.

No action occurs at the ankle joint as the foot begins to rise; ankle extension begins as the center of gravity passes the metatarsophalangeal joints, but the range of this extension is approximately slightly more than half of the metatarsophalangeal action, and therefore the leg is inclined downward by foot action.

The takeoff tracing shown in Fig. 15-18 shows that the force of joint actions will be directed upward more than forward. If the jumper has not lost the momentum of the run, there will be a forward component acting on the body mass, and the resulting angle of projection will be between the horizontal and that suggested by the takeoff position. In the depicted jumper it was calculated to be 33 degrees. Bunn reports that Jesse Owen's angle of projection was between 25 and 26 degrees. Angles of less than 45 degrees are essential for maximum distance, since the center of gravity at landing is lower than at the beginning of flight. (See Chapter 17 for a discussion of optimum projection angle for greatest distance.)

The movement in the air by the arms and legs is for balance and to extend the lower limbs to increase the measured distance of the jump. The lower limbs could be carried in hip-flexed and knee-extended position if the hip flexors were strong enough.

The reach on landing can be longer than in the standing broad jump. A horizontal position of the thighs and a greater degree of knee extension will add to the measured distance. The trunk is hyperextended at midpoint in the flight and is then flexed to prepare for projecting the center of gravity forward at landing. If ankle flexion occurs immediately on contact, the horizontal component of the velocity of projection will carry the body mass forward past the feet. Hip flexion to raise the thighs before landing will also incline the trunk, bringing the center of gravity forward. The arms by swinging forward can aid in carrying the body over the landing contact. The knees are flexed to absorb the shock as landing is completed. (See Chapter 16.)

The flight of the center of gravity cannot be altered after the takeoff. The path is determined by the angle and velocity of projection and by gravitational force once the body is in the air. The only aids to distance that can be made during flight are positioning of the thighs and legs for the reach and of the trunk and arms for carrying the center of gravity forward on landing.

Bedi's investigation of the long jump revealed the following:

1. The jumpers in their run up to the board averaged 26.6 feet per second with the best performers running the fastest.

2. The vertical force averaged 930 pounds with the best jumpers exceeding this amount by more than 100 pounds of force.

3. The braking force was 683 pounds on the average.

4. The largest impulses (force × time) were recorded by the best jumpers.

5. The best long jumper spent 0.11 to 0.12 second on the board, whereas the poorer one spent 0.13 to 0.14 second.

6. The takeoff angle varied from 17 degrees to 25 degrees with the poorest jumper's angle being 17 degrees.

7. The jumpers all had a forward rotation at the takeoff with a large horizontal braking force contributing to this rotational component.

He believes that to jump farther the performers need to do the following:

1. The jumpers should reduce the horizontal braking force at takeoff to minimize the forward rotation and increase horizontal velocity at takeoff in an attempt to reduce wasted energy.

2. It is possible to perform a forward somersault in the air in order to arrive at touchdown with a better landing position, but more vertical force must be generated in the last few milliseconds that the long jumper is on the takeoff board.*

Running high jump

The takeoff for the running high jump is much like that for the running long jump. The differences are those that keep the center of gravity higher to develop a greater vertical component in the flight. This is accomplished mainly by inclinations of the foot and the trunk. In the high jump the foot at the moment

---

*Bedi, J. F.: Angular momentum in the long jump, unpublished doctoral dissertation, Indiana University, May, 1975.

of thrust does not incline as far forward as it does in the long jump. This, as was shown in the description of the standing jump for height, will affect the inclinations of all other segments. As in the standing jump for height, ankle and hip actions serve to maintain the desired direction. The final force is derived from running momentum, from extension of the knee, and from the forceful swing of the free lower limb and the arms. Segmental inclinations of the foot, leg, thigh, and trunk are closer to the vertical and takeoff than in the long jump.

The jump must have a horizontal component to carry the center of gravity across the bar, and the skilled jumper will keep the proportion of this component as small as possible. One method by which this is accomplished is by a diagonal run to approach at a parallel with the bar. This allows space for lifting the free leg parallel with, rather than toward, the bar. Approaching from an oblique angle gives jumpers more latitude to accommodate for errors in spacing, so that they can vary position in crossing the bar.

The height of the center of gravity at takeoff can be estimated. If a jumper is 6 feet tall, the center of gravity in the normal standing position, according to Palmer's formula, would be 40.65 inches above the soles of the feet. In rising to the tip of the toes at takeoff the jumper could raise the center of gravity 7 inches. The position of the arms and the swinging leg could add another 8 inches, bringing the position of the center of gravity 55.65 inches above the ground at takeoff. How high would and could the velocity of the jump carry the center of gravity to enable the jumper to clear the bar at 7.5 feet? If a superior jumper could raise the center of gravity another 30 inches, the attained height would be slightly over 7 feet. Additional height is gained by manipulation of the body segments, which allows the center of gravity to pass under the bar.

This manipulation has been accomplished in various ways since the scissors jump was discarded in competition. One of these is the western roll, in which the trunk is lowered to the horizontal as it reaches bar height; one arm reaches over and is extended below the bar, and the rear thigh and leg are also below the bar. From the high point the trunk rolls over as the rear limb extends, and the leading limb moves below bar level. Recently a dive over the bar with head and chest leading has been developed. This, coupled with the straddle roll form, in which the jumper goes over the bar facing downward, has enabled jumpers to continue to increase their height.

When this style of jumping is used, the center of gravity is located to the rear before the takeoff (Fig. 15-19, *B*). The right (free) leg is swung forward with hip and some knee flexion. As the leg starts upward, there is continued hip flexion, knee flexion, and then full knee extension at the top of the kickup (*C*). Both arms are carried upward at the takeoff with shoulder and some elbow flexion (*D*). The right arm has greater range of movement. The takeoff leg provides force and direction by hip, knee, and ankle extension (*D*). The more vertical the takeoff, the steeper the parabola of flight. Present-day jumpers are emphasizing greater speed during the run, and at the same time they try to take off with an angle as close to 90 degrees as possible.

The roll, or turn, over the bar is accomplished by trunk rotation to the left

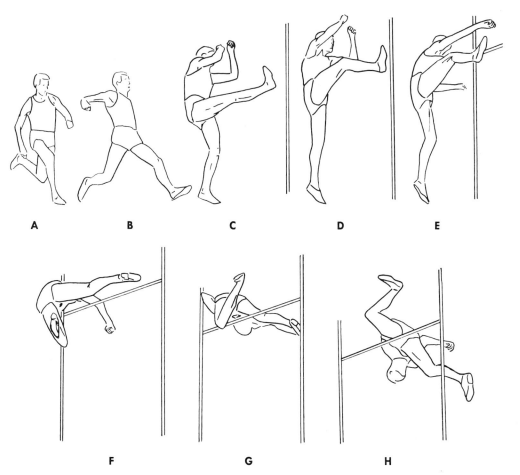

Fig. 15-19. Running high jump.

(left-footed jumper). Neck and trunk flexion at the height of the jump enable the jumper to lift the lower limbs over the bar. As the trunk and lead leg cross the bar, the neck has been in slight rotation to the right. It is moved to the left initiating total trunk rotation to the left accompanied by left hip abduction and knee flexion. After crossing the bar the jumper continues to turn so as to land on the back.

One of us (J. M. C.) has stated his belief that the requirements for world record high jumping are the following (with the last three the most important):

1. Long legs, high center of gravity
2. Enough speed and strength at takeoff to give an upward thrust of considerable magnitude
3. Takeoff foot on the ground long enough for arms, swinging leg, foot, and toe to contribute transference of momentum

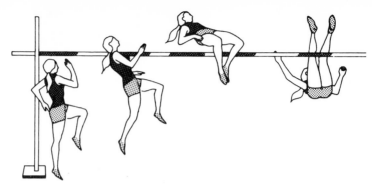

Fig. 15-20. Back flop style of high jumping. Note that the jumper takes off from the ground with her outside leg. Also note that the jumper first executes a scissorlike jump and then twists to roll over the bar on her back. This style is becoming more and more popular with women. It involves less lift and more flexibility than does the straddle style. (From Wakefield, F., and Harkins, D., with Cooper, J. M.: Track and field fundamentals for girls and women, ed. 3, St. Louis, 1973, The C. V. Mosby Co.)

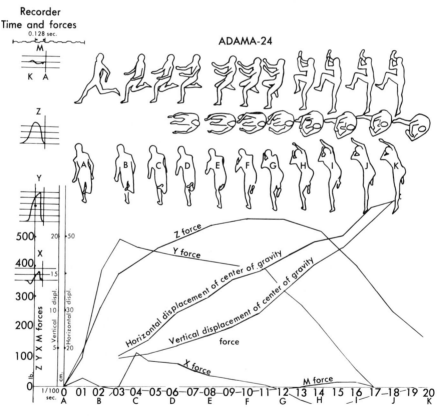

Fig. 15-21. Force-action-time relationships for the jump of a particular jumper, showing the displacement of the center of gravity and the distribution of forces at the takeoff. (From Ward, R. D.: An investigation into the use of computer integration of kinematics, kinetics, and cinematography data in motion analysis, dissertation, Indiana University, Aug., 1971.)

4. Style of crossing the bar like a tumble, so that the center of gravity does not actually cross over the top of the bar but goes beneath it

The Fosbury flop style is shown in Fig. 15-20. The ease of execution and high lift of the hips (center of gravity) possibly makes this mechanically best. (See Hay for greater detail.)

Ward has shown that force, action, and time aspects can be synchronized as shown in Fig. 15-21. Such a study involves using a force plate, three cameras, and an oscillograph recording device.

Pole vault

In the running high and long jumps the momentum of the run rotates the body over the supporting foot. The foot and lower limb serve much the same function as the pole does in the vault. During the run the pole is carried by the front arm in medial rotation, and the shoulder is adducted with some flexion. The elbow is flexed, and the forearm is pronated. In the rear arm there is some shoulder extension, and the elbow is also flexed (Fig. 15-22). A horizontal velocity is imparted to the pole by the run, and, since it is raised upward and pointed downward in the final step, the pole, after contact with the box, will be rotated upward and forward by the horizontal velocity.

At the plant of the pole in the box the right shoulder is laterally rotated and flexed. There is elbow extension. The left arm also has shoulder and some elbow flexion (C). The left hand momentarily releases the pole and then regrasps it. The tracings in Fig. 15-22 were taken from a film in which the performer uses a glass pole.

As the pole is placed on the ground and the final thrust is made by extension of the thigh and plantar flexion of the foot of the supporting limb, the left elbow is extended and the shoulder is flexed. The right elbow extends to retain the grasp on the pole as it rebounds from its compressed position. Note that the hands are spaced well apart. Assisting the thrust of the lower limb is the rapid upward movement of the pole and the swinging right lower limb.

At takeoff the supporting leg, according to Ganslen, is inclined 78 degrees; and, since the trunk remains vertical, the thrust of the supporting joints can be assumed to be close to the vertical. As the pole rotates upward around its ground contact, the body rotates around the hand contact on the pole. The body rotation will be faster than that of the pole, and, as the extended body passes the pole, its speed of rotation will be increased by flexion of the hips and knees.

To elevate the lower part of the body above the hands, first, the hips flex while the knees are flexed (Fig. 15-22, E); the knee position decreases the amount of force needed to flex the hips by moving the center of gravity of the lower limbs closer to the fulcrum (the hip joints). As the thighs approach the vertical, the knees extend to bring the leg in line with the thighs (F). The body's center of gravity is now close to the pole, thereby taking greater advantage of the pole action. In F the trunk has begun to rotate to the left; pelvic rotation will follow, and the right leg will scissor over the left. As the jumper's center of gravity passes the pole, the pulling is converted into a pushing movement, which is achieved by shoulder flexion and elbow extension. This action is completed in one continuous movement with the left hand released from the pole first. The forearms are pronated as the release of each is accomplished. The vaulter should keep the chin down toward the chest in preparing to go over the bar to project the legs as high as possible. The movement of the lower limbs downward after crossing the bar raises the trunk and arms. Elevating the arms still higher helps keep them from striking the bar as they go over. The vaulter must be sure to wait until the pole has almost reached the vertical position before executing the pull-up.

The higher the vaulter places the hands on the pole at the start, the faster he runs, and the steeper the parabola of the path of the center of gravity in flight, the higher he should vault.

Barlow, using rather elaborate electronic equipment, including force plates, special slow motion camera, force transducers, recording oscillograph, and necessary accessories, was able to secure kinematic and kinetic parameters of the pole vaulting of top performers. This data was analyzed by a computer and digitizing system.

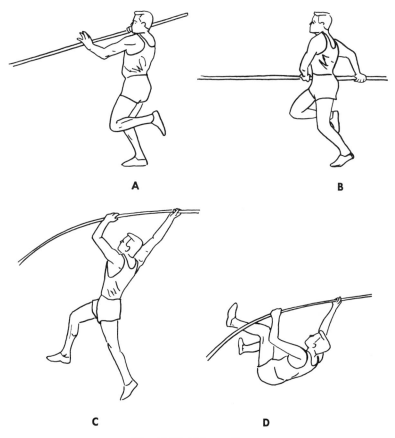

A   **B**

C   **D**

Fig. 15-22. Pole vault.

Some of his findings are as follows:

Kinematic factors

1. The last stride of all vaulters was shortened.

2. The second to last stride was longer than either the third to last or last stride.

3. The best vaulter (who was of world class) took longer strides throughout than any of the other subjects and shortened his last stride the least.

4. All pole plants of those who vaulted 16 feet or higher was initiated in 0.423 second (mean time) as compared with 0.408 second for the less than 16-foot vaulters.

5. Considerable deceleration over the final three strides occurred for those who vaulted less than 16 feet.

6. The best vaulter accelerated longer in the run and decelerated less during the final strides.

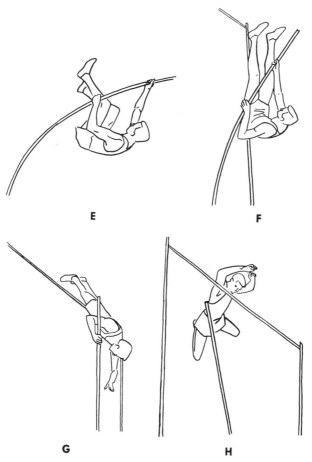

Fig. 15-22, cont'd. Pole vault.

7. Those who vaulted over 16 feet attained a maximum velocity of 28.97 feet per second during the second to last stride, whereas those who vaulted less than 16 feet attained a maximum velocity of 27.26 feet per second under the same conditions.

8. The average takeoff angle for the center-of-gravity projection of all vaulters was 21.9 degrees.

9. The angle of takeoff tended to increase as the height of the cross bar was elevated.

10. When the pole was perpendicular, the top vaulters had no vertical acceleration and the poorer ones negative vertical velocity.

Kinetic factors

1. The average time on the force plate (of the takeoff foot) was 0.122 second.

2. The lowest, or shortest, time was 0.116 second for the top vaulter.

3. The peak vertical striking force at takeoff was an average magnitude of 819 pounds.

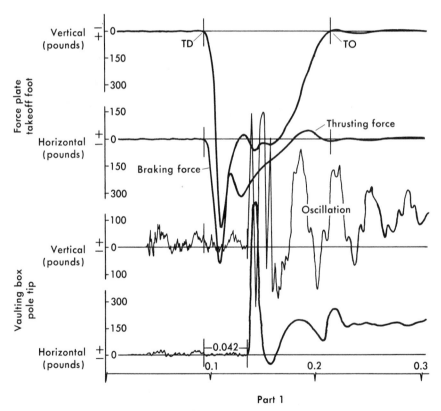

Part 1

Fig. 15-23. Scale-reduced sample of typical recording oscillograph record of forces generated in takeoff and pendular phases of pole vault. (From Barlow, D. A.: Kinematic and kinetic factors involved in pole vaulting, unpublished doctoral dissertation, Indiana University, Aug., 1973.)

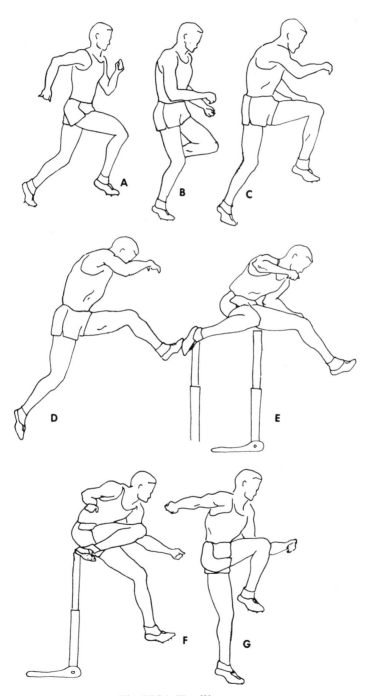

Fig. 15-24. Hurdling.

4. The top performers attained greater vertical force at takeoff than did those who were poorer vaulters.

5. The top vaulters supplied greater braking impulse at takeoff.

6. The vertical extension force tended to increase with the increased height of the cross bar (Fig. 15-23).

The findings of such a study reveal that the pole vaulter, in fact, does jump at the takeoff, attempts to generate considerable vertical force, and runs at close to top sprinting speed. Finally, by studying such data the researcher can find distinguishing factors characteristic of the better vaulters.

Hurdling

The high hurdler is a runner who vaults a series of hurdles. The run must be slightly modified on the approach to each hurdle. The shoulders are flexed and abducted and the scapulae elevated (Fig. 15-24, *A* to *C*). As the body's center of gravity is moved forward by the momentum of the run, the heel is raised (Fig. 15-24, *B* to *D*). At the same time, the knee of the supporting limb extends. Considerable flexion of the hip of the lead limb takes place as the limb is swung forward with the knee extended. (Most hurdlers attempt to prevent the knee from extending completely to a locked position.) The hurdler (Jack Davis) flexes the neck as well as the trunk, so that the center of gravity will not go too high over the hurdle and he will come down to the ground sooner. Note that he starts flexion of the trunk and neck before he leaves the ground *(C)*. The rear leg *(D)* is brought forward by hip flexion. As the thigh is moved forward, it is abducted and rotated medially, bringing the flexed leg close to the horizontal (*E* and *F*).

After the hurdle is cleared, the lead thigh extends to lower the foot, and the leg flexes, thus moving the foot backward with reference to the knee, and at contact will decrease the possibility of backward push *(F* and *G)*. The rear thigh, after the hurdle is cleared, adducts and rotates laterally to bring the foot in line for the next step *(F* and *G)*. After contact body momentum helps to extend the knee of the supporting limb.

The hurdler attempts to raise the center of gravity only high enough to clear the hurdle. Likewise he attempts to get the lead leg down as soon as possible, so that the feet are in contact with the ground, enabling him to run rapidly to the next hurdle.

Dance leap

In the leap the dancer strives for height or distance but also for an alignment of limbs that will give the illusion of floating in air even if in making these alignments some height or distance is sacrificed. In Fig. 15-25 are shown the positions of segments of a skilled dancer at takeoff. The near arm is abducted to shoulder height toward the camera. As the body rises in flight, the front knee is extended, the rear limb is raised toward the back horizontal, and the arm is moved back to the position shown in the midair view. This position is held during flight. It will be noted that on landing the arms and rear limb have changed little; the leading thigh and leg have been flexed to place the foot in contact position (Fig. 15-26).

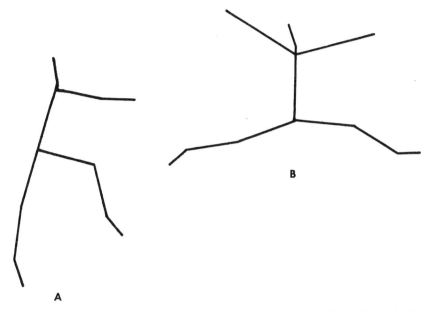

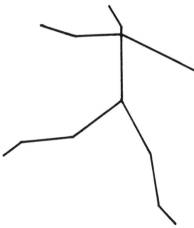

Fig. 15-25. Dance leap. **A,** Takeoff position. The center of gravity is well ahead of last contact point. **B,** Midair position. Horizontal alignment of limbs is held to give an illusion of floating.

Fig. 15-26. Dance leap. Landing position is shown. Rear limb is still close to floating position shown in Fig. 15-25.

SKATING

Although skating can be considered a form of stepping, its mechanics differ in several ways from those of walking. In ice skating the differences are necessitated by two aspects of the situation: (1) the base of support is much smaller (the width of the skate blade compared to that of the shoe or foot) and (2) the supporting surface offers little resistance to a horizontal push (ice compared to ground or floor). In roller skating the base is wider, but the lack of friction between the rollers and the supporting surface affects the mechanics. To improve balance the body's center of gravity is lowered by hip and knee flexion; often the trunk is close to the horizontal. Since friction between skates and supporting surface is negligible, gravitational force cannot be used as a contributing factor in forward progress. The center of gravity must be kept over the supporting foot; it cannot be allowed to fall ahead. If it did, gravity would encounter no resistance as it pushed backward, and balance would likely be lost. In walking, running, and jumping, there is resistance to the backward push, and the body can rotate about the motionless base.

In ice racing while the skater is waiting at the starting line for the starting signal, one of two foot positions is commonly used. In one the skates are placed shoulder width apart, one ahead of the other and both at an angle of 40 degrees (more or less) with the starting line. In the other the front skate is pointed forward (at 90 degrees to the starting line), and the rear skate approaches a parallel with the starting line. Skaters who use the second position believe that it saves a fraction of a second in the start, since the foot need not be lifted and turned as the first step is taken.

At the starting signal the center of gravity is lowered by increasing knee and hip flexion; the weight is shifted to the rear foot, so that the forward one can be lifted slightly for the first step. With this step the rear knee and hip extend. Here for a brief time the center of gravity falls ahead of the supporting foot; this is possible because the angle of the skate resists the backward push of gravity and that of the extension of the rear hip and knee. This extension continues until the rear limb is straight and at an angle of about 45 degrees with the horizontal. Meantime after a short step the front foot has been placed on the ice and angled, as was the rear foot. This type of stepping continues for three or four strides, each increasing in length over the previous one. The arms during the beginning strides move as they do in running, in opposition to the lower-limb movements.

After the starting strides the weight is carried over the front foot; now as the rear foot pushes, it does not affect the equilibrium. Here is seen the advantage of the low center of gravity; as the push from the ice is applied to the body, it is closer to the gravity plane than it would be if the body were erect. After the push, as the supporting foot glides, the rear foot is brought forward; and, as it passes the gliding foot, it takes the weight of the body. The push will have a sideward, as well as a backward, component. This should be minimized by placing the skate as it takes the weight in a forward direction and close to the other foot as it begins the glide.

After the starting strides, mechanics of action change somewhat with the length of the race. Filmstrips prepared in 1962 by Freisinger, 1964 Olympic team coach, show that in the 500-meter race the trunk is slightly above the horizontal, whereas in the longer races it is horizontal. Also in the short-distance race, alternate flexion and extension of the spine are seen. At the end of the push one limb is well back of the gliding foot, and the trunk is fully extended; here trunk and limb balance each other over the supporting limb like two ends of a teeterboard.

As the rear limb swings forward, the spine flexes, again aiding balance. This action is not seen in the longer races.

Arm action in the film was also seen to differ with the distance of the race. In the 500-meter race both arms were seen to swing sideward as well as backward and forward. When the right skate is gliding, the center of gravity must move to the right; here the right arm is abducted to shoulder height and is slightly to the rear of the trunk, and the left arm is in front of and across the body. The arms are reversed when the glide is on the left foot. These films show that in the middle-distance race the left arm is motionless at the side of the body and the hand rests on the lower back. The right arm swings; it is abducted to shoulder height when the glide is on the right skate and is in front of the body and to the left when the glide is on the left foot. It serves a balancing function. In the longer races the arms are motionless, and the hands are clasped behind the back. One observer of the film suggested that in the longer distances there is a glide on both skates for a short period, whereas in the short distances this period of double support does not occur; therefore in the longer distances the balancing effect of the arms might not be needed. An Olympic skater disagreed with this reasoning. She thought that streamlining by lack of arm movement was a major reason and that also less fatigue would occur when arm action was eliminated. She stated that during training she had practiced without arm action to develop balancing adjustments without the use of the arms.

Often the reason for the horizontal position of the trunk is given as a factor in decreasing air resistance. Although this is true, the mechanical advantage of the position should not be overlooked. When the trunk is horizontal, the range of hip extension to the back is increased. This adds to the time during which the push can be applied.

TRAMPOLINE AND DIVING SKILLS

Gaining height. Height is essential in diving and trampoline skills to provide time for the desired movements of body segments while in the air. The more complex the movements, the greater the height must be. Since the force of projection is derived mainly from the rebounding net or board, these surfaces must be depressed as much as possible when great height is desired. Depression is achieved by several means. First, the performer approaches the net or board from a projection. In running dives this is the hurdle that precedes the final landing on the board. On the trampoline the performer uses repeated bounces. When the height of the bounce and the resulting depressions of the net were measured, the following data were obtained from a film of a highly skilled performer:

Height of first bounce—21 inches	Resulting net depression—20 inches
Height of second bounce—45 inches	Resulting net depression—30 inches
Height of third bounce—60 inches	Resulting net depression—31 inches

These measures suggest that after a given height the resulting depression will be relatively less. The depression for any net will be affected by the tension in its springs.

Second, the center of gravity of the body should be directly over the feet as the contact is made to keep the direction of the landing force directly downward.

Third, there is no "give" by the performer as the feet contact the net or board. Ordinarily the jar of landing is decreased by flexion of the ankles, knees, and hips. In dives and on the trampoline the depressing surface takes over the task of eliminating the jolt, and landing is made with full foot contact with flexed ankles, knees, and hips held firmly as the feet land. The arms are extended down and just back of the hips on landing. The relationship of these flexed positions should be such that the center of gravity is over the feet.

Fourth, as the surface depresses, the flexed joints extend, pushing the net or board downward beyond the depth that it would reach were the landing the only force acting on it. On the trampoline the ankle reaches an angle of 90 degrees; the hips and knees extend to bring the legs, thighs, and trunk into a straight line. The arms, at the same time, are swung forward and upward and add to the downward force. In dives the knees are not fully extended; they reserve some of their power for the projection.

When great height is desired, the trampoline performer takes repeated bounces; the diver can use only one landing, and for those dives which require longer time in the air a high diving board is used. He also lands after the hurdle as near the end of the board as safety permits.

Projectional direction. From the low point of depression the performer rides upward on the rebounding surface. During this time the center of gravity develops a velocity equal to that of the canvas or board, and at the departure point this is increased by ankle extension and some further shoulder flexion and in dives by the remaining amount of possible knee extension. The direction that the center of gravity has during flight is determined by the position of the center of gravity in relation to the feet at the final thrust. The diver must have some forward lean to enter the water a few feet from the board. The position of the entry will depend on the lean. Beginning divers are likely to lean too far forward as they attempt a straight front dive; they concentrate on clearing the board rather than on gaining height, and, consequently, as they enter the water, their bodies approach a horizontal, rather than a vertical, line. Since the center of gravity follows a parabolic curve, the time of flight from takeoff until the hips enter the water is a measure of the height attained. Block has suggested that in working with women the beginner be given a distance goal of 5 to 8 feet from the board as the desirable entry and that the diver attempt to develop a projection that would have a minimum time of 1.1 seconds. Such projections would mean that the center of gravity would have an inclination of 22 to 30 degrees beyond the perpendicular at takeoff and a velocity of 13 to 14 feet per second. These goals, experimentally, were found to be within the capacity of beginning college women divers. Groves found with an expert male diver that the lean for various dives ranged from 20 to 34 degrees at takeoff and that the height reached by the center of gravity ranged from 2.4 to 4.6 feet.

On the trampoline no forward component of velocity is needed, and the

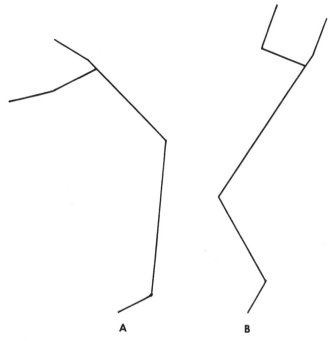

Fig. 15-27. A, Takeoff position from the trampoline of highly skilled college man for forward somersault. **B,** Takeoff position from the trampoline for backward somersault. Position of the center of gravity determines the direction of total body rotation.

center of gravity can be in a line that is perpendicular to the final thrust. In bounces to gain height this will be done to convert the rebounding force as much as possible into an upward projection.

Rotations and twists in flight. As the performer leaves the canvas or board, the position of the center of gravity also starts the body rotations in the sagittal or transverse planes or both. The amount of lean depends on the amount of rotation desired during flight. The performer riding upward on the rebounding surface has the desired body rotations in mind and makes adjustments to place the center of gravity in the needed relationship to the final thrust. In Fig. 15-27 are shown line tracings at takeoff of an expert performer planning to execute forward and backward somersaults during flight. In the forward movement the center of gravity has been carried ahead of the toes by hip and shoulder flexion. The thrust will start the rotation in a counterclockwise direction. For the backward movement knee flexion has carried the center of gravity back of the toes, and rotation in a clockwise direction will be started. Once the body is in flight, joint actions will add to the speed of rotation of the segments. Reuschlein measured on film the rotation of body parts of an expert performer executing a forward somersault in the pike position. The degrees of rotation in space of the trunk and the lower limbs and the changes in the hip angle could be measured.

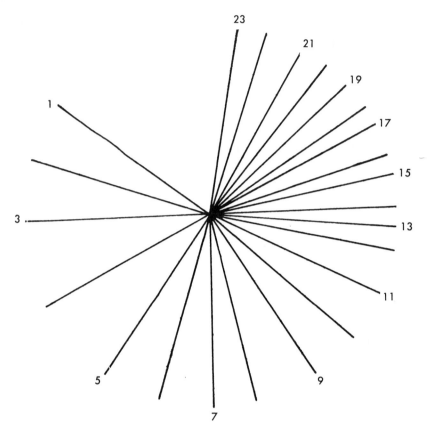

Fig. 15-28. Trunk inclination during forward somersault from the trampoline of highly skilled college man: line **1**, inclination at takeoff; line **23**, inclination at landing. Time interval between any two lines is 0.0474 second. Note that the trunk moves fastest between lines **3** and **5**, where gravitational force is most helpful.

The trunk, slightly above the horizontal at the beginning of flight, must rotate counterclockwise until it reaches the 12 o'clock position—more than 270 degrees (Fig. 15-28). The lower limbs, starting near the 6 o'clock position, must rotate more than 360 degrees counterclockwise (Fig. 15-29). In the first 0.284 second the trunk rotated 110 degrees and the limbs 61 degrees to bring the trunk close to the 6 o'clock position. The limbs approached the 3 o'clock position. During this time there was 49 degrees of flexion in the hip, showing that the entire body rotated 61 degrees. The trunk movement downward was assisted by gravitational pull.

In the next 0.521 second the limbs rotated faster than the trunk. They moved through 228 degrees and the trunk through 135 degrees. Again the difference was due to hip joint action, which measured 93 degrees of extension. In the remaining time before landing, 0.285 second, the trunk moved through 53 degrees and the limbs 72 degrees; the hips extended 29 degrees. The positions of the trunk and limbs are the result of total body rotation and hip joint actions.

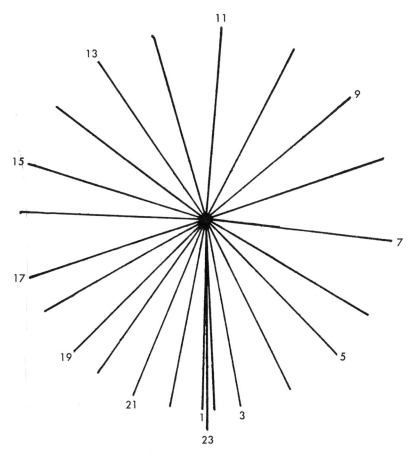

Fig. 15-29. Inclination of lower limbs with knees extended in forward somersault shown in Fig. 15-28. Note that speed is greatest between lines **6** and **8**, where the trunk is closest to the vertical. (See Fig. 15-28.) Time between all lines is 0.0474 second.

The positions of the arms and head will affect the movements of the lower limbs and trunk. They were not analyzed in this study.

If greater speed of rotation is desired, the body will assume a tuck position to shorten the length of the moment arms. While the body is in midair, the speed of rotation will be decreased by extending the limbs and the trunk, as is done as the body enters the water.

In twists the movement is also started as the body leaves the board or canvas by shifting the weight to one foot. In midair the arms or lower limbs or both are moved to the side to accentuate the movement.

In Fig. 15-30 are shown the approach steps, the hurdle, landing on the board, depression of the board, and the takeoff for a dive. On the step preceding the hurdle *(A)* the forward knee is flexed to place the thigh in position for the force-producing phase; the shoulders are hyperextended, and the hands are back of the

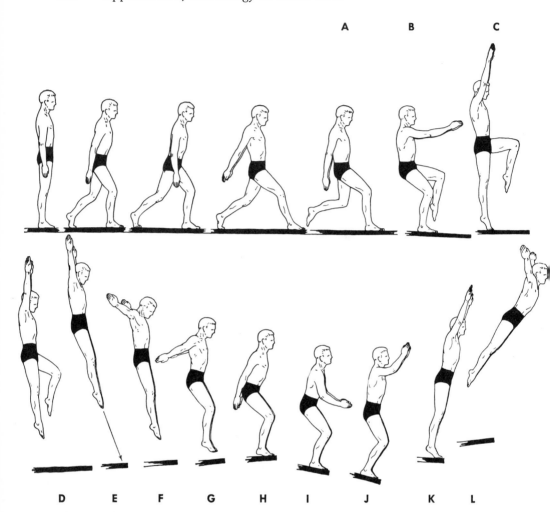

Fig. 15-30. Approach and takeoff for running dive. (From Armbruster, D. A., Sr., Allen, R. H., and Billingsley, H. S.: Swimming and diving, ed. 6, St. Louis, 1973, The C. V. Mosby Co.)

hips. From *A* to *C* are seen the force-producing joint actions and those which direct the line of force. Force is directed by the inclinations of the leg and the trunk. From *A* to *B*, the leg is moved forward by ankle flexion; from *B* to *C*, backward by ankle extension. The trunk is maintained in vertical position by hip extension as the thigh moves forward. Force is produced (*B* to *C*) by knee and ankle extension, by the forward swing of the free lower limb, and by arm movement from horizontal to vertical. (See Fig. 15-31.)

While the body is in flight during the hurdle, the lower limbs are brought together with extended hip, knee, and ankle (*E*). From *F* to *G* preparation for landing is made by flexion at the hip, knee, and ankle, accompanied by downward movement of the arms. The head is flexed to keep the eyes on the target—the end of the board. *(F).*

As the board is depressed *(H to J)* by the force of body impact, the body's center of gravity can be seen to have moved from a position back of the feet to one closer to them. This has been done by ankle flexion, slight knee extension, and more than 90 degrees of shoulder flexion, which moves the arms forward and upward.

From *J* to *K,* projection force is developed by board and joint actions. The board moves upward through some 20 degrees. (From the body position in flight [*L*], it can be seen that the board was beyond the horizontal at takeoff.) Body mechanics will be similar to those described in this chapter in the discussion on mechanics of the stepping pattern. The major contribution will be the lever that acts at the knee joint to move the thigh through some 60 degrees of extension. Ankle extension will contribute to the force: gravitational force will raise the rear part of the foot, and, when the weight has been taken from the foot as the body moves upward, the foot will be further extended by action of the ankle extensor muscles; foot extension, whatever the force, will push against the board. Leg and trunk inclinations have been adjusted by extension at the ankle and hip to direct the force.

Note that, because the body's center of gravity is ahead of the last contact point, the upward and backward direction of the board's force at takeoff has started body rotation in the sagittal plane; this rotation will be increased by joint actions during flight.

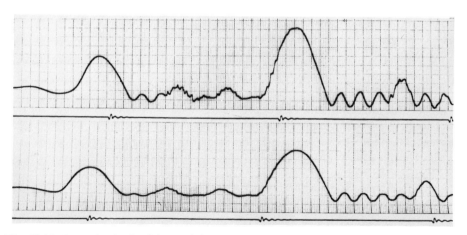

Fig. 15-31. Records obtained in studying the force exerted on the board in a dive. First rise in each graph shows the force exerted on the board in the takeoff for the hurdle; second large rise, that for the takeoff for the dive. Lines below each graph record time. (Courtesy Kinesiology Research Laboratories, University of Wisconsin.)

RELATIONSHIPS OF BODY AND WATER WEIGHTS

If the human body, either stationary or moving, is supported by water, the mechanical problems that it encounters differ from those encountered when it is supported by a more rigid surface and when surrounded by air. When the body is supported by the ground or a floor, those surfaces are usually more than strong enough to resist the weight of the body and any additional force applied by moving body segments. When the supporting surface is water, this surface is unable to support the body; it gives way, and the body sinks, wholly or partially. It will sink until the weight of the displaced water equals the weight of the body. If the displaced water equals the weight of the body before the latter is completely immersed, the body will float. The first recognition of this weight relationship is attributed to Archimedes (287-212 B.C.), who said, "A body immersed in a fluid is buoyed up by a force equal to the weight of the displaced fluid." This concept is known as Archimedes' principle.

The weight of a body compared to that of an equal amount of water is known as the *specific gravity* of the body:

$$\text{Specific gravity} = \frac{\text{Weight of body}}{\text{Weight of equal amount of water}}$$

Human bodies differ in specific gravity; those with greater proportions of bone and muscle will be heavier. However, all are close to a specific gravity of 1, some slightly less and some slightly more.

The specific gravity of a given body can be determined by various methods. If the body is a regular geometric solid, its dimensions can be measured and its volume calculated. If the volume is known, the body weight can be compared to the weight of an equal volume of water.

If the body is irregular in shape, it can be submerged to determine the weight of the water that it displaces. If the body sinks, its weight can be determined while the body is completely submerged. The loss of weight when submerged is the weight of the displaced water.

$$\text{Specific gravity} = \frac{\text{Body weight}}{\text{Loss of weight in water}}$$

If the body does not sink or does not sink readily, additional weight may be attached to it to ensure complete submersion. The submerged weight of the attached mass should be determined. The loss of body weight in the water will be the total weight of the submerged body and attached mass minus the weight of the mass when under water. The formula just given for bodies that sink readily can be applied to determine specific gravity.

In measuring twenty-seven college women Rork and Hellebrandt found that after full inspiration the mean specific gravity was 0.9812, ranging from 0.9635 to 1.0614; when the lungs were deflated, the average was 1.0177. Only five subjects had a specific gravity less than 1 on full expiration. According to these authors, their findings compare favorably with those reported by previous investigators. It is to be expected that in general the specific gravity of women will be less than that of men and that of children will be less than that of adults, especially at ages when the trunk is a greater proportion of the total body mass.

FLOATING POSITION IN WATER

Persons whose specific gravity is less than 1 will float with some part of the body above the surface of the water. The position of the body as it floats will depend on the relationship of the center of gravity of the body to the center of weight of the displaced water. In most individuals the lower limbs will sink because they are heavier than the water that they displace. However, the chest, which displaces water weighing more than this portion of the body, will float. The lungs assist in flotation by causing a balloonlike effect. The center of weight of the water displaced by the total body will therefore be nearer the head than is the center of gravity of the body. As the lower limbs sink, the spine will be arched, and the center of gravity will move toward a vertical line passing through the center of weight of the displaced water. When these two centers are in the same vertical line, the downward rotation of the lower limbs will cease.

Rork and Hellebrandt presented the following formula for determining the distance between the centers when the body is in a horizontal position: $X = \dfrac{fd}{B}$.
X represents the distance between the centers; f the force required to hold the lower limbs in a horizontal line, a measure obtained from a scale attached at the ankles; d, the height of the center of gravity (Chapter 7); and B, the body weight minus f.

Since in the adult the center of gravity is farther from the head than is the center of weight of the water, any changes in relative position of body segments that move the center of gravity closer to the head will bring the centers closer together. Raising the arms overhead in line with the trunk would do so as would flexing the knees. For floating, the head, as well as all other body segments, should be resting in the water. The center of buoyancy of a body is also a factor in flotation.

Since muscle is heavier than fat, clearly a heavily muscled person will sink lower in the water than will a fatter person of the same size. This difference in body composition determines the extent of immersion in the water.

FORCES ACTING DURING LOCOMOTION IN WATER

Resisting forces. As the body moves through water, its progress is resisted by this medium. Karpovich states that, as investigations on plane and ship models have shown, this resistance consists mainly of three factors: skin resistance, eddy resistance, and wave-making, or frontal, resistance. The opposing force of frontal resistance is the greatest of these. Also it has been found that a looser-fitting suit offers more resistance than does a tighter-fitting suit. In observing the drag, Karpovich found less resistance in the prone position than in gliding on the back. This finding has been disputed by some. Counsilman found that the prone position offers less resistance than does the side position and that, if the body is rolled

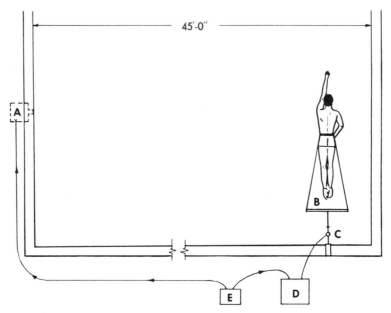

Fig. 15-32. Diagrammatic representation of a situation used in measuring the force exerted by a swimmer. **A,** Camera; **B,** tethering apparatus attached to swimmer's waist and to strain gauge, **C; D,** force is amplified before reaching recording device, **E.** (Courtesy Pennsylvania State Biomechanics Laboratory.)

by an external force, the resistance increases and is still greater with a self-rolling position. However, all top swimmers roll their bodies to some extent. There evidently are advantages to the roll that are greater than those lost through resistance. Among them are the following: (1) the arm is closer to the line of the body rather than to the side, and, consequently, its pull is more effective; (2) the recovery of the arm is facilitated; and (3) the breathing position is improved. Because of the body roll often the legs cross as the kick is executed. This allows the opposite arm and foot to work together. The feet kick "down and out" to counteract the effect of the one-arm recovery in a cycle (Fig. 15-32).

A crossover kick may be due to a lack of good shoulder mobility that causes the swimmer to scythe (cut across at an angle) with the arms, rather than lifting them over the water with a high elbow. This high-elbow position shortens the radius of rotation and improves efficiency in the expenditure of mechanical energy.

In observing the effect of the speed of the body on resistance, Alley found that, when the body is in the prone position, resistance increased up to approximately 2 feet per second. At speeds between 2 and 5 feet per second, the lower limbs were lifted toward the body line. This action, of course, decreased the resistance. When the speed reached 6 feet per second, a noticeable bow wave added to the resistance. These observations were made while dragging the body

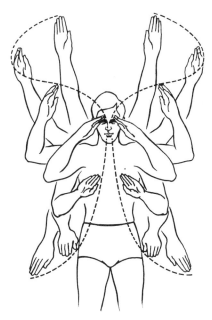

Fig. 15-33. Swimmer using free style. Effective force is demonstrated as this champion swimmer continually moves his hands to stimulate an airfoil to maintain laminar flow. This is an application of Bernoulli's principle of the airfoil. (Modified from Counsilman, J. E.: The science of swimming, Englewood Cliffs, N.J., 1968, Prentice-Hall, Inc.; drawn by Paul Hutinger.)

through the water without changing limb positions. During swimming further resistance will be caused by the arms and legs. The limbs not only increase the cross section of the body surface but also in the recovery, strokes may move against the water in a direction opposite to that of the propelling push.

Propelling forces. The aim of a good swimmer should be to push a large amount of water a short distance because of Bernoulli's law, since water is a liquid and will move quickly away from the applied force. This is why good swimmers constantly are pitching their hands to find "new" water, so as to continue to apply a force directly backward. Whatever the stroke the propelling push against the water is made by the arms, the hands, and the feet. The latter two, which are at the end of the levers of the upper and lower limbs, should be held at an angle that will provide the greatest push against the water. In arm strokes the hand position with reference to the arm can be changed as the arm moves, so that the hand is kept pushing directly backward with a sculslinglike action, which helps the swimmer to apply a constant force against the water (Fig. 15-33). The foot position with reference to the leg can also be varied, but this coordination is more difficult. A frequent observation is that many beginners in executing the flutter kick without the arm stroke will move backward instead of forward. The difference in direction of movement of the body in the water results from the position of the foot with reference to the leg. As Cureton has shown, the foot

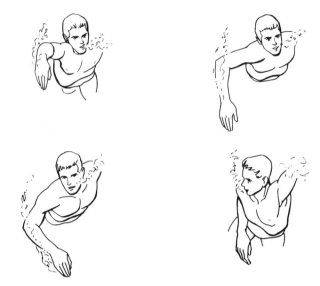

Fig. 15-34. Crawl stroke.

position can be such that it pushes backward on the downstroke as well as on the upstroke. As the hand and foot apply force, the resistance arm of the lever comprises the entire limb, and the fulcrum is at the shoulder or the hip joint. The distal segment, the foot in particular, can provide another lever, in this case acting at the ankle joint.

Because the hand can so readily be placed in a position to apply maximum force, it is to be expected that its contribution to forward movement will be greater than that of the foot. In fact, the feet exert little push in long-distance swimming. Karpovich found that in the crawl stroke good swimmers derived 70% of the push from the arms and 30% from the legs. Poor swimmers derived 77% from the arms. In the breaststroke, however, the legs are effective; it has been said that they contribute as much as 50% of the propelling force. In the crawl stroke the hand is more effective if the elbow is flexed (Fig. 15-34). In this position the moment arm (distance between the shoulder and the hand) is shortened, and the shoulder muscles are more effective; in addition, the application of force is closer to the body and will have less sideward effect.

The roles of lift and drag as applied to bodies moving through water have been discussed by Brown and Counsilman and by Farell; they have related their concepts to swimming. Brown and Counsilman contend that the best swimmers make better use of lift and that lift is one of the most important factors in creating a champion swimmer.

Scheuchenzuber found the following in his study:

1. Taller swimmers seemed to perform at a top level more often than did shorter swimmers.

2. Swimmers with greater palmar area were superior to those with less.

3. The greatest depth of the swimmers' fingertips was reached prior to their arms' reaching a position perpendicular to the longitudinal axis of the body.

4. The mean peak force of the palmar-dorsal pressure was found to occur after 54.7% of the total time of the stroke had elapsed, commencing with the entry of the hand into the water.

5. Superior swimmers exhibited greater hydrodynamic lift in their movements than did less capable ones, but all subjects used this principle to some extent.

SUGGESTED READINGS

Cooper, J. M.: Kinesiology of the high jump, Biomechanics I, First International Seminar, Zurich, 1967.

Counsilman, J. E.: The science of swimming, Englewood Cliffs, N.J., 1968, Prentice-Hall, Inc.

Counsilman, J. E.: The application of Bernoulli's principle to human propulsion in water, Bloomington, Ind., 1971, Indiana University Press.

Hildebrand, M.: How animals run, Sci. Am. **202**:148, May, 1960.

Howell, A. B.: Speed in animals, Chicago, 1944, University of Chicago Press.

Morton, D. J., and Fuller, D. D.: Human locomotion and body form, Baltimore, 1952, The Williams & Wilkins Co.

Scheuchenzuber, H. J., Jr.: Kinetic and kinematic characteristics in the performance of tethered and non-tethered swimming of the front crawl arm stroke, unpublished doctoral dissertation, Indiana University, Aug., 1974.

See Bibliography for additional references.

STOPPING
MOVING
OBJECTS

CHAPTER 16 Catching, falling, and landing

MECHANICS OF STOPPING MOVING OBJECTS

Among the variety of motor skills that human beings perform is the ability to stop a moving object. The object may be external, such as a ball, or it may be the performer's own body, as in landing from a height. The pattern of joint actions varies with the situation, but in all situations the mechanical principles are the same. If the stop is skillfully made, the momentum of the moving object is decreased gradually by joint actions. These actions are such that the object is permitted to continue its motion as its velocity is gradually decreased. If the object is contacted with the hands and the arms are out to meet it, the joint actions are those of a pulling pattern, usually extension of the upper arm and flexion of the forearm. Although the joint actions in pulling and stopping are the same, the source of energy differs. The momentum of the oncoming object moves the segments in the direction in which the object was moving; at the same time muscular effort resists that motion. As the upper arm is extended by the force of the object, the shoulder flexors resist; as the forearm is flexed, the elbow extensors resist. In pulling, the object to be moved resists while shoulder extensors and elbow flexors contract. Likewise when the body lands from a height, the momentum of the center of gravity tends to flex ankle, knee, and hip joints. These actions are resisted by the extensor muscles at the joints.

The common skills used to stop moving objects are catching, falling, and landing from a height or after a projection of the body.

CATCHING

Catching is the act of reducing the momentum of an object in flight to the point of zero or near zero velocity and retaining possession of it at least momentarily. This is accomplished by use of the hands, body, feet, and auxiliary pieces of equipment. The momentum of the object is transferred to that of the receiving mechanism. When an object is light in weight and traveling slowly, a human being can easily stop it. However, if the object is heavy or is traveling at great speed or both, the transfer of momentum must be gradual to prevent injury to the hands or other parts of the body and for the receiver to control the object once in possession of it.

When one part or parts of the body, such as the hands, are held rigid at the

276

moment that a fast-moving object comes in contact with it, the part must absorb the full force of the impact. In sports the momentum of an object being caught is decreased by increasing the distance at which it is caught; this process is known as *giving,* or *recoiling,* with the object until it is traveling slowly enough to be controlled accurately.

If the object to be caught is heavy, such as a large medicine ball, or is traveling unusually fast, such as a fast ball thrown by a baseball pitcher, to dissipate its momentum over a long distance may be difficult and will take more time than can be allowed during the process of playing a particular game. The more practical procedure is to increase the mass (inertia) of the stopping mechanism and decrease the distance over which it travels. For example, the baseball catcher dissipates the momentum of the ball thrown by the pitcher by placing the body directly in front of the path of the oncoming ball. He assumes a stance whereby the feet are placed in a stride position with the knees bent and center of gravity low; this is the best posture to recoil from the force (momentum of the ball), and at the same time it offers as much of the body to absorb the momentum of the ball as possible.

The receiver must be careful not to make unnecessary body motions when running to receive an object. Unnecessary up-and-down movements (raising and lowering the center of gravity and thereby moving the head and eyes up and down through a vertical plane) may cause the receiver to lose track of the path of flight of the object. Outstretching the arms (shoulder flexion and elbow extension) while running may cause the receiver to slow down because he is not using the arms properly in the run and also is projecting the center of gravity too far forward. It also may tense the arms and cause him to drop the ball.

A ball is not caught with the fingers; rather it is received first against the middle of the palm of the hand (made into the form of a cup), and then the fingers close around it, preventing it from escaping (Fig. 16-1). If it is caught against the rigid heel of the hand, it likely would rebound too quickly from the hand to be caught and could cause injury to the hand.

The effective catcher (receiver in any sport or endeavor) has loose, flexible hands to catch the object and to dissipate its momentum gradually. Correct body posture is also essential. Placing the hands in the best possible position is another requirement for success. For example, a ball traveling in flight at a height below the waist is caught with the fingers pointing downward. In all instances the hands are placed so that they have a basketlike quality. Seldom does a good performer not make use of two hands, even though the actual catch is made with one hand. The object (such as a ball) may rebound out of one hand if the momentum is not properly dissipated. The use of both hands aids in trapping the object.

Large objects thrown with great speed, such as a football (which is also thrown with a spin), are caught and then quickly cradled (Fig. 16-2); that is, the receiver pins the football against the body as soon as possible to prevent its escape because of the reaction. If the arms do not have to be extended fully for the catch, the receiver, in this instance, should not do so. In the flexed position

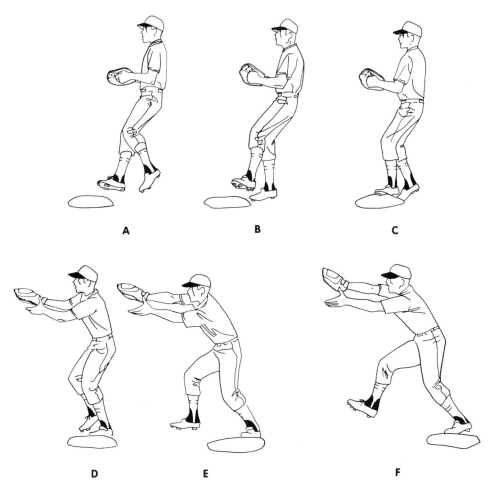

Fig. 16-1. First baseman moving to contact base and reaching to meet ball; as the ball is drawn toward the body, its momentum is dissipated.

the arm muscles can withstand the force of the impact and more easily cradle the ball. Although it is large, a basketball is round and usually traveling at less speed than a football; consequently, this object may be caught by the hands alone. In baseball the first baseman moves the arms from shoulder extension flexion and from elbow flexion to extension. The legs are in a flexed position to help stabilize the body. (See Fig. 16-1.) The objective is to dissipate the momentum of the ball over as long a distance as possible. (The ball, of course, travels a shorter distance to the first baseman if the elbows are extended.) A glove is used to augment the catching surface and to protect the hand by attenuating the blow.

The momentum gained during the catch may be used in starting the next movement. If the next action is to be a throw, the ball is drawn back during the

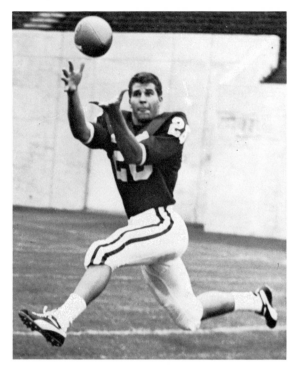

Fig. 16-2. Catching a football.

catch in preparation for throwing. Whenever possible the receiver should move the body into position for the next action as the catch is made to reduce still further the time required for the complete movement. Also the momentum of the body and the reconverted momentum of the ball (since it seldom comes to a complete rest but usually continues in a small angular path as the arm is moved to throw) may be used in moving the ball in the new direction.

FALLING

Falling done properly involves a gradual reduction in the momentum of the body when it comes in contact with the floor, ground, or other surface.

Principles and techniques of protection in falling. Four general principles and techniques of protection in falling may be listed. *First* is the sit-down-and-roll technique. The center of gravity is lowered, and the action in falling is such that the weight of the body is distributed over a large area. If the fall is vertical, the momentum should be transferred from the vertical to the horizontal as soon as possible to reduce the force of the fall. The *second* technique is to protect the bony projections of the body and to employ the fleshy parts as striking surfaces. The *third* principle is that extended levers offer a greater potential range of motion that do flexed ones. Therefore when the legs or arms strike the surface in falling, they should be prepared for the contact by being placed in extension. The force of the fall can be taken up then by a gradual flexion of the legs or arms. The *fourth* technique is during a fall in which the landing is made on the feet to maneuver to bring the center of body weight near a position above the feet to utilize the shock-absorbing action of the ankles, knees, and hips.

The recovery from a stumble is mainly reflexive. Both the righting reflex and equilibrium reactions (built-in) are activated. As the toe trips over an obstacle and the body starts to fall forward, reflex and equilibrium reactions set in. Normally the head and trunk are extended to counteract the forward momentum. The shoulders are often abducted to assist in regaining balance.

If a person starts to fall to the right side, for example, he usually elevates and abducts the shoulder and extends the elbows (with arms out to the sides). The body is shifted to the left to help check the momentum to the right. The side of the buttocks is offered as the landing surface. The legs are flexed to decrease the force of the blow and to lower the center of gravity so that the distance of the fall is reduced. A rotation of the trunk may take place so that the momentum of the fall is dissipated in two directions—opposite and to the rear. Protective extension of the arms is often used to help dissipate the momentum of the fall.

LANDING

Landing is a type of fall that enables the performer to strike a surface without incurring injury to the body parts if possible. In the act of landing in the long jump (Fig. 16-3) the jumper wants to land not only so as to dissipate

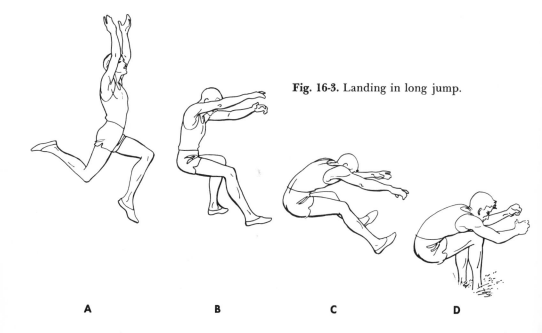

Fig. 16-3. Landing in long jump.

A   B   C   D gradually the force of the ground reacting against him but also so that the feet strike the pit at the farthest distance possible from the takeoff board. As he prepares to land, the jumper flexes the hips to add to the distance (Fig. 16-3, *C*). Just before landing, the knees must flex to bring the feet to a contact position that will gain as much distance as possible and that, although ahead of the body's center of gravity, will not be so far ahead that the body will fall backward. The desired forward movement will be facilitated by hip flexion and continued knee flexion on landing. These actions lower the center of gravity and thus shorten the distance between it and the ankle joint, which will be the axis as the body moves forward by rotating around the base. During flight the body had a forward, as well as a downward, momentum, and the forward one now provides the force for the body rotation. The hip flexion, by moving the trunk forward, also aids at landing by moving the center of gravity forward. (See Bedi on somersault style.)

SUGGESTED READINGS

Bedi, J. F.: Angular momentum in the long jump, unpublished doctoral dissertation, Indiana University, May, 1975.

Broer, M. R.: Efficiency of human movement, Philadelphia, 1966, W. B. Saunders Co.

Bunn, J. W.: Scientific principles of coaching, Englewood Cliffs, N. J., 1955, Prentice-Hall, Inc.

See Bibliography for additional references.

PART IV General information

CHAPTER 17 Projections

PROJECTILES

Projection of an object or of oneself is the outcome—the product—of many motor skills. Since the velocity and the angle of projection imparted to the projectile by the performer determine the degree of skill, the instructor who can measure them has a device that can profitably be added to instructional procedures. For example, if greater velocity is desired, changes in joint action can be suggested. If velocity is measured before and after the changes have been made, the instructor can evaluate suggestions and the learner has had the opportunity to experience the effect of some lever action, thereby adding to understanding of body mechanics.

Since air resistance is negligible when the body projects itself and when it projects many objects, the path of flight of these projectiles is determined by two forces: the force imparted by body levers and the force of gravity. If the time of flight is known, the effect of gravity can be determined. The following discussion applies only to those projections for which air resistance is neglible; it does not apply to projectiles such as the javelin, discus, badminton bird, or balls that are spinning rapidly.

Effect of gravity

The effect of gravity on unsupported objects is the same regardless of the weight of the object. The constant acceleration of gravitational force pulls the object downward a distance that equals in feet 16.1 t^2, in which t represents the time in seconds during which gravity has been acting on the object. In 1 second an object would be pulled downward 16.1 feet (16.1×1^2); in 0.5 second the distance would be 4.025 feet (16.1×0.5^2). If the velocity and direction imparted by body levers are known, the path of flight can be determined. In Fig. 17-1 the horizontal line represents the projection of an object by means of force imparted by the body, a velocity of 80 feet per second in a horizontal direction. Each dot represents an additional 8 feet in flight and also an additional 0.1 second of time. The effect of gravity at each time interval is represented by the vertical lines. The lower ends of the vertical lines mark the path of flight resulting from the two forces. The path of flight can be determined in like manner whenever the velocity and direction imparted by body force to an object are known.

285

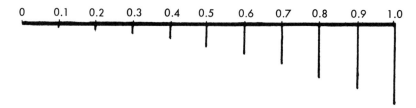

Fig. 17-1. Gravitational effect at each 0.1 second on an object projected horizontally at 80 feet per second. Each 0.4 inch represents 8 feet.

Determination of velocity and angle

When the body projects itself or an object, neither the velocity nor the angle of projection is known. However, information can be obtained in such situations, and with this information velocity and angle can be determined. The needed items of information are (1) the starting point of flight, (2) the end point in its relation to the start—that is, the horizontal distance from the starting point and the vertical distance between the two points—and (3) the time of flight.

Velocity. If a ball resting on the ground (starting point) were kicked and landed 80 feet from the starting point (horizontal distance 80 feet, vertical distance 0 feet) in 2.1 seconds (time), the effect of gravity during this time would be 71.001 feet (16.1 × 2.1²). Had gravity not pulled the ball downward, it would then have been 71 feet above the landing point. The horizontal distance, 80 feet, and the vertical line, 71 feet, form two sides of a right-angled triangle. The path that the ball would travel had gravity not pulled it down is that connecting the starting point and the upper end of the 71-foot vertical, the hypotenuse of the triangle. Its length is the square root of the sum of the squares of the sides (80² + 71²), or 107 feet, the distance that the ball would have been projected by the force imparted by the body. This is 50.9 feet per second (107 ÷ 2.1).

Had the ball landed on a downslope 20 feet below the starting point and had the horizontal distance and the time been the same, the calculations would differ. The vertical line of gravitational force would be the same length, but the lines of the triangle would be 80 feet horizontally and 51 feet vertically (71 − 20). The length of the hypotenuse in this case would be the square root of the 51² + 80², 94.87 feet, and the velocity 45.18 feet. Had the ball hit a wall at a height 20 feet above the starting point and 80 feet away from it in the same time, the vertical line completing the triangle would be 91 feet in length (71 + 20), the hypotenuse 121.16 feet, and the velocity 57.69 feet per second. These examples show that the measure of the horizontal distance of a throw or a jump is not a valid measure of the force exerted by the body levers.

Other mathematic calculations can be used to determine the length of the hypotenuse, and they are presented in the next paragraph.

Angle. Once the horizontal and the vertical distance of the triangle have been determined, the angle of projection can be found by calculation and reference to the values of natural trigonometric functions. The vertical length of the triangle divided by the horizontal length is the value for the tangent. In the first illustration 71 ÷ 80 = 0.8875, the tangent of an angle of 41° 35′; the downslope tangent value is 0.6375, and the angle is 32° 31′; in the third situation the tangent value is 1.1375, and the angle is 48° 41′.

• • •

With trigonmetric relationships the measures of angles and velocities can be obtained in many ways; those which require the least calculation can be used. As one example the angles of projection might have been determined before the velocities. When the angle is known, another trigonometric value might be used to determine the length of the hypotenuse, which is equal to the length of the vertical side divided by the sine of the angle. In the first of the situations the sine of an angle of 41° 35′ is 0.6637: 71 ÷ 0.6637 = 107. In the downslope the angle was 32° 31′; the sine value is 0.5375, and 51 ÷ 0.5375 = 94.8. In the last situation the sine value is 0.751, and 91 ÷ 0.751 = 121.

In teaching situations in which velocities of projections are measured frequently, instructors have prepared tables that give the velocity and angle for specific distance and time measures. These measurements are usually based on a given vertical height, and although not accurate to a fine degree they are sufficiently so to measure individual progress and to determine group averages.

Although velocity can be measured satisfactorily for most class situations, investigators often want a method of measurement that will be accurate to a finer degree. Research needs frequently promote the development of new devices. The need for a precise measure of the velocity of projectiles led to the development of the velocimeter shown in Fig. 17-2, which records the time during which a projectile travels 1 meter horizontally. This instrument is easily portable and can be set up in less than 5 minutes without tools. As shown in Fig. 17-2, *B,* it can be used indoors; it is equally efficient out of doors in full daylight. The large area between the stands supporting the valance enables it to be used to measure a variety of throwing and kicking skills and the velocity of batted balls, such as those used in tennis, golf, and baseball.

Location of high point of flight

If an object is projected horizontally or downward, the highest point of its flight will be the starting point. If it is projected upward, gravity will immediately decrease vertical velocity, and the high point will be reached when the downward velocity imparted by gravity is equal to that of the upward velocity imparted by the body. The velocity caused by gravitational force is always 32.2 t (the time value in seconds). Thus the high point is reached when vertical velocity − 32.2 t = 0. The time to the high point is vertical velocity ÷ 32.2.

In the first situation in kicking (p. 286), the velocity was 50.9 feet per second, and the angle was 41° 35′. It is now convenient to consider this velocity as the hypotenuse of a triangle. It has a vertical and a horizontal component. The vertical component is the hypotenuse times the sine of the angle—in this case 50.9 × 0.6637 = 33.78. The high point will be reached when t = 33.78 ÷ 32.2, or

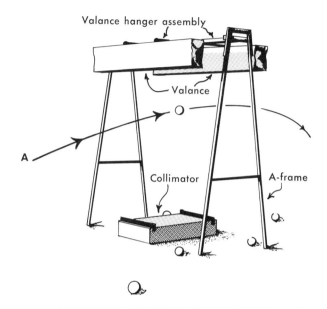

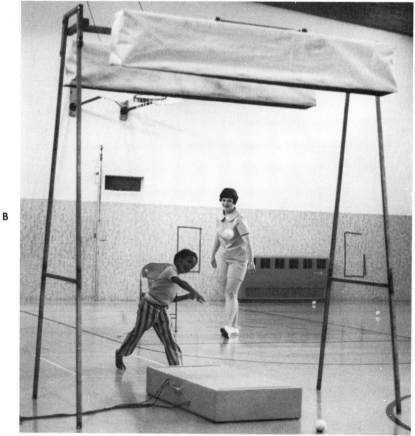

Fig. 17-2. A, Velocimeter, a device to measure precise horizontal velocity of projectiles. **B,** Velocimeter used indoors to measure the velocity of a ball thrown by a child. (Courtesy Kinesiology Research Laboratories, University of Wisconsin.)

1.049 + . The time for total flight was 2.1 seconds, and the high point is reached midway in flight. This will always be the case when the vertical distance between the beginning and end of flight is zero.

When the vertical distance between the beginning and end of flight is not zero, the time to the high point will not be half the flight time. In the downslope situation, the vertical component of the velocity imparted by the body is 0.5375 × 45.2 = 24.29 feet per second. The time to the high point is 24.9 ÷ 32.2 = 0.754 second. In this situation the drop after the high point continues after the level of the starting point is reached. In the third situation the vertical component of velocity is 0.751 × 57.69 = 43.32 feet per second. The time to the high point is 43.32 ÷ 32.2 = 1.345 seconds. Here the drop does not reach the level of the starting point.

The horizontal distance to the high point can be calculated with the cosine value of the velocity imparted by the ball. The distance from the starting point will be the horizontal component of the velocity multiplied by the time to the high point. When the projection velocity in each of the three kicking situations is multiplied by the cosines of the angles, the horizontal components are as follows:

1. (Cosine 0.7479) × 50.9 = 38.068 feet per second
2. (Cosine 0.8432) × 45.2 = 38.112 feet per second
3. (Cosine 0.6602) × 57.69 = 38.086 feet per second

The horizontal distance to the high point in each case is as follows:

1. 38.068 × 1.05 (time to high point) = 39.97 feet
2. 38.112 × 0.754 (time to high point) = 28.74 feet
3. 38.086 × 1.345 (time to high point) = 51.23 feet

If the exact height of the high point is desired, it is obtained by multiplying the vertical velocity by the time to the high point and subtracting from the product, the 16.1 t^2 value for this time.

The processes described can be used to determine the position of the projectile at any time in its flight. When the projection has a downward component, the 16.1 t^2 value is added, instead of subtracted, in determining the height, and the resulting sum would be subtracted from the starting height.

Knowledge of velocity, angle, and position at any time in flight can be applied to many situations and will enable the instructor to set specific goals for development of skill in a given situation. One illustration is that of developing skill in a tennis serve. Most beginners are likely to direct the ball upward; yet a velocity of 80 to 90 feet per second can be achieved by the average adult. Suppose that the height at which the ball is impacted is 8 feet and the ball has a velocity of 80 feet per second. The net is approximately 40 feet from the impact, and the ball would reach it in 0.5 second. The 16.1 t^2 value for this time is 4.025 feet, so that, as the ball reaches the net, it would be 3.975 feet above the ground, thus clearing the net by 0.975 foot. The ball would reach the ground when the 16.1 t^2 value was 8 feet; $8 = 16.1\ t^2$; $t^2 = \dfrac{8}{16.1} = 0.4969$; $t = 0.704$ second. The horizontal distance would be 80 × 0.704 = 56.32 feet, which is well within the service court.

Angle, velocity, and ball position have been applied by Mortimer in determining the projection most likely to make a basket from the free throw line when the starting point is 5 feet above the floor. She recommends a velocity of 24 feet per second and an angle of 58 degrees.

OPTIMUM PROJECTION ANGLE FOR GREATEST DISTANCE

A projection angle of 45 degrees is often recommended as the optimum when the greatest possible distance is desired. This is true only when the vertical distance between the starting point and the end of the flight is zero. Bunn has shown this in discussing the projection of the shot put.

When the vertical distance between the start and the end of flight and the velocity of projection are known, the angle that results in the greatest distance is one in which the following applies:

$$\text{Sine}^2 = \frac{\text{Velocity}^2}{2 \ (\text{velocity}^2 - gh)}$$

In this formula, g is 32.2, and h is the vertical distance between the start and end of flight. If the start is higher than the end, h will be a minus quantity.

Bunn gives a table of the distances that the shot put would reach if projected at angles from 37 through 44 degrees when released at a height of 7 feet at velocities from 20 to 50 feet per second. If the shot were given a velocity of 30 feet per second, the determination of the optimum angle would be as follows:

$$\text{Sine}^2 = \frac{30^2}{2 \ [30^2 - (32.2 \times -7)]}$$

In this case the end of the flight is below the starting point, and h has a minus value.

$$\text{Sine}^2 = \frac{900}{2 \ (900 + 225.4)}$$

$$\text{Sine}^2 = \frac{900}{2250.8} = 0.39985$$

In this case the sine = 0.6323, which is the value for an angle of 39° 13′. For a 39-degree angle and for a 40-degree angle Bunn's table gives a distance of 34.42 feet, the longest for the angles included in his table.

In jumping for distance the center of gravity is higher at the beginning of flight than it is at landing. At the beginning of flight the body is extended, the arms are raised, and in an adult 6 feet tall, the height of the center of gravity can be estimated as 3 plus feet. If the landing is made with the thighs horizontal and some inclination of the legs, it will be assumed for this illustration that the center of gravity is 1.5 feet lower than it was at the beginning of flight. If the velocity of projection is 16 feet per second, the optimum angle for greatest distance will be one in which the following applies:

$$\text{Sine}^2 = \frac{16^2}{2\,[16^2 - (32.2 \times -1.5)]}$$

$$\text{Sine}^2 = 0.4206$$

In this case the sine = 0.6485. This is the value for an angle of 40° 26′.

If the velocity is 12 feet per second and the other measures remain the same, the optimum angle is 37° 43′. If the positions of the center of gravity are determined at the beginning and end of flight, as they can be from film, the value of h can be more accurately determined. The velocity of the center of gravity can also be determined from these film measures (Chapter 7). In calculating the angle of projection in better-than-average performers we have found that this angle is less than 45 degrees; this is another example of the body's making necessary adjustments without the person's being aware that it is doing so.

SUMMARY OF CALCULATIONS

For ready reference the calculations discussed in this chapter and others that are related and useful are summarized here.

Range is the horizontal distance between the starting and landing point; time means the time in flight.

1. Horizontal velocity = Range ÷ Time.
2. In determining vertical velocity (V. vel.) consideration must be given to the vertical distance (VD) between the starting and the landing point. When VD is 0:
   V. vel. = 16.1 t² ÷ Time
3. When the starting point is higher than the landing point:
   V. vel. = (16.1 t² − VD) ÷ Time

Note that, if 16.1 t² is less than VD, the minus quantity indicates that the projection is below the horizontal.

4. When the starting point is lower than the landing point:
   V. vel. = (16.1 t² + VD) ÷ Time
5. For the projection velocity (Proj. vel.):
   a. When the horizontal velocity (Horiz. vel.) and vertical velocity components are known:
      (Proj. vel.)² = (Horiz. vel.)² + (V. vel.)²
   b. When the angle of projection is known:
      Proj. vel. = V. vel. ÷ Sine, or
      Proj. vel. = Horiz. vel. ÷ Cosine.
6. The angle of projection can be determined by use of trigonometric relationships.
   For the angle of projection:
   a. Tangent of the angle = V. vel. ÷ Horiz. vel.
   b. Sine of the angle = V. vel. ÷ Proj. vel.
   c. Cosine of the angle = Horiz. vel. ÷ Proj. vel.

7. The high point (h.p.) of the projection can be located by finding first the time to the high point.
   Time to high point = V. vel. ÷ 32.2
8. The distance of the high point above the starting point = (V. vel. × Time to h.p.) − 16.1 (time to h.p.)²
9. The horizontal distance from the starting to the high point = Horiz. vel. × time h.p.

The relationships used in finding the high point can be used to locate the projectile at any time and at any point in flight. For example, a tennis ball was projected from a height of 7 feet and 40 feet from the net at a velocity of 50 feet per second and at an angle of 10 degrees above the horizontal. Where was the ball when it reached the net? The horizontal and vertical velocity components must be known. They can be found by rearranging the equations in 5b:

V. vel. = Proj. vel. × Sine
Horiz. vel. = Proj. vel. × Cosine

For an angle of 10 degrees the sine is 0.173; the cosine is 0.984. In the described tennis situation the numerical values are as follows:

V. vel. = 50 × 0.173, or 8.65 feet per second
Horiz. vel. = 50 × 0.984, or 49.2 feet per second

Following is the time to the net:

40 ÷ 49.2, or 0.81 second

During this time the vertical velocity has moved the ball upward; gravitational force has moved it downward. The combined effect will be as follows:

(8.65 × 0.81) − 16.1 (0.81)²
7.00 − 10.573, or 3,573 feet

At the time that the ball reaches the net it will be 3.573 lower than the starting point, or 3.427 feet above the ground and 0.427 foot above the net, which is 3 feet in height.

The question might also arise as to where the ball would be at a given time, such as 0.5 second after the flight began. From the starting point it would travel horizontally as follows:

49.2 × 0.5, or 24.6 feet

Vertically it would travel as follows:

(8.65 × 0.5) − 16.1 (0.5)²
4.325 − 4.025, or 0.3 foot

In 0.5 second the ball would be 0.3 foot higher than, and 24.6 feet from, the starting point.

REFERENCE TABLES

For the convenience of persons who determine projection velocity and angle, two tables are included here. Table 17-1 gives the values of four trigonometric

Table 17-1. Natural trigonometric functions*

Degrees	Sine	Tangent	Cotangent	Cosine	Degrees
0	0.0000	0.0000	—	1.000	90
1	0.0174	0.0174	57.29	0.9998	89
2	0.0349	0.0349	28.63	0.9993	88
3	0.0523	0.0524	19.08	0.9986	87
4	0.0697	0.0699	14.30	0.9975	86
5	0.0871	0.0874	11.43	0.9961	85
6	0.1045	0.1051	9.514	0.9945	84
7	0.1218	0.1227	8.144	0.9925	83
8	0.1391	0.1405	7.115	0.9902	82
9	0.1564	0.1583	6.313	0.9876	81
10	0.1736	0.1763	5.671	0.9848	80
11	0.1908	0.1943	5.144	0.9816	79
12	0.2079	0.2125	4.704	0.9781	78
13	0.2249	0.2308	4.331	0.9743	77
14	0.2419	0.2493	4.010	0.9703	76
15	0.2588	0.2679	3.732	0.9659	75
16	0.2756	0.2867	3.487	0.9612	74
17	0.2923	0.3057	3.270	0.9563	73
18	0.3090	0.3249	3.077	0.9510	72
19	0.3255	0.3443	2.904	0.9455	71
20	0.3420	0.3639	2.747	0.9396	70
21	0.3583	0.3838	2.605	0.9335	69
22	0.3746	0.4040	2.475	0.9271	68
23	0.3907	0.4244	2.355	0.9205	67
24	0.4067	0.4452	2.246	0.9135	66
25	0.4226	0.4663	2.144	0.9063	65
26	0.4383	0.4877	2.050	0.8987	64
27	0.4539	0.5095	1.962	0.8910	63
28	0.4694	0.5317	1.880	0.8829	62
29	0.4848	0.5543	1.804	0.8746	61
30	0.5000	0.5773	1.732	0.8660	60
31	0.5150	0.6008	1.664	0.8571	59
32	0.5299	0.6248	1.600	0.8480	58
33	0.5446	0.6494	1.539	0.8386	57
34	0.5591	0.6745	1.482	0.8290	56
35	0.5735	0.7002	1.428	0.8191	55
36	0.5877	0.7265	1.376	0.8090	54
37	0.6018	0.7535	1.327	0.7986	53
38	0.6156	0.7812	1.279	0.7880	52
39	0.6293	0.8097	1.234	0.7771	51
40	0.6427	0.8391	1.191	0.7660	50
41	0.6560	0.8692	1.150	0.7547	49
42	0.6691	0.9004	1.110	0.7431	48
43	0.6820	0.9325	1.072	0.7313	47
44	0.6946	0.9656	1.035	0.7193	46
45	0.7071	1.000	1.000	0.7071	45
Degrees	**Cosine**	**Cotangent**	**Tangent**	**Sine**	**Degrees**

*For degree values at the left use headings at the top of the table; for degree values at the right refer to the bottom of the table.

Table 17-2. Gravity distance*

Time	0.00	0.01	0.02	0.03	0.04	0.05	0.06	0.07	0.08	0.09
0.0	0.000	0.001	0.006	0.014	0.025	0.040	0.057	0.078	0.013	0.13
0.1	0.161	0.194	0.231	0.272	0.315	0.362	0.412	0.465	0.521	0.58
0.2	0.644	0.710	0.779	0.851	0.927	1.006	1.088	1.173	1.262	1.35
0.3	1.449	1.547	1.648	1.745	1.861	1.972	2.086	2.204	2.324	2.44
0.4	2.576	2.706	2.840	2.976	3.116	3.260	3.387	3.556	3.709	3.86
0.5	4.025	4.187	4.353	4.524	4.694	4.870	5.048	5.230	5.416	5.60
0.6	5.796	5.980	6.188	6.290	6.584	6.802	7.014	7.227	7.444	7.66
0.7	7.889	8.116	8.346	8.579	8.816	9.056	9.299	9.545	9.795	10.04
0.8	10.304	10.573	10.825	11.091	11.360	11.632	11.970	12.186	12.468	12.75
0.9	13.041	13.332	13.627	13.925	14.226	14.530	14.838	15.148	15.462	15.77
1.0	16.100	16.432	16.750	17.080	17.414	17.750	18.090	18.433	18.779	19.12
1.1	19.481	19.837	20.196	20.558	20.923	21.292	21.664	22.039	22.417	22.79
1.2	23.184	23.602	23.963	24.357	24.755	25.156	25.560	25.967	26.378	26.79
1.3	27.209	27.629	28.052	28.469	28.899	29.342	29.778	30.208	30.660	31.10
1.4	31.556	32.008	32.464	32.922	33.384	33.850	34.318	34.790	35.265	35.74
1.5	36.225	36.709	37.197	37.688	38.172	38.680	39.180	39.684	40.192	40.70
1.6	41.216	41.732	42.252	42.776	43.307	43.832	44.365	44.901	45.440	45.98
1.7	46.529	47.078	47.630	48.187	48.745	49.306	49.861	50.439	51.011	51.58

t									
1.8	52.164	52.745	53.329	53.917	54.508	55.102	55.660	56.310	56.903	57.51
1.9	58.121	58.734	59.361	59.907	60.593	61.220	61.849	62.482	63.118	63.75
2.0	64.400	65.046	65.644	66.346	67.002	67.960	68.322	68.987	69.206	70.326
2.1	71.001	71.679	72.360	73.044	73.732	74.422	75.116	75.813	76.514	77.217
2.2	77.924	78.634	79.347	80.064	80.783	81.566	82.232	82.962	83.694	84.430
2.3	85.169	85.911	86.657	87.405	88.157	88.912	89.671	90.432	91.197	91.965
2.4	92.736	93.510	94.288	95.069	95.854	96.640	97.431	98.224	99.021	99.823
2.5	100.625	101.432	102.341	103.054	103.871	104.690	105.503	106.339	107.168	108.000
2.6	108.836	109.675	110.517	111.362	112.211	113.262	113.917	114.780	115.637	116.502
2.7	117.369	118.240	119.114	119.992	120.872	121.756	122.643	123.534	124.437	125.024
2.8	126.224	127.127	128.034	128.943	129.856	130.772	131.692	132.614	133.540	134.469
2.9	135.401	136.336	137.275	138.217	139.162	140.110	141.062	142.016	142.974	143.936
3.0	144.900	145.868	146.828	147.802	148.790	149.770	150.754	151.781	152.731	153.724
3.1	154.721	155.721	156.724	157.730	158.740	159.752	160.768	161.787	162.810	163.835
3.2	164.864	165.896	166.931	167.970	169.021	170.056	171.104	172.157	173.210	174.268
3.3	175.168	176.393	177.480	178.531	179.605	180.682	181.763	182.846	183.933	185.023
3.4	186.116	187.212	188.312	189.415	190.521	191.630	192.742	193.858	194.977	196.100
3.5	197.125	198.354	199.585	200.620	201.759	202.901	204.045	205.193	206.344	207.498
3.6	208.656	209.817	210.981	212.148	213.319	214.492	215.669	216.849	218.033	219.219
3.7	220.409	221.602	222.798	223.998	225.200	226.406	227.615	228.828	230.043	231.262
3.8	232.484	233.709	234.938	236.169	237.404	238.642	239.884	241.128	242.376	243.627
3.9	244.881	246.138	247.399	248.663	249.930	251.200	252.474	253.750	255.030	256.314
4.0	257.600									

*Distance in feet through which freely falling objects move in a given time, calculated as distance $= \tfrac{1}{2}g\,t^2$ ($g = 32.2$).

functions for 0 to 90 degrees. Since function values from 90 to 135 are the same as those from 0 to 45 and those from 135 to 180 are the same as those from 45 to 90, the table includes values from 0 to 180 degrees. This covers the range of all projections that a person might make. Table 17-2 gives the distance that gravity will move a freely falling object downward for every 0.01 second from 0 to 4 seconds, a range that includes the flight time of most objects that a person could project.

SUGGESTED READINGS

Mortimer, E. M.: Basketball shooting, Res. Q. Am. Assoc. Health Phys. Educ. 22:234, 1951.
Tricker, R. A. R., and Tricker, B. J. K.: The science of movement, New York, 1967, American Elsevier Publishing Co., Inc.
Verwiebe, F. L.: Does a ball curve? Am. J. Physics 10:119, 1942.

See Bibliography for additional references.

CHAPTER 18 Spin and bounce of balls

The ball is the most frequently used implement in sports. These balls vary in size, shape, mass, and construction. Diameters range from a ½-inch marble to a 10-foot push ball. Practically all balls used in sports are spheres with exception of the football and the lawn bowling ball. Balls vary in mass from the light ping-pong ball to the heavy shot or hammer. Balls are constructed from several types of material such as rubber, leather, wood, celluloid, brass, lead, ivory, glass, agate, clay, and plastic. They may be hollow or solid and may contain substances that vary the weight and reaction of the ball. The cover may be smooth, fuzzy, dimpled, ribbed, or ridged. The ball may be ringed with metal or have holes for gripping. Each separate characteristic affects the manner in which the ball is delivered, the way it passes through space or along a surface, and how it reacts to the objects that it strikes. In addition, the handling of the ball further affects its behavior in space or on the surface and the way that it reacts to the objects with which it comes in contact.

The ball to be used for each game is prescribed by the rules, and, because the characteristics of the ball are fixed the player need not consider the relative merits of balls of different sizes, shapes, and types of construction. The player is concerned only with the action of the ball that has been prescribed for the game that is being played. The action of the ball is affected first by the force and second by the spin applied.

EFFECTS OF THE DIRECTION OF APPLIED FORCE

The force that a performer applies to a ball usually puts the ball in motion. If the force is applied through the center of gravity of the ball, the resulting motion will be linear. The direction of the linear motion may be horizontal or vertical, or it may have vertical and horizontal components. In situations in which the ball is moving through the air, the force of gravity changes the vertical velocity, and the direction of motion becomes curvilinear rather than linear. The effect of gravity on a projectile is discussed in Chapter 17.

EFFECT OF SPIN ON A BALL IN FLIGHT

The manner in which any ball passes through space and reacts to objects depends on the effect of the amount of spin of the ball. A ball thrown with a great deal of spin will move more slowly than another thrown at the same force but with only a slight spin. The reduction in speed because of the great

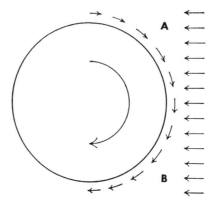

Fig. 18-1. Rapidly spinning ball encounters more resistance at **A** than at **B** and in flight will curve toward **B**.

amount of spin results in a lessening of the force of the ball in flight. The reason that the spin reduces speed is that a spinning ball offers more resistance to the air through which it travels.

A spinning ball seeks the line of least resistance in its flight through the air. A rapidly spinning ball creates a greater friction on one side of the ball than on the other. As a result the flight of the ball is curved. This phenomenon is illustrated in Fig. 18-1. The extent of the curve when various balls are delivered with a common speed and rate of spin depends on the shape and mass of the ball. Light balls, such as ping-pong and tennis balls, curve widely. In heavy ones, such as medicine balls, the curve is too slight to be noticeable. Verwiebe has measured the cure of the baseball by having the pitched ball pass through five screens of fine thread placed at equal intervals between the pitcher's rubber and home plate. By measuring the different points on the screens where the ball passed through, he was able to follow the path of the ball. He found that a baseball could be thrown in a curved path. A slow pitch broke into a curve sooner and wider than a faster pitch. A curve as wide as 6 inches was measured.

The direction and amount of the curve of a thrown ball depends on the direction and amount of spin and the speed of the ball. One thrown with a spin from right to left will curve to the left as it follows the line of least resistance. In golf this is known as a *hook* and is caused when a right-handed golfer strikes the ball with the outside of the clubhead ahead of the inside of the clubhead. In a baseball pitch this is an *outcurve* when pitching to a right-handed batter. The right-handed pitcher delivering an outcurve throws the ball so that the fingers against the right side of the ball twist the ball from right to left.

The ball spinning from left to right will curve toward the right as it follows the line of least resistance. In golf the *slice* is caused by striking the ball with the heel of the clubhead ahead of the outside of the clubhead, imparting a spin to the right. In baseball this is the *incurve* and results from the push of the pitcher's index finger against the left side of the ball.

Top spin causes the ball to fall rapidly. In this case since the line of resistance is in the same direction as the force of gravity, the effect of the spin on the curve is pronounced. A golf ball hit with a top spin drops quickly to the fairway and rolls a considerable distance.

A *backspin,* or undercut, will diminish the rate of falling of the ball. If the speed and rate of backspin result in an upward component greater than the force of gravity, the ball will continue to rise upward until the speed of the spin is diminished. A fast ball in baseball may be thrown with a slight backspin by holding two fingers on top of the ball and allowing the fingers to slide downward as the ball is pushed forward. The fast ball appears to maintain a horizontal flight during the 60-foot flight from the pitcher to the catcher.

EFFECT OF SPIN ON ROLLING BALLS

A rolling ball with a top spin, at the point of contact, pushes back against the surface on which it is rolling, and therefore the resulting forward push of the surface increases the forward velocity of the ball. Consequently, a ball with a top spin rolls farther than it would if it had no spin. Conversely, a ball spinning from bottom to top exerts a forward push against the surface, and the backward push from the surface will decrease the forward velocity of the roll. Thus a ball with a backspin does not roll as far as it would if it had no spin.

EFFECT OF SPIN ON BOUNCING BALLS

A ball that has no spin will rebound from a smooth surface at the same angle that it had when it hit the surface. If the approach is at an angle of 90 degrees, the rebound will be at the same angle; if the approach angle is 45 degrees, the rebound will be at an angle of 45 degrees with the surface. This is because all contacting parts of the ball push against the resisting surface with equal force. If the ball has rotatory motion, the contacting parts can push against the surface with different amounts of force.

A ball with a top spin rebounds at a lower angle than it would if it had no spin; a ball with a backspin rebounds at a higher angle. A ball spinning to the right or left rebounds in the direction of spin.

SUGGESTED READINGS
Broer, M. R.: Efficiency of human movement, Philadelphia, 1966, W. B. Saunders Co.
Ketlinski, R.: How is a curve ball thrown? Ath. J. **51**:12, 1971.
Verwiebe, F. L.: Does a ball curve? Am. J. Physics **10**:119, 1942.

See Bibliography for additional references.

CHAPTER 19 Hints for understanding and improving movement

Knowledge of the structure and function of certain parts of the human anatomy are especially beneficial to persons who are interested in how one accomplishes and may improve the effectiveness of one's movements. Keep in mind that the bones act as levers and are thus the moving parts of the body. The muscles are the energy-producing elements; they also act as covering and protection for the greater portion of the bony area. The tendons and ligaments help hold the bones together. This concept must be kept in mind. A joint is most likely to be dislocated when bony contact is decreased. Bony contact is least at the midpoint of the range of the joint's movement. With a force greater than can be borne by a joint the greatest damage will be done to one stabilized by bone and ligaments. Various areas of the body, their potential for action, and precautionary measures to avoid injury are discussed in this chapter.

1. The skull is made up of twenty-one bones. The mandible (lower part of the face), which is a movable bone, is part of the head. Although the twenty-one other bones are held together tightly, they can be separated by a blow. A football player who uses the head to block an opponent or uses it in attempting to drive over a tackler must strike the opponent with the frontal bone of the skull (frontal eminence and top front part). In this position the head is a perpendicular continuation of the body. If the head is turned a few degrees off the perpendicular (to one side), the player tends to follow the head; thus it is much easier to be pushed aside, injury is more likely to occur, and forward momentum is lessened. Moving the neck gently from side to side prior to a physical performance tends to improve balance in action and helps relieve muscle tension. The awareness of body position is thus greatly increased. The mandible, the movable bone of the head, is connected to the skull in such a manner that it can be driven into the brain from a blow such as might be sustained in boxing. The boxer must protect himself by keeping the chin down against the chest in moving about exchanging blows with the opponent. If a blow is received with the chin down, there is less chance that the condyles will be driven up into the brain.

2. Because at the shoulder the bones are held together only by surrounding muscles, this area must be protected from blows. A football player must be careful when blocking with the shoulder to have the protection of all the avail-

able muscles. This means not only that the arms should be across the body with the hands against the middle of the chest, so that the deltoideus muscles are used as protectors, but also that the chest and back muscles that attach to the humerus, such as the pectoralis muscles and latissimus dorsi, aid in protecting or holding the humerus in the best position to prevent injury. Dislocated shoulders (acromioclavicular separation) often result when the arm is in a poor position, that is, extended away from the body when a blow is received.

On the other hand, the anatomy of the shoulder is such that the humerus swings from a movable base. The base is formed by the scapula and clavicle together with the muscles and ligaments that form the capsule within which the ball-shaped head of the humerus fits into the concavity of the glenoid fossa of the scapula. The radius of the glenoid fossa is smaller than that of the head of the humerus. Conversely, the humeral head is considerably larger than that of the glenoid surface, but the radius of curvature of the glenoid fossa is greater than that of the humeral head. A fibrocartilaginous ring enlarges the articular surface further, so that the head of the humerus is allowed great freedom of movement. Also the capsular ligament is firm at the distal portion and loose at the proximal part to permit freedom of movement. This great freedom of movement enables people to play many sports that involve a quick, wide range of arm movements. This great freedom of arm movement depends on strong musculature to keep the joint intact if strenuous demands are made on it.

The best position of the shoulder for withstanding a blow is with the humerus held downward and rotated medially because the head of the humerus is tied into the glenoid fossa by the capsular ligament, which is reinforced above by the coracohumeral and coracoacromial ligaments. These ligaments are not adequate to keep the shoulder joint in normal position when undue forces from the outside act on it. The protective support of the shoulder joint, then, is dependent mainly on the tonus of the surrounding muscles.

In addition to the deltoideus, the latissimus dorsi, the levator scapulae, the pectoralis muscles, and the teres major, the long head of the biceps brachii passes through the capsular sac, acting to strengthen the joint further. The long head of the triceps arises from a prominence immediately below the glenoid surface of the scapula.

The hand can be extended farthest from the shoulder when the arm, with extended forearm, is abducted 135 degrees because the humerus moves farther out of its socket at this point. A basketball player on defense often places one arm in this position to attempt to block an opponent's pass or shot better. A basketball player who wishes to have the highest reach in a jump leans to the opposite side to bring the abducted arm to the vertical position.

The range of motion of the shoulder-arm complex is large in forward and sideward movements and restricted in backward movements. With the elbow extended from 90 degrees of abduction the arm can be moved backward in the transverse plane 30 degrees beyond the body line. The arm can be carried sideward and upward only to the vertical with the humerus medially rotated. With outward rotation, which swings the scapula forward and opens the face of the glenoid fossa and also swings the greater tubercule forward and away from the costal surface of the scapula, the arm can be elevated past the vertical from 20 to 30 degrees. With the elbow flexed 90 degrees and the shoulder rotated medially rarely can the arm be abducted beyond the horizontal; with the shoulder rotated laterally abduction can be continued beyond the vertical.

3. The motions of the arm affect the velocity and accuracy of a movement. Medial rotation of the arm (extended elbow and shoulder flexed) during shot-putting, throwing, and striking furnishes much more power to the movement than does an outward rotation of this limb. Effective use of the latissimus dorsi (arm muscle with origin on the back) and the pectoralis major (arm muscle with origin on the chest) must be made by this rotation, especially in throwing actions and rope climbing. Chinning and lifting are strongest with the palms of the hands help upward in a forearm-supinated position.

The tendon of the long head of the biceps is inserted into the bicipital tuberosity of the radius. When the radius and ulna are uncrossed with the forearm in supination, the biceps pulls directly against the radius, and all of its power is directed toward flexion. The contraction of the biceps produces no rotational force against the forearm when the hand is in supination. This is the strongest position for elbow flexion. However, when the radius is rotated across the ulna with the palm of the hand in pronation, the tendon of the biceps is wrapped around the shaft of the radius. In this position, part of the power of the contraction of the biceps is applied toward supinating the forearm and the remainder toward flexing the elbow. The strongest action of the biceps in flexing the elbow is with the palm held in supination and with the elbow half flexed. This position should be employed in turning a screw when a screwdriver is used. The insertion of the brachialis is into the anterior surface of the ulna. The brachialis pulls directly in flexing the elbow. The brachioradialis is another flexor of the elbow. Because it is inserted into the lower end of the radius, its effort arm is long, and it has a better mechanical advantage than does the biceps. The action of the brachioradialis is strongest when the forearm is in pronation because in this position the perpendicular distance from the axis of motion is greatest. These results have been found in laboratory situations.

Extension of the elbow is accomplished by the three heads of the triceps and the anconeus. The action of the flexors is approximately one and one-half times stronger than that of the extensors in most people. However, because of their great use of the extensors, gymnasts have been shown to have developed these muscles to equal the strength of the flexors. The action of these anterior flexors of the elbow is coordinated with that of the triceps and supinators, which cross the posterior portion of the elbow. All act together in movements that involve combinations of flexion or extension and rotation of the forearm.

Pure supination of the forearm is a more powerful movement than is pronation (when the arm is in a flexed position). However, in many overarm movements, such as throwing a ball, the medial rotation of the humerus is accompanied by pronation of the forearm.

4. The contribution of the action of the wrist, hand, and fingers to the

performance of certain movements is self-evident. The action that can be made with the human hand and fingers, especially the thumb grasp, is one of the factors that has set the human being apart from other mammals. The main muscles that help determine the strength of wrist and finger actions are attached above or below the elbow or both (Appendix C, Table C-1). Consequently, the size of the hand is not correlated positively with the strength exhibited by it.

The many bones that compose the wrist (eight small carpal bones arranged in two rows and closely held together by ligaments), hand (five metacarpals), fingers (three phalanges to each finger) and thumb (two phalanges) have the potential for a great range of motion. These twenty-six bones, each in turn moving through its own range of motion, have an accumulated action like that of a whip crack. The great shooter in basketball, the top hitter in baseball, and the top passer in football are so relaxed that these bones appear to "rattle around" as action takes place. The key here is that these performers know how to relax the muscles that might restrict the joint action.

The wrist strength in flexion is nearly double that of extension, and the power of extension is lessened when the wrist is in the flexed position. The hand of the opponent in jujitsu can be rendered nearly helpless if the wrist is held in flexion.

During extreme flexion of the wrist, it is almost impossible to curl the fingers strongly in full flexion. This is because the finger extensors, passing over the wrist joint, are too short to allow full finger flexion. A similar situation exists when the wrist is hyperextended, the range of hyperextension of the fingers is restricted because the length of the finger flexors passing over the wrist limits the movement. An involuntary adjustment to this relationship between finger and wrist action can be seen; when the fingers are voluntarily flexed, as in making a fist, the action is likely to be accompanied by wrist extension.

5. The proper function of the hip is important in movement. The articulation between the head of the femur and the acetabulum of the hip bone is a ball-and-socket joint. This hip joint permits movements of flexion, extension, abduction, adduction, circumduction, and medial and lateral rotation of the thigh. It is generally believed that the limit to which dancers, high jumpers, and high hurdlers can flex and abduct the thighs is determined for the most part by the flexibility of the ligaments and muscles, not normally by the arrangement of the bones of the hip joint. For the most part the integrity of the joint is maintained by the pressure of the atmosphere against the partial vacuum in the hip joint. This is contrasted with the shoulder, in which the integrity of the joint is dependent on the musculature that surrounds it.

Since many of the large muscles that move the femur and have their origin on the pelvis have medial rotation as a secondary function to such actions as adduction, and flexion, medial rotation of the thigh is a strong action. When great power is needed, such as when a fullback in football charges through the line, medial rotation of the thigh is used. Of course, the foot is turned slightly inward as a result of this movement. Also the knee is often flexed. However, when a performer such as a sprinter tries too hard when running, he may find that the primary and secondary functions of the large muscles of the hip tend to neutralize one another and he "ties up." The six lateral rotators of the hip (which are situated between the posterior portion of the pelvis and the greater trochanter of the femur) are then activated and cause the hip to turn outward. The runner's stride is shortened when the hips and feet point outward. The legs move more slowly, and he performs at far from his optimum. These lateral rotators are the piriformis, obturator externus, obturator internus, gemellus superior, gemellus inferior, and quadratus femoris. This group of small muscles has lateral rotation as its special action. Medial rotation is a secondary function of some of the large muscles, as mentioned previously.

Runners and jumpers have special need of the gluteal muscles—the gluteus maximus, gluteus medius, and gluteus minimus. They function most strongly in extension. The powerful gluteus maximus does not function strongly either until the hip is flexed (with the trunk inclined forward to a 45-degree angle to be most effective), bringing the gravitational line in front of the hip, or until a strong resistance from the supporting surface is encountered, such as in running, jumping, climbing, and lifting. The gluteus maximus is also brought into strong action during the crouch start in sprinting. Persons who are climbing up a hill flex the trunk to activate the gluteus maximus. Elderly people incline the trunk forward while climbing stairs, as do bicyclists, for the same reason.

It is amazing how the body is designed so that the most effective use may be made of its parts. The several joints of the upper and lower limb enable a performer to transfer momentum from one joint to another. (The flea has five joints in the legs and is able to jump many times its own height.)

6. The knee joint and the actions that it may accomplish are unusual. It is free yet firm, stable yet versatile, and massive yet shapely. The absorption of stresses and strains, most of which are imposed on it from the upper body, is only a secondary function. The primary function of knee action is to impart motion to the lower leg in kicking and to the thigh in locomotion.

The knee joint, situated between the hip and ankle joint in the long, weight-bearing lower extremity, meets the rotatory stresses imparted by the femur by means of strong ligaments that bind the bones together. The knee joint is surrounded by fascia, tendons, and ligaments. The anterior portion of the knee joint is bound by the capsular and patellar ligaments. They allow an extreme range of motion to be accomplished in flexion of the knee. The posterior aspects of the knee are joined by the short popliteal ligament, which checks hyperextension of the joint. Sideward displacement is prevented medially by the tibial and laterally by the fibular collateral ligaments. In the middle of the knee joint lie the anterior and posterior cruciate ligaments, crossing each other like the lines of the letter X. The anterior cruciate ligament checks inward rotation. Outward rotation tends to uncross and relax the cruciate ligaments. These ligaments bind the femur and tibia together and prevent extreme motion of the tibia forward and backward and inward in rotation.

Participation in modern dance and football seems to put undue stress on the cruciate ligaments. Frequently the ligaments are not able to withstand the stress that occurs in these activities, and a knee injury results.

The relatively small surfaces of the head of the tibia are deepened for articulation with the large condyles of the femur by two semilunar fibrocartilages called *menisci*. These two crescent-shaped cartilages are thickest at the edges, attached to the outside of the joint, and free at the inside borders. The upper and lower surfaces of each semilunar meniscus are concave and are invested with a smooth synovial membrane, which serves to lubricate the knee joint. Motion in the knee is thus an articulation between the condyles of the femur and the upper surfaces of the semilunar menisci and the condyles of the tibia and the lower surfaces of the menisci. The knee is designed for two separate functions. When the leg is flexed less than 20 degrees, the joint is stable because of the restrictions of the surrounding ligaments. When the knee is flexed beyond 20 degrees, the posterior reinforcing ligaments are relaxed because the condyles are closed together in the rear. The knee joint then becomes loose and free for axial functions. However, the flexed knee is not adapted to heavy weight-bearing functions.

Each meniscus covers approximately the peripheral two thirds of the corresponding articular surface of the tibia. The semilunar menisci are commonly torn or loosened by a severe blow or twist that may occur in strenuous activity such as football, in a fall, or in a blow from some external object. If one meniscus is removed surgically, the other becomes the major weight-bearing surface, and its susceptibility to injury is increased. The removal of both semilunar menisci does not necessarily restrict the strength or range of movement of the knee joint. In giving way to the blow or twist the menisci absorb some of the force. With the menisci removed this factor of safety is absent, and a severe blow or twist of the limb is more likely to damage the surrounding ligaments or to shatter the articulating surfaces of the bones.

The patella, one of the sesamoid bones in the body, lines within the tendon of the quadriceps femoris muscle. The patella is fastened to the tibia by the heavy patellar ligament. The angle of pull of the quadriceps is improved by the patella, and it is a protective shield defending the upper front of the knee joint. During flexion the patella occupies the deep groove between the two condyles of the femur. When the knee is extended by the action of the quadriceps, the patella is drawn strongly upward through the long recess (groove) in the front part of the femur. With the pulling up of the patella by the strong contraction of the quadriceps muscle in, for example, a kicking action, the pads that lie beneath the tedon lift up the synovial lining of the joint capsule. Thus the lining is pulled out of the way of the closing in of the bones (femur and tibia), and impingement between the condyles of the joint is prevented. Bursae above and below the patella act as protective cushions and elevate the patellar tendon, which improves its position mechanically to act.

7. The action of the foot and its relationship to the lower leg are worth considering. The lower leg differs in structure a great deal from the forearm because of its weight-bearing function. The lower leg does not have the great

rotational motility of the forearm. The tibia is the major heavy weight-supporting bone of the lower leg. The tibia is enlarged at each end to form the articulation at the upper end with the femur and at the lower end with the talus (or astragalus) of the foot.

The hinge joint formed by the articulation of the tibia and fibula with the talus has practically no side-to-side motion because the projecting processes from the tibia and fibula reach down past the joint and embrace the talus tightly.

Although the axes through both the knee and ankle joint are horizontal in the normal upright standing position, these axes are not parallel to each other. With the knee joint in a frontal plane the axis of the ankle joint runs from posterolateral to anteromedial. Because of this arrangement it is natural for plantar flexion of the foot to be accompanied by lateral displacement and for dorsiflexion to be accompanied by medial movement of the foot. Thus coaches and teachers should expect that in running, walking, kicking, and jumping movements the toes will point slightly to the outside rather than straight ahead in the direction of the movement.

The long base of support offered by the foot makes possible a wide range of movements of the upper body without the balance of the body being seriously affected. The rear of the foot projects about 3 inches behind the center of the line of support and about 7 inches in front. It is therefore much more difficult to topple the body forward than to topple it backward.

The extra length added to the leg by the extension of the foot increases the effectiveness of the leg action in walking, running, jumping, and kicking. Even the simple act of reaching upward is increased by about 3 inches by rising on the toes. Not only is the extra length of the foot an advantage to leg movements, but the musculature of the foot is also an additional source of power in performance.

The kinesthetic sensations arising from the muscles and tendons of the foot aid in maintaining balance. When the feet are numbed by poor circulation or get too cold, these sensations are lost, and the ability to maintain balance is impaired.

The foot is an arch supported by two pillars, the ball and the heel of the foot. One pillar is anterior and the other posterior to the keystone of the arch, the talus, which bears the weight of the body. The arch serves as a half-elliptic spring that acts to absorb the shock when the body lands on the feet. The force of the shock is dissipated as the arch is flattened during walking. The force is also lessened by distributing it over a larger foot area through the arch. If the foot were flat, the force of landing would be transmitted directly to the small area immediately under the ankle: injury could result. The arch also places the toes in a good position for gripping the ground.

The range of motion in the tarsometatarsal segment of the foot is approximately 10 to 20 degrees in dorsiflexion and 30 degrees in plantar flexion (dorsi-extension). Swimmers and ballet dancers develop considerably more flexibility in this segment to be good performers. Tarsometatarsal mobility is also useful in walking, running, and jumping, since it adds to the total range of motion.

The first metatarsal bone of the foot supports nearly one third of the weight of the body in standing, and at times during running and jumping it bears more than half the weight load. The metatarsals are the long lever arms of the foot machine. The longer these levers, the greater is the linear range of movement and also the greater is the speed that can be developed if the power source is adequate for the load to be moved.

In walking the forepart of the foot moves upward in dorsiflexion during the forward swing to clear the ground. The foot moves downward in plantar flexion after the heel strikes the ground to grip the ground and push off with the toes. Since the great toe carries at least one third of the load during the forward propulsion phase of walking and running, it should be strongly activated to increase the effectiveness of the movement.

Morton mentions structural stability in relation to the present arched conformation of the foot. He states that "structural stability is manifested in the foot's arched contour, even in individuals under complete anesthesia. As the foot will resist any forcible effort to flatten it under such circumstances, this rigid arch is obviously not dependent upon the muscles."* However, he states that "foot balance is dependent upon the interrelated presence of both structural (bones and ligaments) and postural (muscle) stability, . . . and any appreciable defect in either element will be manifested by an unbalanced posture, irrespective of the integrity of the other element."*

During the act of walking, according to Morton, the body weight is transferred from the heel along the axis of balance, which is near the center longitudinal line of the foot, and thence medially toward the great toe. The bottom of the foot contains large pads that serve to cushion the weight-bearing focal points. The plantar surface of the toes aids in gripping the ground during walking, running, and jumping.

*Morton, D. J.: The human foot, Morningside Heights, N.Y., 1942, Columbia University Press.

SUGGESTED READINGS
Basmajian, J. V.: Muscles alive, ed. 2, Baltimore, 1967, The Williams & Wilkins Co.
Grant, J. C.: A method of anatomy, Baltimore, 1965, The Williams & Wilkins Co.
Hollinshead, W. H.: Functional anatomy of the limbs and back, ed. 2, Philadelphia, 1960, W. B. Saunders Co.
Morton, D. J.: The human foot, Morningside Heights, New York, 1942, Columbia University Press.
Smout, C. G., and McDowall, R. J.: Anatomy and physiology for students of physiotherapy, occupational therapy and gymnastics, Baltimore, 1956, The Williams & Wilkins Co.
Steindler, A.: Kinesiology of the human body under normal and pathological conditions, Springfield, Ill., 1955, Charles C Thomas, Publisher.
Thompson, C. W.: Manual of structural kinesiology, ed. 7, St. Louis, 1973, The C. V. Mosby Co.
Wells, K.: Kinesiology, ed. 5, Philadelphia, 1971, W. B. Saunders Co.

See Bibliography for additional references.

CHAPTER 20 Coefficients of elasticity and friction

COEFFICIENT OF ELASTICITY

The coefficient of elasticity (restitution) of a body is its ability to regain its original size and conformation after a given force has distorted its shape. All materials are elastic. Five kinds of stress—tension, compression, bending, twisting, and shearing—tend to deform given materials. The builder selects materials and a shape that will best resist the particular kind of stress that will be applied or that is anticipated; for example, bricks resist compression and nothing else. Steel resists any of the stresses just named quite well. Balls and other similar sports equipment, although yielding to each of these stresses, most often are subjected to compression. In the place-kick the toe of the shoe of the kicker often distorts the ball as much as one third of its original shape. The baseball is temporarily flattened against the bat as much as one fourth. A golf ball may be distorted as much as one tenth or more and a tennis ball up to one-half of its original shape.

The word *strain* is used in mechanics to describe the deformation that takes place when an object is distorted. The word *stress* always refers to the forces acting on the bodies being distorted. *Strain* refers to the effect that stress produces.

$$\text{Strain} = \frac{\text{Elongation}}{\text{Original length}} = \frac{E}{L}$$

$$\text{Stress} = \frac{\text{Force applied}}{\text{Area of cross section}} = \frac{F}{A}$$

$$\text{Young modulus } (y) = \frac{\text{Stress}}{\text{Strain}} = \frac{\dfrac{F}{A}}{\dfrac{E}{L}} = \frac{F}{A} \times \frac{L}{E} = \frac{FL}{AE}$$

Hooke's law states that *strain* is proportional to *stress*. Since elasticity refers to that property which enables a body to recover its original shape or volume, a scrutiny of certain types of material may be interesting. Rubber, for example, is not perfectly elastic and therefore does not return to its original shape if distorted to the maximum. In fact, high-tempered steel and spring brass are much more elastic than is rubber. All gases act as perfectly elastic substances; for example, gas is used in pneumatic tires. Liquids are also perfectly elastic but difficult to compress. The inside of the best golf balls has a liquid core.

This concept explains why a small boy can hit a tennis ball farther than a hard ball (baseball). The tennis ball can be compressed to the point at which it is considerably distorted, but the bat cannot be swung fast enough to distort the baseball sufficiently to cause it to rebound off the bat as far as the tennis ball rebounds off the racket. Golf instructors recommend that some women and small men not purchase an expensive golf ball because they will not be able to compress an expensive ball (because of its liquid center) to the same degree that they can a cheaper ball, which has only a rubber center.

Handball players sometimes following a procedure that has a bearing on this discussion. They soak in hot water a "stale" handball. The heat causes a rearrangement of molecules to take place inside the handball, which will then bounce for a while as much as when it was new. Handball players also sometimes soak their hands in hot water to help prevent them from becoming bruised. The fluid in the hands is brought to the surface and helps the skin to withstand blows.

COEFFICIENT OF FRICTION

Friction is the resistance that opposes every effort to slide or roll one body over another. Friction may be a hindrance or a help in sports performance. Some general facts about friction include the following:

1. Static, or starting, friction is greater than moving or sliding friction.

2. Although many factors are involved, generally friction depends on the velocity, load, condition, and nature of the two surfaces that are interacting with each other.

3. In most practical sports situations friction tends not to depend much on the velocity of the sliding surfaces. However, starting friction is decidedly greater than sliding friction. Also friction, usually, decreases to some extent with increasing speed.

4. Friction depends on the nature and condition of the contacting surfaces because (a) friction is less when the surfaces are smooth and hard, (b) with dry surfaces friction is approximately the same regardless of the size of the area of contact, whether it be on the end or on the side, and (c) friction is approximately proportional to the area of contact with well-lubricated surfaces.

The force needed to overcome friction is nearly proportional to the normal, or perpendicular, force with which the surfaces are pressed together, as follows:

$$\text{Coefficient of friction} = \frac{\text{Force of friction}}{\text{Normal force}}$$

Force of friction = Coefficient of friction × Normal force

Another way to present this is as a ratio, as follows: the force pressing the surfaces together is represented by H (normal force) and R (force needed to overcome friction): therefore $\frac{R}{H} = B$. The smaller B is, the less friction is created. On the other hand, the larger B is, the more the surfaces cling together, and the larger the force that will be required to cause slippage. Sometimes it is advantageous to produce surfaces that have a high coefficient of friction; at other times it is advantageous to do just the opposite. Some examples of each are presented in the following paragraphs.

Sprinters lean forward at the start of a race to reduce the friction that their feet make against the ground. Ashes are put on automobile tires for driving on snow to increase friction so that sufficient traction against the snow can be secured.

In wet weather a small amount of silica sand placed on the hands of a football passer may enable him to throw the football more accurately. The coefficient of friction will be increased. However, wet, wrinkled socks inside a football player's shoes do the same thing and are likely to cause blisters.

Basketball players attempting to play on a floor that has been covered with wax for a dance may have to make the soles of their shoes irregular by cutting them with a knife so that there is sufficient friction between the soles and the floor surface to enable them to move. Ping-pong paddles that have a rough, irregular surface enable the players to put more spin on the ball because of the increased friction.

Surfaces such as the new, unsmooth cement rings used for shot-putting and discus throwing prevent the performer from slipping too fast as he goes around and across the ring. Cleats and spikes on athletic shoes have the same effect. However, the placement of the cleats and spikes may affect the amount of friction created.

When the problem of slippage is too great and the surfaces cannot be changed, the performer will have to keep the center of gravity more nearly over the base of support. He will have to take short steps, avoid too much body lean, and may have to drop the center of gravity as low as possible by squatting. In this way he will be able to remain in a playing posture and to perform at reasonable efficiency.

Because of the condition of a surface (for example, slick and wet), it is possible to "spin the wheels" too fast, and the coefficient of friction will be insufficient for the object, such as a car or a person, to move forward successfully. The two surfaces must be in contact with each other long enough for traction to take place. Moving at a lower speed enables this to occur.

SUGGESTED READINGS

Black, N. H.: An introductory course in college physics, New York, 1941, Macmillan, Inc.
Gamow, G., and Cleveland, J. M.: Physics: foundations and frontiers, Englewood Cliffs, N.J., 1960, Prentice-Hall, Inc.

See Bibliography for additional references.

PART V

Appendixes

APPENDIX A Principles of movement

1. A body at rest tends to remain at rest, whereas a body in motion tends to continue in motion with constant speed in the same straight line unless acted on by an outside force (law of inertia). The body at rest tends to resist being set into motion, but after it is in motion, whether linear or angular, the body will tend to continue until another force stops it (Newton's first law of motion).

2. The velocity of a body can be changed (accelerated) only when acted on by an outside force. The produced acceleration is proportional to and in the direction of that force (Newton's second law).

3. Every force is accompanied by an equal and opposite force (Newton's third law).

4. To change the direction of flight some force must be acting.

5. In swinging exercises if the radius of movement between the center of rotation and the center of weight is shortened on the upswing and lengthened on the downswing, the angular velocity will be accelerated.

6. When the body is being supported by the arms, the center of the weight of the body should be as nearly as possible directly over the base of support (hands).

7. In vaulting exercises the center of weight is moved ahead in the direction of the motion.

8. In many exercises on the rings, parallel bars, or horizontal bar that involve pull-ups and push-ups to various positions, there should not be any pause between the moves. Movement should be continuous throughout the feat.

9. To execute swinging suspension movements properly, force must be exerted when the body is directly under the point of support. The performer pulls toward the center of rotation (along the line of the radius), thus increasing the acceleration of the angular velocity. The center of weight rises fast, and this coupled with a shortening of the radius enables the performer to move rapidly.

10. To mount properly a piece of apparatus on which the performer will be doing angular motions, the center of rotation must be brought as close as possible to the center of support at the proper moment. This is called *timing*. Following are examples of proper mounting:

    a. On the flying rings the performer attempts the mount at the end of the swing because at this moment gravity is momentarily neutralized by the upward momentum and no centrifugal force has to be counteracted. (However, only still rings are used in Olympic competition.)

313

    b. On the bars the performer should usually attempt to mount (in swinging exercises) as the center of weight passes a point directly below the point of support.

    c. In certain exercises the momentum of a part may be transferred to the whole body. In the uprise on the bars the leg momentum carries the trunk and legs high above the piece, and the special move is done just before the leg and trunk have completed their swing.

    11. In many swinging movements the weight of the body when beneath the bar is pulled directly upward toward it to reduce the effort that the arms have to make to support the body weight.

    12. Many activities involve the use of both linear and angular momentum that are delicately integrated. Perhaps the discus throw is the most notable example.

    13. An implement adds length to a lever arm. The action of a joint (arm, leg, or wrist) may give added distance to the movement.

    14. The summation of forces may take place in a given direction if the forces are added successively at the point of greatest velocity of the previous force.

    15. If a blow or fall is distributed over a larger area or is allowed to dissipate over a longer time or distance or both, the effect is lessened.

    16. An individual unsupported in the air is unable to raise or lower the center of gravity as he travels through space. However, the body or body appendages may be rotated.

    17. Among the forces that one has to contend with in moving are air, water, friction, and gravity. An attempt should be made to minimize their effects in some instances and in others to use them to advantage.

    18. The top performers in rotation movements such as somersaults turn very rapidly. They have learned to complete their turn(s) in the time that is available while they are in the air.

Patterns of motion and rhythmic patterns of selected sports

PATTERNS OF MOTION

Vigorous movements of the body and limbs that occur in sports actions reveal some interesting phenomena. However, to understand the concepts enumerated in this appendix better, certain terms should be defined. According to Dorland *facilitation* in this setting has the following meanings: "the promotion or hastening of any natural process; the reverse of inhibition; specifically, the effect of a nerve impulse acting across a synapse, and resulting in an increase in the efficacy of subsequent impulses in that nerve fiber, or impulses in other convergent nerve fibers, in exciting the postsynaptic element."* *Proprioceptive* refers to the process by which the tissues (muscles included) receive stimulation. *Neuromuscular* pertains to the nerves and muscles. *Proprioceptive neuromuscular facilitation* may be defined as the methods used to stimulate the proprioceptors (Chapters 4 and 5) so that the response of the neuromuscular system is increased in time or intensity or both.

Knott and Voss have said, "The mass movement patterns of facilitation are spiral and diagonal in character. This is in keeping with the spiral and rotatory characteristics of the skeletal system of bones, and joints, and the ligamentous structures. This type of motion is also in harmony with the typographical alignment of the muscles from origin to insertion and with the structural characteristics of the individual muscles."†

Logan and Wallis state, "One of the major reasons that movements are diagonal when one extremity is used to impart force to an object is that the diagonally opposite extremity is involved in maintaining balance. This is particularly true in throwing. Another reason that diagonal movements are the rule is that pendular levers revolving on multiaxis articulations involve angular momentum; that is, as an attempt is made to move an extremity through a range in one plane of motion, there is a tendency for the lever to describe a circle. There-

---

*Dorland's illustrated medical dictionary, ed. 25, Philadelphia, 1974, W. B. Saunders Co.
†Knott, M., and Voss, D.: Proprioceptive neuromuscular facilitation, ed. 2, New York, 1969, Harper & Row, Publishers.

315

fore, the lever moves in an arc which usually becomes diagonal since the joint is moving through space."* These authors have called this diagonal pattern *serape*.

Knott and Voss have stated further, "There are two diagonals of motion for each of the major parts of the body."† The head and neck, upper trunk, and lower trunk and limbs make up the major portions of the body. Each of these diagonals of motion is composed of two patterns, one being a major component of flexion or of extension. Therefore each of the major parts has two flexion and two extension patterns, and each diagonal is antagonistic to the other. The major components, in turn, combine with two other components. The motions are then flexion or extension, motion toward and across the midline of the body (adduction) or motion across and away from the midline (abduction), and rotation (external rotation-supination and inversion and internal pronation and eversion).

Some examples of the diagonal patterns of facilitation are the action of the neck along with the head and upper trunk. This region has patterns of movement that may be described as flexion or extension plus the possibility of rotation to either the right or left, as Knott and Voss point out. The right shoulder or upper extremity in a tennis serve, for example, (for a right-handed person), is flexed and extended and adducted and abducted during the course of the action. (See Chapter 9.)

In the lower extremity, hip and knee flexion and extension are combined with adduction and abduction and with external and internal rotation in many actions in sports. Usually plantar flexion of the ankle and foot goes with hip extension, and dorsiflexion goes with hip flexion.

In the follow-through in many activities, especially throwing, the right shoulder will approach the left hip in its action as it is extended, adducted, and internally rotated with the elbow extended.

The left shoulder, in turn, is horizontally abducted and externally rotated with the elbow flexed.

The reason that athletes in preparation for an action move the body to the extreme opposite rotary position is to put the main muscles to use in maximum stretch because at this position the muscles will contract through the greatest range. The little extra movement at the last moment by the athlete to put the muscles even more in a stretch facilitates further the activation of the stretch reflex mechanism.

RHYTHMIC PATTERNS OF SELECTED SPORTS

The sounds made by performers in action in sports competition were recorded on a tape recorder. These sounds were then transcribed into musical scores. Subsequently the performers repeated their actions, and the music was tested against their movements and necessary corrections made. In most instances the foot

---

*Logan, G., and Wallis, E.: Recent findings in learning and performance, unpublished material, Los Angeles, Oct., 1960.
†Knott, M., and Voss, D.: Proprioceptive neuromuscular facilitation, ed. 2, New York, 1969, Harper & Row, Publishers.

Baseball — pitching

These musical scores include pertinent action only; the completion of the performance is not included.

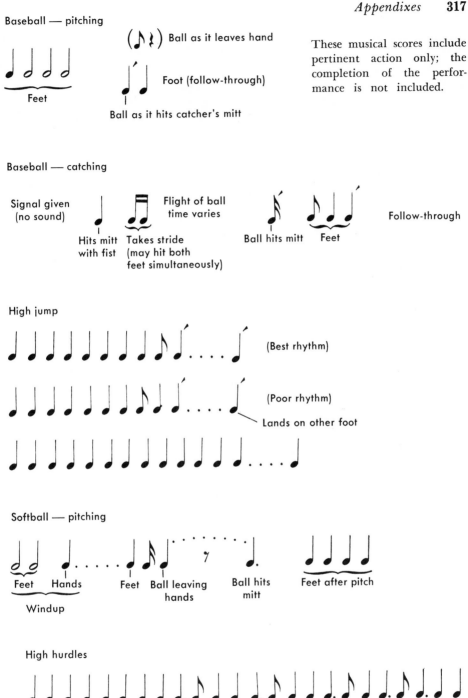

Baseball — catching

High jump

Softball — pitching

High hurdles

Punching bag

(Regular rhythm — very fast)

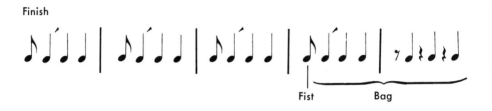

Fist   Bag

These musical scores include pertinent action only; the completion of the performance is not included.

Finish

Fist   Bag

Tumbling — back handspring and backflip

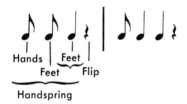

Hands   Feet
Feet   Flip
Handspring

Discus — two performers varied

Uneven

Step Toe-tap   Feet

Even

Basketball

Setup   (♪) Swish of ball in basket

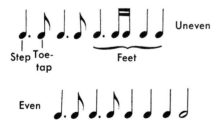

Foot   Foot   Takeoff   Landing
Ball

sounds were the most audible and the ones used in recording the action. The musical sounds have been used to help beginners learn to make the supposedly correct foot movements at the proper rate and with the right emphasis.

Performing with better players has been known to improve the effectiveness of poorer players. On the other hand, the effectiveness of a better performer may decrease if he picks up the rhythm of a poorer performer. Some of the musical scores of the sounds made by performers in selected sports are presented in the accompanying illustrations.

GENERAL COMMENTS AND OBSERVATIONS

1. Every performer has a certain individual composite rhythm.
2. Each segment of each performer's body has a rhythm all its own.
3. The complete rhythm of movement is hard to record.
4. In some sports, such as boxing or batting in baseball, the opponent tries to "feel" one's rhythm.
5. The rhythm of a performer is not smooth and even in tempo. It is often uneven but consistent in pattern.
6. Usually the tempo (speed) of movement is one of the biggest single factors in distinguishing the good from the poor performer.
7. Most performers do not know what their rhythm is and only subconsciously recognize it.
8. There seems to be a rhythmic pattern that is best for an individual to use, and also this pattern may be best in general for all good performers.
9. As people discover better and more effective ways to accomplish a task (perform a skill), they may develop different rhythmic patterns from the ones now used by top performers. (Additional information on this subject may be found in the article by Cooper and Andrews in *Quest*.)

SUGGESTED READINGS
Cooper, J. M., and Andrews, E. W.: Rhythm as a linguistic art: signs, symbols, sounds, and motion, Quest **23**:61, Winter, 1975.
Glasgow, R. B.: Fundamentals of physical education, Philadelphia, 1932, Lea & Febiger.

Skeletal movement
terminology; muscle
attachments

SKELETAL MOVEMENT TERMINOLOGY

The basic movements of the skeleton, of which the anatomic standing position is the beginning position, are as follows:

Flexion—action of two adjacent segments approaching one another
Extension—action away from flexion
Hyperextension—a segment extended beyond its normal starting position in extension
Adduction—movement toward the midline of the body
Abduction—movement in the frontal plane away from the midline of the body
Circumduction—movement of a segment in a conelike or circular motion
Rotation—movement of a segment in a rotatory action about its own longitudinal axis; outward rotation of the forearm so that the palm of the hand is turned upward, called *supination;* inward rotation of the forearm, called *pronation;* eversion and inversion—movements of the foot outward and inward; elevation and depression—movements of the shoulder girdle occurring in sternoclavicular joint

The student of kinesiology will be better able to understand how the human body moves and what its joint limitations are if he has a clear concept of joint action. In addition to helping in the analysis of human movement, this information may be of use in understanding joint injuries and abnormalities. The various types of joints are as follows:

1. The gliding joint (arthrodial), in which the bones glide over one another or one or more bones glide over another bone, is best illustrated by the articulating surfaces of the vertebrae and the tarsal and carpal bones. Most of the movement between any two surfaces is extremely small but may be large in respect to a total segment, such as the whole foot. Each small movement is added to the next one to get a wide range of movement.

2. The hinge joint (ginglymus), in which one surface is round with a knoblike end that fits into another concave surface and the action is hingelike and usually in only one plane about a single axis, is exemplified by the elbow joint as it moves in flexion and extension.

3. The ball-and-socket joint (enarthrodial) has the capacity to move in many

planes and three axes. Many actions, such as extension, flexion, circumduction, rotation, abduction, and adduction, are accomplished by this type of joint.

4. The condyloid joint (ovoid) has movement similar to the ball-and-socket joint but occurring in only two planes, forward and backward and from side to side. The articulations between the carpal bones of the wrist and the metacarpals of the fingers are examples of this joint.

5. The saddle joint, in which flexion, extension, abduction, and circumduction may be accomplished, is an unusual joint found only in the thumb and in the articulation between the carpal and metacarpal joints.

6. The pivot joint (trachoid) permits movement in one plane about one axis. An example of the movement accomplished by this joint is rotation of the radius in the forearm.

MUSCLE ATTACHMENTS

The proximal and distal attachments of the muscles of the upper and lower limbs are presented in Tables C-1 and C-2.

The order of listing muscles in Tables C-1 and C-2 is that used in Tables 5-1 and 5-2; that is, first, the muscles that have primary action on the most proximal segment are listed alphabetically (for the upper limb those acting on the shoulder girdle and for the lower limb those acting on the thigh). Next are listed alphabetically those muscles that have primary action on the next most proximal segment (for the upper limb those acting on the upper arm and for the lower limb those acting on the leg). This method of listing continues; the last alphabetical lists are of those acting on the fingers and the toes.

Table C-1. Attachments of muscles of upper limb

Muscle	Proximal attachment	Distal attachment
Levator scapulae	Transverse processes of atlas and axis; posterior tubercles of transverse processes of third and fourth cervical vertebrae	Vertebral border of scapula between medial angle and triangular smooth surface at root of spine
Pectoralis minor	Upper margins and outer surfaces of third, fourth, and fifth ribs near their cartilage; aponeuroses covering intercostales	Medial border and upper surface of coracoid process of scapula
Rhomboideus major	Spinous processes of second, third, fourth, and fifth thoracic vertebrae; supraspinal ligament	Lower part of triangular surface at root of spine of scapula; to inferior angle with arch connected to vertebral border by thin membrane
Rhomboideus minor	Lower part of ligamentum nuchae; spinous processes of seventh cervical and first thoracic vertebrae	Base of triangular smooth surface at root of spine of scapula

Continued.

Table C-1. Attachments of muscles of upper limb—cont'd

Muscle	Proximal attachment	Distal attachment
Serratus anterior	Outer surfaces and superior borders of upper eight or nine ribs; aponeuroses covering intervening intercostales	Ventral surface to vertebral border of scapula
Subclavius	First rib and its cartilage at their junction in front of costoclavicular ligament	Groove on undersurface of clavicle between costoclavicular and conoid ligaments
Trapezius	External occipital protuberance and medial third of superior nuchal line of occipital bone from ligamentum nuchae, spinous process of seventh cervical and spinous processes of all thoracic vertebrae, and corresponding portion of supraspinal ligament	Superior fibers—posterior border of lateral third of clavicle; middle fibers—medial margin of acromion and superior lip of posterior border of spine of scapula; inferior fibers—converge into aponeurosis inserted into tubercle at apex of smooth triangular surface on medial end of spine
Coracobrachialis	Apex of coracoid process in common with biceps brachii; intermuscular septum between two muscles	Into impression at middle of medial surface and border of body of humerus between origins of triceps brachii and brachialis
Deltoideus	Anterior border and upper surface of lateral third of clavicle; lateral margin and upper surface of acromion and lower lip of posterior border of spine of scapula as far back as triangular surface at its medial end	Deltoid prominence on middle of lateral side of body of humerus
Infraspinatus	Medial two thirds of infraspinous fossa; ridges on its surface; infraspinous fascia, which covers it	Middle impression on greater tubercle of humerus
Latissimus dorsi	Spinous processes of lower six thoracic vertebrae; posterior layer of lumbodorsal fascia, by which it is attached to spines of lumbar and sacral vertebrae; supraspinal ligament; posterior part of crest of ilium; external lip of crest of ilium lateral to margin of sacrospinalis; three or four lower ribs	Bottom of intertubercular groove of humerus, extending higher on humerus than tendon of pectoralis major
Pectoralis major	Anterior surface of sternal half of clavicle; half breadth of anterior surface of sternum as low down as attachment of cartilage of sixth or seventh rib; cartilages of all true ribs; aponeurosis of obliquus externus abdominis	Crest of greater tubercle of humerus

Table C-1. Attachments of muscles of upper limb—cont'd

Muscle	Proximal attachment	Distal attachment
Subscapularis	Medial two thirds of subscapular fossa; lower two thirds of groove on axillary border of bone; some fibers from tendinous laminae that intersect muscle and are attached to ridges on bone; others from aponeurosis that separates muscle from teres major and long head of triceps brachii	Lesser tubercle of humerus and front of capsule of shoulder joint
Supraspinatus	Medial two thirds of supraspinous fossa; strong supraspinous fascia	Highest of three impressions on greater tubercle of humerus
Teres major	Oval area on dorsal surface of interior angle of scapula; fibrous septa interposes between muscle and teres minor and infraspinatus	Crest of lesser tubercle of humerus
Teres minor	Dorsal surface of axillary border of scapula for upper two thirds of its extent and from two aponeurotic laminae, one of which separates it from infraspinatus, the other from teres major	Lowest of three impressions on greater tubercle of humerus; directly into humerus immediately below this impression
Anconeus	Back of lateral epicondyle of humerus	Side of olecranon and upper fourth of dorsal surface of body of ulna
Biceps brachii	Long head, from supraglenoid tuberosity at upper margin of glenoid cavity; short head from apex of coracoid process in common with coracobrachialis	Rough posterior portion of tuberosity of radius
Brachialis	Lower half of front of humerus extending below to within 2.5 cm. of margin of articular surface; from intermuscular septa more extensively from medial than lateral	Tuberosity of ulna and rough depression on anterior surface of coronoid process
Brachioradialis	Upper two thirds of lateral supracondylar ridge of humerus and from lateral intermuscular septum, being limited above by groove for radial nerve	Lateral side of base of styloid process of radius
Triceps brachii	Long head, infraglenoid tuberosity of scapula; lateral head, posterior surface of body of humerus and lateral border of humerus and lateral intermuscular septum; medial head, posterior surface of body of humerus below groove for radial nerve, extending from insertion of teres major to within 2.5 cm. of trochlea, medial border of humerus, and back of whole length of medial intermuscular septum	Posterior portion of upper surface of olecranon; band of fibers continues downward on lateral side over anconeus to blend with deep fascia of forearm

Continued.

Table C-1. Attachments of muscles of upper limb—cont'd

Muscle	Proximal attachment	Distal attachment
Pronator quadratus	Pronator ridge on lower part of volar surface of body of ulna; medial part of volar surface of lower fourth of ulna; strong aponeurosis that covers medial third of muscle	Lower forth of lateral border and volar surface of body of radius; deeper fibers into triangular area above ulnar notch of radius
Pronator teres	Humeral head immediately above medial epicondyle, tendon common to origin of other muscles, intermuscular septum between it and flexor carpi radialis, the antibrachial fascia; ulnar head, medial side of coronoid process of ulna	Rough impression at middle of lateral surface of body of radius
Supinator	Lateral epicondyle of humerus; radial collateral ligament of elbow joint and annular ligament; ridge on ulna that runs obliquely downward from dorsal end of radial notch; tendinous expansion that covers surface of muscle	Lateral edge of radial tuberosity and oblique line of radius as low down as insertion of pronator teres; back part of medial surface of neck of radius; dorsal and lateral surfaces of body of radius midway between oblique line and head of bone
Flexor carpi ulnaris	Humeral head, medial epicondyle of humerus; ulnar head, medial margin of olecranon and upper two thirds of dorsal border of ulna and intermuscular septum between it and flexor digitorum sublimis	Pisiform bone and prolonged from it to hamate and fifth metacarpal bones by pisohamate and pisometacarpal ligaments; transverse carpal ligament
Flexor carpi	Medial epicondyle by common tendon; elbow joint fascia; intermuscular septa between it and pronator teres laterally, palmaris longus medially, and flexor digitorum sublimis beneath	Base of second metacarpal bone and slip to base of third metacarpal bone
Extensor carpi radialis brevis	Lateral epicondyle of humerus; radial collateral ligament of elbow joint; strong aponeurosis that covers it; intermuscular septa between it and adjacent muscles	Dorsal surface of base of third metacarpal bone on radial side
Extensor carpi radialis longus	Lower third of lateral supracondylar ridge of humerus; lateral intermuscular septum; common tendon of origin of extensor muscles of forearm	Dorsal surface of base of second metacarpal bone on radial side
Extensor carpi ulnaris	Lateral epicondyle of humerus by common tendon; dorsal border of ulna in common with flexor carpi ulnaris and flexor digitorum profundus; deep fascia of forearm	Prominent tubercle on ulnar side of base of fifth metacarpal bone

Table C-1. Attachments of muscles of upper limb—cont'd

Muscle	Proximal attachment	Distal attachment
Palmaris longus	Medial epicondyle of humerus by common tendon; intermuscular septa between it and adjacent muscles; antibrachial fascia	Central part of transverse carpal ligament; palmar aponeurosis
Abductor digiti quinti	Pisiform bone; tendon of flexor carpi ulnaris	Ulnar side of base of first phalanx of little finger; ulnar border of aponeurosis of extensor digiti quinti proprius
Abductor pollicis brevis	Transverse carpal ligament; tuberosity of navicular; ridge of greater multangular	Radial side of base of first phalanx of thumb; capsule of metacarpophalangeal articulation
Abductor pollicis longus	Lateral part of dorsal surface of body of ulna; interosseus membrane; middle third of dorsal surface of body of radius	Radial side of base of first metacarpal bone
Adductor pollicis	From capitate bone; bases of second and third metacarpals; intercarpal ligaments; sheath of tendon of flexor carpi radialis	Ulnar side of base of first phalanx of thumb; lateral portion of flexor brevis and abductor policis brevis
Extensor digiti quinti proprius	From common extensor tendon; intermuscular septa between it and adjacent muscles	Joins expansion of extensor digitorum communis on dorsum of first phalanx of little finger
Extensor digitorum communis	Lateral epicondyle of humerus; intermuscular septa between it and adjacent muscles; antibrachial fascia	Second and third phalanges of fingers
Extensor indicis proprius	Dorsal surface of body of ulna below origin of extensor pollicis longus; interosseus membrane	Joins tendon of extensor digitorum communis, which belongs to index finger
Extensor pollicis brevis	Dorsal surface of body of radius below that muscle; interosseus membrane	Base of first phalanx of thumb
Extensor pollicis longus	Lateral part of middle third of dorsal surface of body of ulna below origin of abductor pollicis longus; interosseus membrane	Base of last phalanx of thumb
Flexor digiti quinti brevis manus	Convex surface of hamulus of hamate bone; volar surface of transverse carpal ligament	Ulnar side of base of first phalanx of little finger
Flexor digitorum profundus	Upper three fourths of volar and medial surfaces of ulna; depression on medial side of coronoid process; upper three fourths of dorsal border of ulna; ulnar half of interosseous membrane	Bases of last phalanges
Flexor digitorum sublimis	Humeral head, medial epicondyle of humerus, ulnar collateral ligament of elbow joint, intermuscular septa between it and adjacent muscles; ulnar head, medial side of coronoid process; radial head, oblique line of radius	Sides of second phalanx about its middle

Continued.

Table C-1. Attachments of muscles of upper limb—cont'd

Muscle	Proximal attachment	Distal attachment
Flexor pollicis brevis	Lateral portion, lower border of transverse carpal ligament and lower part of ridge on greater multangular bone; medial portion, ulnar side of first metacarpal bone	Lateral portion, radial side of base if first phalanx of thumb; medial portion, ulnar side of base of first phalanx
Flexor pollicis longus	Grooved volar surface of body of radius; adjacent part of interosseous membrane; medial border of coronoid process or medial epicondyle of humerus	Base of distal phalanx of thumb
Interossei dorsales	Each of four muscles arising by two heads from adjacent sides of metacarpal bone of finger into which muscle is inserted	Bases of first phalanges; aponeuroses of tendons of extensor digitorum communis
Interossei volares	Each of three muscles arises from entire length of metacarpal bone of one finger	Side of base of first phalanx; aponeurotic expansion of extensor communis tendon to same finger
Lumbricales manus	First and second from radial sides and volar surfaces of tendons of index and middle fingers respectively; third from contiguous sides of tendons of middle and ring fingers; fourth from contiguous sides of tendons of ring and little fingers	Into tendinous expansion of extensor digitorum communis, covering dorsal aspect of finger after passing to radial side of corresponding finger
Palmaris brevis	Transverse carpal ligament and palmar aponeurosis	Into skin on ulnar border of palm of hand
Opponens pollicis	Ridge on greater multangular; transverse carpal ligament	Whole length of metacarpal bone of thumb on radial side
Opponens digiti quinti manus	Convexity of hamulus of hamate bone; contiguous portion of transverse carpal ligament	Whole length of metacarpal bone of little finger along its ulnar margin

Table C-2. Attachments of muscles of lower limb

Muscle	Proximal attachment	Distal attachment
Adductor brevis	Outer surface of inferior ramus of pubis	Line leading from lesser trochanter to linea aspera and into upper part of linea aspera
Adductor longus	Front of pubis at angle of junction of crest with symphysis	Linea aspera between vastus medialis and adductor magnus, with both of which it usually blends
Adductor magnus	Small part of inferior ramus of pubis; inferior ramus of ischium; outer margin of inferior part of tuberosity of ischium	Linea aspera and upper part of its medial prolongation below; adductor tubercle on medial condyle of femur
Gemelli	Outer surface of spine of ischium; upper part of tuberosity of ischium	With obturator internus into medial surface of greater trochanter
Gluteus maximus	Posterior gluteal line of ilium, rough portion of bone, including crest immediately above and behind it; posterior surface of lower part of sacrum and side of coccyx; aponeurosis of sacrospinalis, sacrotuberous ligament, fascia of gluteus medius	Iliotibial band of the fascia lata; gluteal tuberosity between vastus lateralis and adductor magnus
Gluteus medius	Outer surface of ilium between iliac crest and posterior gluteal line above and anterior gluteal line below; gluteal aponeurosis covering its outer surface	Oblique ridge that runs downward and forward on lateral surface of trochanter
Gluteus minimus	Outer surface of ilium between anterior and inferior gluteal lines; behind from margin of greater sciatic notch	Anterior border of greater trochanter
Gracilis	Anterior margins of lower half of symphysis pubis and upper half of pubic arch	Upper part of medial surface of body of tibia below condyle
Iliacus	Upper two thirds of iliac fossa; inner lip of iliac crest; behind, from anterior sacroiliac and iliolumbar ligaments and base of sacrum; in front, reaching anterior superior and inferior iliac spines and notch between them	Lateral side of tendon of psoas major; some fibers being prolonged onto body of femur about 2.5 cm. below and in front of lesser trochanter
Obturator externus	Rami of pubis, interior ramus of ischium; medial two thirds of outer surface of obturator membrane; tendinous arch that completes canal for passage of obturator vessels and nerves	Trochanteric fossa of femur
Obturator internus	Inner surface of anterolateral wall of pelvis; pelvic surface of obturator membrane except in posterior part; tendinous arch that completes canal for obturator vessels and nerve; to a slight extent from obturator fascia that covers muscle	Forepart of medial surface of greater trochanter above trochanteric fossa

Continued.

Table C-2. Attachments of muscles of lower limb—cont'd

Muscle	Proximal attachment	Distal attachment
Pectineus	Pectineal line and to slight extent from surface of bone in front of it; between iliopectineal eminence and tubercle of pubis; from fascia covering anterior surface of muscle	Rough line leading from lesser trochanter to linea aspera
Piriformis	Front of sacrum by three fleshy digitations attached to portions of bone between first, second, third, and fourth anterior sacral foramina; margin of greater sciatic foramen; anterior surface of sacrotuberous ligament	Upper border of greater trochanter behind, but often partly blended with, common tendon of obturator internus and gemelli
Psoas major	Anterior surfaces of bases and lower borders of transverse processes of all lumbar vertebrae; sides of bodies and intervertebral fibrocartilages of last thoracic and all lumbar vertebrae by five slips, each of which is attached to the adjacent upper and lower margins of two vertebrae and to intervertebral fibrocartilage; series of tendinous arches that extend across constricted parts of bodies of lumbar vertebrae between slips	Lesser trochanter of femur
Psoas minor	Sides of bodies of twelfth thoracic and first lumbar vertebrae; fibrocartilage between them	Pectineal line and iliopectineal eminence; iliac fascia
Quadratus femoris	Upper part of external border of tuberosity of ischium	Upper part of linea quadrata, that is, line extending vertically downward from intertrochanteric crest
Sartorius	Anterosuperior iliac spine and upper half of notch below it	Upper part of medial surface of tibia nearly as far forward as anterior crest; behind tendon of gracilis; capsule of knee joint; fascia on medial side of leg
Tensor fasciae latae	Anterior part of outer lip of iliac crest; outer surface of anterior superior iliac spine and part of outer border of notch below it between gluteus medius and sartorius; deep surface of fascia lata	Between two layers of iliotibial band of fascia lata about junction of middle and upper thirds of thigh
Biceps femoris	Long head, on back of tuberosity of ischium and lower part of sacrotuberous ligament; short head, lateral lip of linea aspera within 5 cm. of lateral condyle and lateral intermuscular septum	Lateral side of head of fibula and by small slip into lateral condyle of tibia

Table C-2. Attachments of muscles of lower limb—cont'd

Muscle	Proximal attachment	Distal attachment
Semimem-branosus	Upper and outer impression on tuberosity of ischium above and lateral to the biceps femoris and semitendinosus	Horizontal groove on posterior medial aspect of medial condyle of tibia; back part of lateral condyle of femur; fascia of popliteus muscle; tibial collateral ligament and fascia of leg
Semitendinosus	Lower and medial impression on tuberosity of ischium by tendon common to it and biceps femoris; from aponeurosis that connects two muscles 7.5 cm. from their origin	Upper part of medial surface of body of tibia nearly as far forward as its anterior crest
Popliteus	Depression at anterior part of groove on lateral condyle of femur; to small extent from oblique popliteal ligament of knee joint	Medial two thirds of triangular surface above popliteal line on posterior surface of body of tibia
Rectus femoris	Anterior inferior iliac spine; groove above brim of acetabulum	Base of patella
Vastus medialis	Lower half of intertrochanteric line, middle supracondylar line, tendons of adductors longus and magnus, and medial intermuscular septum	Medial border of patella and quadriceps femoris tendon, an expansion going to capsule of knee joint
Vastus intermedius	Front and lateral surfaces of body of femur in its upper two thirds and from lower part of lateral intermuscular septum	Deep part of quadriceps femoris tendon, which is inserted in base of patella
Vastus lateralis	Upper part of intertrochanteric line, anterior and inferior borders of greater trochanter, lateral lip of gluteal tuberosity, and to upper half of lateral lip of linea aspera	Lateral border of patella, blending with quadriceps femoris tendon
Articularis genu	Anterior surface of lower part of body of femur	Upper part of synovial membrane of knee joint
Gastrocnemius	Medial head, depression at upper and back part of medial condyle and from adjacent part of femur; lateral head, impression on side of lateral condyle and from posterior surface of femur immediately above lateral part of condyle; both heads, subjacent part of capsule of knee	Unites with tendon of soleus and forms with it tendo calcaneus, which is inserted into middle part of posterior surface of calcaneus
Peroneus brevis	Lower two thirds of lateral surface of fibula; medial to peroneus longus; intermuscular septa that separates it from adjacent muscles	Tuberosity at base of fifth metatarsal bone on lateral side
Peroneus longus	Head and upper two thirds of lateral surface of body of fibula; deep surface of fascia; intermuscular septa between it and muscles on front and back of leg	Lateral side of base of first metatarsal and lateral side of first cuneiform

Continued.

Table C-2. Attachments of muscles of lower limb—cont'd

Muscle	Proximal attachment	Distal attachment
Peroneus tertius	Lower third or more of anterior surface of fibula; lower part of interosseous membrane; intermuscular septum between it and peroneus brevis	Dorsal surface of base of metatarsal bone of little toe
Plantaris	Lower part of lateral prolongation of linea aspera; oblique popliteal ligament of knee joint	With tendo calcaneus into posterior part of calcaneus
Soleus	Back of head of fibula; upper third of posterior surface of body of bone; popliteal line; middle third of medial border of tibia; tendinous arch placed between tibial and fibular origins of muscle	Tendo calcaneus into middle part of posterior surface of calcaneus
Tibialis anterior	Lateral condyle and upper half or two thirds of lateral surface of body of tibia; adjoining part of interosseous membrane; deeper surface of fascia; intermuscular septum between it and extensor digitorum longus	Medial and under surfaces of first cuneiform bone; base of first metatarsal bone
Tibialis posterior	Posterior surface of interosseous membrane except for its lowest part; lateral portion of posterior surface of tibia between commencement of popliteal line above and junction of middle and lower thirds of body below; upper two thirds of medial surface of fibula; deep transverse fascia; intermuscular septa separating it from adjacent muscles	Tuberosity of navicular bone; sustentaculum tali of calcaneus; three cuneiforms; cuboid; and bases of second, third, and fourth metatarsal bones
Abductor digiti quinti	Lateral process of tuberosity of calcaneus; undersurface of calcaneus between two processes of tuberosity; forepart of medial process; plantar aponeurosis; intermuscular septum between it and flexor digitorum brevis	With flexor digiti quinti brevis into fibular side of base of first phalanx of fifth toe
Abductor hallucis	Medial process of tuberosity of calcaneus; laciniate ligament; plantar aponeurosis; intermuscular septum between it and flexor digitorum brevis	Tibial side of base of first phalanx of great toe
Adductor hallucis	Oblique head, bases of second, third, and fourth metatarsal bones and sheath of tendon of peroneus longus; transverse head, plantar metatarsophalangeal ligaments of third, fourth, and fifth toes and transverse ligament of metatarsus	Lateral side of base of first phalanx of great toe, fibers of two heads blending

Table C-2. Attachments of muscles of lower limb—cont'd

Muscle	Proximal attachment	Distal attachment
Extensor digitorum brevis	Forepart of upper and lateral surfaces of calcaneus; lateral talocalcanean ligament; common limb of cruciate crural ligament	Dorsal surface of base of first phalanx of great toe; lateral sides of tendons of extensor digitorum longus of second, third, and fourth toes
Extensor digitorum longus	Lateral condyle of tibia; upper three fourths of anterior surface of body of fibula; upper part of interosseous membrane; deep surface of fascia; intermuscular septa between it and tibialis anterior on medial side and peronei on lateral side	Second and third phalanges of four lesser toes
Extensor hallucis longus	Anterior surface of fibula for about middle two fourths of its extent medial to origin of extensor digitorum longus; interosseous membrane to similar extent	Base of distal phalanx of great toe; base of proximal phalanx
Flexor digitorum longus	Posterior surface of body of tibia from immediately below popliteal line to within 7 or 8 cm. of its lower extremity; fascia covering tibialis posterior	Bases of last phalanges of second, third, fourth, and fifth toes
Flexor digiti quinti brevis	Base of fifth metatarsal bone; sheath of peroneus longus	Lateral side of base of first phalanx of fifth toe
Flexor digitorum brevis	Medial process of tuberosity of calcaneus; central part of plantar aponeurosis; intermuscular septum between it and adjacent muscles	Sides of second phalanx of each of lesser toes
Flexor hallucis brevis	Medial part of undersurface of cuboid bone; contiguous portion of third cuneiform; prolongation of tendon of tibialis posterior	Medial and lateral sides of base of first phalanx of great toe
Flexor hallucis longus	Inferior two thirds of posterior surface of fibula with the exception of 2.5 cm. at its lowest part; lower part of interosseous membrane; intermuscular septum between it and peronei laterally and from fascia covering tibialis posterior medially	Base of last phalanx of great toe
Interossei dorsales pedis	Surfaces of adjacent metatarsal bones	Bases of first phalanges; aponeurosis of tendons of extensor digitorum longus
Interossei plantares	Bases and medial sides of bodies of third, fourth, and fifth metatarsal bones	Medial sides of bases of first phalanges of same toes; aponeuroses of tendons of extensor digitorum longus

Continued.

Table C-2. Attachments of muscles of lower limb—cont'd

Muscle	Proximal attachment	Distal attachment
Lumbricales pedis	From tendons of flexor digitorum longus as far back as their angles of division; each of four muscles springing from two tendons except first	Expansions of tendons of extensor digitorum longus on dorsal surfaces of first phalanges
Quadratus plantae	Lateral head, lateral border of inferior surface of calcaneus in front of lateral process of its tuberosity, long plantar ligament; medial head, medial concave surface of calcaneus	Two heads joining to be inserted into lateral margin and upper surface and undersurface of tendon of flexor digitorum longus; slips usually sent to tendons going to second, third, and fourth toes

APPENDIX D Scheuchenzuber's center-of-gravity computer program*

JOE SCHEUCHENZUBER
Program—BODY C/G PROGRAM
Language—FORTRAN

Purpose

The purpose of this program is to compute present body center-of-gravity data, given the available segmental end points. The program also includes the options of a plot of the movement of the segments and calculations of the velocity and acceleration for the center of gravity from frame to frame. The latter option should be used only for gross estimations because of the limitations of using film analysis for computing kinetic data.

Program input for each set of frames
Card 1
    Col.   1-2   Number of sets of data to be processed (any number)
Card 2
    Col.   1-3   Number of frames in set (up to 50)
    Col.   6-11   Multiplier for this set
                  Form XX.XXXX or free form with decimal punched
    Col. 16-25 Data type to be used in computation for this set of data
                  Form (one of the following)
                  DEMPSTER = Dempster
                  B AND F   = Braune and Fischer
                  CLAUSER = Clauser
                  HARLESS = Harless
                  BSTEIN (F) = Bernstein (female data)
                  BSTEIN (M) = Bernstein (male data)
    Col. 30-34 Weight of the subject for this set
                  Form XXXX.X or free form with decimal punched
    Col. 39-43 Weight of object for this set (if any) (none needed)
                  Form XXX.XX or free form with decimal punched
    Col. 48-53 Frame rate for the set
                  Form XXXXX.X or free form with decimal punched

---

*Additional information regarding this type of computer program can be obtained from the Biomechanics Laboratory of the School of Health, Physical Education and Recreation, Indiana University, Bloomington, Ind. 47401.

333

Col. 60   Punch 1 if printed segmental c.g. data is wanted.

Col. 61   Punch 1 if punched deck of segmental c.g. data is wanted.

Col. 62   Punch 1 if a printer plot of body c.g. data is wanted.

Col. 63   Punch 1 if a printer plot of right-side segmental c.g. data is wanted.

Col. 64   Punch 1 if a printer plot of left-side segmental c.g. data is wanted.

Col. 65   Punch 1 if velocity and acceleration data for body c.g. is wanted.

Program input for each frame (see figure)

Card 1

Col. 1   Punch 0 if top of head was taken on this frame.

        Punch 1 if c.g. for head was taken on this frame.

        Punch 2 if estimated body c.g. was taken on this frame.

Col. 4-10   Coordinate of X zero point

        Form XXXX.XXX or free form with decimal punched

Col. 11-17   Coordinate of Y zero point

        Form XXXX.XXX or free form with decimal punched

Col. 18-22   Number of frame analyzed (as counted from first frame)

        (actual frame number)

Seg.	Col.	Card 2 (X for segments below) Card 3 (Y for segments below)
1	1-4	Top of head or head c.g. or estimated body c.g.
2	5-8	Sternal notch or blank if not available
3	9-12	Crotch or blank if not available
4	13-16	Right shoulder
5	17-20	Right elbow
6	21-24	Right wrist
7	25-28	Right finger (Leave blank if not available.)
8	29-32	Left shoulder
9	33-36	Left elbow
10	37-40	Left wrist
11	41-44	Left finger (Leave blank if not available.)
12	45-48	Right hip
13	49-52	Right knee
14	53-56	Right ankle
15	57-60	Right toe (Leave blank if not available.)
16	61-64	Left hip
17	65-68	Left knee
18	69-72	Left ankle
19	73-76	Left toe (Leave blank if not available.)
20	77-80	Object—estimated c.g. of object (if any) or blank

Form: Each coordinate's form is XX.XX or free form with decimal punched

For each additional frame return to top of page.

For next set of frames return to Card 2 under Program input for each set of frames.

When punching data, note that Form XXX.XX means that the decimal is implied between the third and fourth digit and must not be punched unless necessary for change in magnitude of data.

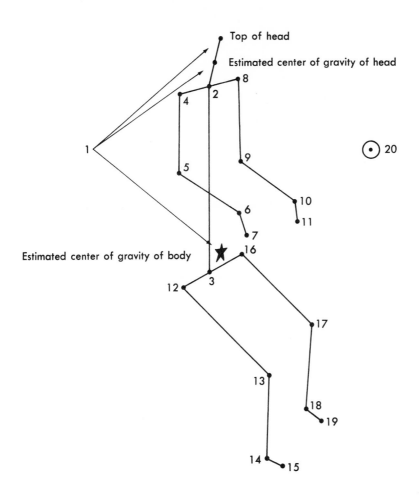

Bibliography

Adrian, E. D.: The physical background of perception, London, 1947, Oxford University Press.

Adrian, M. J.: An introduction to electrogoniometry, Kinesiology Review, p. 12, 1968.

Adrian, M., Tipton, C. M., and Karpovich, P.: Electrogioniometry manual, Springfield, Mass., 1965, Springfield College.

Alley, L. E.: An analysis of water resistance and propulsion in swimming the crawl stroke, Res. Q. Am. Assoc. Health Phys. Educ. 23:253, 1952.

Alt, F., editor: Advances in bioengineering and instrumentation, New York, 1966, Plenum Press.

Amar, J.: The human motor, Dubuque, Iowa, 1972, W. C. Brown Co.

Anderson, T. M.: Human kinetics and analysing body movements, London, 1951, William Heineman Medical Books, Ltd.

Anson, B. J.: Morris' human anatomy, New York, 1966, McGraw-Hill Book Co.

Aristotle: Parts of animals, movements of animals, and progression of animals, Cambridge, Mass., 1945, Harvard University Press.

Armbruster, D. A., Sr., Allen, R. H., and Billingsley, H. S.: Swimming and diving, ed. 6, St. Louis, 1973, The C. V. Mosby Co.

Atwater, A. E.: Movement characteristics of the overarm throw: a kinematic analysis of men and women performers, dissertation, University of Wisconsin, 1970.

Baird, J. E.: Energy costs of women during walking, thesis, University of Southern California, 1959.

Bard, P.: Medical physiology, ed. 11, St. Louis, 1961, The C. V. Mosby Co.

Barham, J. N., and Thomas, W. L.: Anatomical kinesiology, New York, 1969, Macmillan, Inc.

Barham, J. N., and Wooten, E. P.: Structural kinesiology, New York, 1973, Macmillan, Inc.

Barlow, D. A.: Kinematic and kinetic factors involved in pole vaulting, unpublished doctoral dissertation, Indiana University, Aug., 1973.

Barlow, D. A., and Cooper, J. M.: Mechanical considerations in the sprint start, Athletic Asia 2:27, Aug., 1972.

Barthelemy, N. R.: A mechanical analysis of the backhand drive in tennis, thesis, University of Wisconsin, 1953.

Bartlett, F. C.: The measurement of human skill, Br. Med. J. 1:835, 1947.

Basmajian, J. V.: New views of muscular tone and relaxation, Can. Med. Assoc. J. 77:293, 1957.

Basmajian, J. V.: Primary anatomy, Baltimore, 1964, The Williams & Wilkins Co.

Basmajian, J. V.: Muscles alive: their functions as revealed by electromyography, ed. 2, Baltimore, 1967, The Williams & Wilkins Co.

Basmajian, J. V., and Bentzon, J. W.: An electromyographic study of certain muscles of the leg and foot in the standing position, Surg. Gynecol. Obstet. 98:662, 1954.

Bates, B. T.: The development of a computer program with application to a film analysis: the mechanics of female runners, unpublished dissertation, Indiana University, Aug., 1973.

Batterman, C.: Mechanics of the crawl stroke, Swimming World 7:4, 1966.

Beck, M. C.: The path of the center of gravity during running in boys grades one to six, dissertation, University of Wisconsin, 1965.

Bedi, J. F.: Angular momentum in the long jump, unpublished dissertation, Indiana University, May, 1975.

Beevor, C.: The Croonian lectures on muscular movements, delivered before the Royal College of Physicians of London, London, 1903, Macmillan, Ltd.

Bernstein, N.: The coordination and regulation of movement, Oxford, 1967, Pergamon Press.

Bleustein, J. L., editor: AMF, Inc., mechanics and sport, New York, 1973, The American Society of Mechanical Engineers.

Blievernicht, D. L.: A multidimensional timing device for cinematography, Res. Q. 38:146, 1967.

Blievernicht, J. G.: Accuracy in the tennis forehand drive—a cinematographic analysis, Res. Q. Am. Assoc. Health Phys. Educ. 39:776, 1968.

Block, J.: Teaching the running front dive through progressive goals, thesis, University of Wisconsin, 1952.

Bowen, W. P.: The action of muscles in bodily movement and posture, Springfield, Mass., 1912, The F. A. Bassette Co.

Bowen, W. P., and McKenzie, R. T.: Applied anatomy and kinesiology, Philadelphia, 1919, Lea & Febiger.

Bowen, W. P., and Stone, H. A.: Applied anatomy and kinesiology: the mechanism of muscular movement, ed. 6, Philadelphia, 1949, Lea & Febiger.

Bowne, M. E.: The relationship of selected measures of acting body levers to ball throwing velocities, dissertation, University of Wisconsin, 1956.

Boyd, I. A., et al.: The role of the gamma system in movement and posture, New York, 1964, Association for the Aid of Crippled Children.

Braun, G. L.: Kinesiology: from Aristotle to the twentieth century, Res. Q. Am. Assoc. Health Phys. Educ. 12:163, 1941.

Braune, W., and Fischer, O.: Ueber den Schwerpunkt des menschlichen Körpers mit Rüchsicht auf die Austrustung des deutschen Infanteristem, Abh. D. K. Sachs Ges. Wiss. 15:2, 1889.

Breen, J. L.: What makes a good hitter? JOHPER 38:36, April, 1967.

Brennan, L. J.: A comparative analysis of the golf drive and seven iron shot with emphasis on pelvic and spinal rotation, thesis, University of Wisconsin, 1968.

Bresnahan, G. T.: A study of the movement pattern in starting the race from a crouch position, Res. Q. Am. Assoc. Health Phys. Educ. 5 (1) (supp.):5, 1934.

Briggs, D. W.: Impulse characteristics and the effect they have on center of gravity displacement during execution of the men's 3000 meter steeplechase water jump, unpublished dissertation, Indiana University, 1976.

Broer, M. R.: Efficiency of human movement, Philadelphia, 1966, W. B. Saunders Co.

Broer, M. R.: An introduction to kinesiology, Englewood Cliffs, N. J., 1968, Prentice-Hall, Inc.

Broer, M. R., and Houtz, S. J.: Patterns of muscular activity in selected sports skills, Springfield, Ill., 1967, Charles C Thomas, Publisher.

Brooke, J. D., editor: Human movement—a field of study, Lafayette, Ind., 1973, Balt Publishers.

Brouha, L.: Physiology of training, including age and sex differences, J. Sports Med. Phys. Fitness 2:1, 1962.

Brown, G. M.: Relationship between body types and static posture of young adult women, Res. Q. Am. Assoc. Health Phys. Educ. 31:403, 1960.

Brown, P. T.: The effect of three levels of warm-up on the reaction time and speed of movement of the baseball swing, unpublished doctoral dissertation, June, 1971.

Brown, R. M., and Counsilman, J.: The role of lift in propelling the swimmer. In Cooper, J. M., editor: Proceedings of the C.I.C. Symposium on Biomechanics, Chicago, 1971, The Athletic Institute.

Brunnstrom, S.: Comparative strengths of muscles with similar functions, Phys. Ther. 26:59, 1946.

Bunn, J. W.: Scientific principles of coaching, Englewood Cliffs, N. J., 1955, Prentice-Hall, Inc.

Canna, D. J., and Loring, E.: Kinesiography, Fresno, Calif., 1955, The Academy Guild Press.

Cavagna, G. A., Margaria, R., and Arcelli, E.: A high speed motion picture analysis of work performed in sprint running, Encyclop. Cinemat. 5:309, 1965.

Cavagna, G. A., Sailene, F. B., and Margaria, R.: Mechanical work in running, J. Appl. Physiol. 19:249, 1964.

Clark, W. E.: The anatomy of work. In Floyd, W. F., and Welford, A. T., editors: Symposium on human factors in equipment design, London, 1954, H. K. Lewis & Co., Ltd.

Clarke, H. H.: Recent advances in measurement and understanding of volitional muscular strength, Res. Q. Am. Assoc. Health Phys. Educ. 27:263, 1955.

Clauser, C. E., McConville, J. T., and Young, J. W.: Weight, volume, and center of mass of segments of the human body, AMRL-TR-69-70, Wright-Patterson Air Force Base, Ohio, Aug., 1969.

Cleaveland, H. G.: The determination of the center of gravity in segments of the human body, thesis, University of California, 1955.

Clouse, F. C.: A kinematic analysis of the development of the running pattern of pre-school boys, dissertation, University of Wisconsin, 1959.

Cochran, A., and Stobbs, J.: The search for the perfect swing, Philadelphia, 1968, J. B. Lippincott Co.

Cohen, J. S.: The field hockey pass: a cinematographic analysis, thesis, University of Wisconsin, 1969.

Collins, M. R.: The effect of stride length on efficiency in distance running, thesis, University of Southern California, 1951.

Collins, M. R.: Research on sprint running, Athletic J. 32:30, 1952.

Collins, P. A.: Body mechanics of the overarm and sidearm throws, thesis, University of Wisconsin, 1960.

Comstock, H. M.: Fundamentals of the bent-arm backstroke, Swimming World 5 (4):9, 1964.

Cooper, J. M.: Kinesiology of high jumping. In Wartenweiler, J., Jokl, E., and Hebbelinck, M., editors: Proceedings of the First International Seminar on Biomechanics, New York, 1968, S. Karger, AG.

Cooper, J. M.: Kinematic and kinetic analysis of the golf swing. In Nelson, R. C., and Morehouse, C. A., editors: Biomechanics IV, Baltimore, 1974, University Park Press.

Cooper, J. M., and Andrews, E. W.: Rhythm as a linguistic art: signs, symbols, sounds, and motions, Quest 23:61, Jan., 1975.

Cooper, J. M., Lavery, J., and Perrin, W.: Track and field for coach and athlete, Englewood Cliffs, N. J., 1970, Prentice-Hall, Inc.

Cooper, J. M., and Siedentop, D.: The theory and science of basketball, ed. 2, Philadelphia, 1975, Lea & Febiger.

Cooper, L.: Aristotle, Galileo, and the tower of Pisa, Ithaca, N. Y., 1935, Cornell University Press.

Corey, E. J.: Studies in the dynamics of histogenesis. Experimental, surgical and roentgenographic studies in the architecture of human cancellous bone, the resultant of back pressure vectors of muscle action, Radiology 13:127, 1929.

Counsilman, J. E.: Forces in two types of crawl strokes, Res. Q. Am. Assoc. Health Phys. Educ. 26:2, 1955.

Counsilman, J. E.: The science of swimming, Englewood Cliffs, N. J., 1968, Prentice-Hall, Inc.

Croskey, M. I., et al.: The height of the center of gravity in man, Am. J. Physiol. 61:171, 1922.

Cureton, T. K.: Mechanics and kinesiology of the crawl flutter kick, Res. Q. Am. Assoc. Health Phys Educ. 1 (4):87, 1930.

Cureton, T. K., Jr., and Wickens, J. S.: The center of gravity in the human body in the antero-posterior plane and its relation to posture, physical fitness, and athletic ability, Res. Q. Am. Assoc. Health Phys. Educ. 6 (2) (supp.):93, 1935.

Darwin, C.: The origin of species, Cambridge, Mass., 1964, Harvard University Press.

Dawson, P. M.: The physiology of physical education, Baltimore, 1935, The Williams & Wilkins Co.

Della, D. G.: Individual differences in foot leverage in relation to jumping performance, Res. Q. Am. Assoc. Health Phys. Educ. 21:11, 1950.

Dempster, W. T.: Space requirements of the seated operator, WADC Techn. Rep., Washington, D. C., July, 1955, U.S. Department of Commerce.

Dittmer, J. A.: A kinematic analysis of the development of the running pattern of grade school girls and certain factors which distinguish good from poor performance at the observed ages, thesis, University of Wisconsin, 1962.

Dobbins, D. A.: Loss of triceps on an overarm throw for speed, thesis, University of Wisconsin, 1970.

Duchenne, G. B.: Physiology of motion, Philadelphia, 1949, J. B. Lippincott Co.

Duvall, E. N.: Kinesiology, the anatomy of motion, Englewood Cliffs, N. J., 1959, Prentice-Hall, Inc.

Dyson, G.: The mechanics of athletics, ed. 5, London, 1970, University of London Press, Ltd.

Ekern, S. R.: An analysis of selected measures of the overarm throwing patterns of elementary school boys and girls, dissertation, University of Wisconsin, 1969.

Elftman, H.: The force exerted on the ground in walking, Arbeitsphysiologie 10:485, 1938.

Elftman, H.: The function of the arms in walking, Hum. Biol. 11:4, 1939.

Elftman, H.: The work done by muscles in running, Am. J. Physiol. 129:672, 1940.

Ellfeldt, L., and Metheny, E.: Movement and meaning: development of a general theory, Res. Q. Am. Assoc. Health Phys. Educ. 29:264, 1958.

Evans, F. G.: Stress and strain in bones, Springfield, Ill., 1957, Charles C Thomas, Publisher.

Evans, F. G., editor: Biomechanical studies of the muscular-skeletal system, Springfield, Ill., 1961, Charles C Thomas, Publisher.

Eyraud, K. C.: A quasi-dynamic simulation of a parallel ski turn initiation, thesis, University of Wisconsin, 1969.

Fahie, J. J.: Galileo, his life and works, London, 1903, J. Murray Co.

Farell, C.: Drag of bodies moving through fluids. In Cooper, J. M., editor: Proceedings of C.I.C. Symposium on Biomechanics, Chicago, 1971, The Athletic Institute.

Fay, T.: The origin of human movement, Am. J. Psychiatry 111:644, 1955.

Feldenkrais, M.: Body and mature behaviour, London, 1949, Routledge & Kegan Paul, Ltd.

Felton, E.: A kinesiological comparison of good and poor performers in the standing broad jump, thesis, University of Wisconsin, 1960.

Fenn, W. O.: Work against gravity and work due to velocity changes in running, Am. J. Physiol. 93:433, 1930.

Fenn, W. O.: Electrolyte changes in cat muscle during stimulation, Am. J. Physiol. 121:595, 1938.

Fisk, C. S.: The dynamic function of selected muscles of the forearm: an electromyographical and cinematographical investigation, unpublished doctoral dissertation, Indiana University, 1976.

Flatten, E. K.: A study of the relationship between amplitude scores by gymnastic judges and measured by cinematographic techniques, unpublished doctoral dissertation, Indiana University, Oct., 1974.

Fortney, V.: Trends and traits in the action of the swinging leg in running, thesis, University of Wisconsin, 1963.

Foster, M.: Lectures on the history of physiology, Cambridge, Mass., 1970, Harvard University Press.

Fox, M. G., and Young, O. G.: Placement of the gravity line in anteroposterior posture, Res. Q. Am. Assoc. Health Phys. Educ. 25:277, 1954.

French, J. D.: The reticular formation, Sci. Am. 196:54, May, 1957.

Froelich, A.: Observations of the velocity of the hand, thesis, University of Wisconsin, 1959.

Fulton, J. F., editor: Textbook of physiology, Philadelphia, 1955, W. B. Saunders Co.

Fung, Y. C., Perrone, N., Ankliker, M., editors: Biomechanics, its foundations and objectives, Englewood Cliffs, N.J., 1974, Prentice-Hall, Inc.

Galen, C.: On the natural faculties, New York, 1916, G. P. Putnam's Sons.

Gans, C.: Biomechanics: an approach to vertebrate biology, Philadelphia, 1974, J. B. Lippincott Co.

Ganslen, R. V.: Mechanics of the pole vault, Athletic J. 21:20, 1941.

Gardner, E. B.: The neuromuscular base of human movement: feedback mechanisms, JOHPER 36:61, Oct., 1965.

Gardner, E. B.: Proprioceptive reflexes and their participation in motor skills, Quest 12:1, 1969.

Garrett, G. E.: Methodology for assessing individuality: a comparative approach, dissertation, Purdue University, 1970.

Garrett, R. E., Widule, C. J., and Garrett, G. E.: Computer-aided analysis of human motion, Kinesiology Review, p. 1, 1968.

Gartmann, H.: Man unlimited, New York, 1957, Pantheon Books, Inc.

Gellhorn, E.: Physiological foundations of neurology and psychiatry, Minneapolis, 1953, University of Minnesota Press.

Gelner, J.: Accuracy in the tennis forehand drive—a cinematographic analysis thesis, University of Wisconsin, 1965.

Gesell, A.: The embryology of behavior, New York, 1940, Harper & Row, Publishers.

Gesell, A., and Thompson, H.: Infant behaviour: its genesis and growth, New York, 1934, McGraw-Hill Book Co.

Glassow, R. B.: Fundamentals of physical education, Philadelphia, 1932, Lea & Febiger.

Glassow, R. B., and Broer, M. R.: A convenient apparatus for the study of motion picture film, Res. Q. Am. Assoc. Health Phys. Educ. 9 (2):41, 1938.

Glassow, R. B., and Kruse, P.: Motor performance of girls age 6 to 14 years, Res. Q. Am. Assoc. Health Phys. Educ. 31:3, 1960.

Glassow, R. B., and Mortimer, E. M.: Soccer-speedball guide, Washington, D. C., 1966, American Association for Health, Physical Education, and Recreation.

Goldthwaite, J. E., et al.: Essentials of body mechanics in health and disease, ed. 5, Philadelphia, 1952, J. B. Lippincott Co.

Gollnick, P. D., and Karpovich, P. V.: Electrogoniometric study of locomotion and some athletic movements, Washington, D. C., 1961, Report to the U. S. Army Medical and Development Command, Office of Surgeon General.

Gowitzke, B. A.: Kinesiological and neurophysiological principles applied to gymnastics, Kinesiology Review, p. 22, 1968.

Gray, J.: How animals move, London, 1960, Cambridge University Press.

Groves, R., and Camaione, D. N.: Concepts in kinesiology, Philadelphia, 1975, W. B. Saunders Co.

Groves, W. H.: Mechanical analysis of diving, Res. Q. Am. Assoc. Health Phys. Educ. 21:132, 1950.

Halverson, L.: A comparison of the performance of kindergarten children in the takeoff phase of the standing broad jump, dissertation, University of Wisconsin, 1958.

Hart, I.: The mechanical investigations of Leonardo da Vinci, London, 1925, Chapman & Hall, Ltd.

Hasselkus, B. R.: Variations in the postural sway related to aging in women, thesis, University of Wisconsin, 1974.

Hawley, G.: Anatomical analysis of sports, New York, 1940, A. S. Barnes & Co., Inc.

Hay, J. G.: The biomechanics of sports techniques, Englewood Cliffs, N. J., 1973, Prentice-Hall, Inc.

Haycroft, J. B.: Animal mechanics. In Schafer's textbook of physiology, vol. 2, New York, 1900, Macmillan, Inc.

H'Doubler, M. N.: Dance: a creative art of experience, Madison, Wis., 1957, University of Wisconsin Press.

Heath, T. L.: The works of Archimedes, Cambridge, England, 1897, Cambridge University Press.

Heath, T. L.: Archimedes. In Encyclopaedia Britannica, vol. 2, London, 1954, Encyclopaedia Britannica International, Ltd.

Hellebrandt, F. A.: Standing as a geotropic reflex, Am. J. Physiol. 121:471, 1938.

Hellebrandt, F. A.: The physiology of motor learning, Cereb. Palsy Rev. 10:9, 1958.

Hellebrandt, F. A., Brogdon, E., and Tepper, R. H.: Posture and its cost, Am. J. Physiol. 129:773, 1940.

Hellebrandt, F. A., and Franseen, E. B.: Physiological study of the vertical stance of man, Physiol. Rev. 23:220, 1943.

Hellebrandt, F. A., Hellebrandt, E. T., and White, C. H.: Methods of recording movement, Am. J. Phys. Med. 39:178, 1960.

Hellebrandt, F. A., Houtz, S. J., Partridge, M. J., and Walters, C. E.: Tonic neck reflexes in exercises of stress in man, Am. J. Phys. Med. **35**:144, 1956.

Hellebrandt, F. A., Rarick, G. L., Glassow, R., and Carns, M. L.: Physiological analysis of basic motor skills, Am. J. Phys. Med. **40**:14, 1961.

Hellebrandt, F. A., Riddle, K. S., and Fries, E. C.: Influence of postural sway on stance photography, Physiotherapy Rev. **22**:88, 1942.

Hellebrandt, F. A., Riddle, K. S., Larsen, E. M., and Fries, E. C.: Gravitational influences on postural alignment, Physiotherapy Rev. **22**:149, 1942.

Hellebrandt, F. A., Schade, M., and Carns, M. L.: Methods of evoking tonic neck reflexes in normal subjects, Am. J. Phys. Med. **41**:90, 1962.

Hellebrandt, F. A., Tepper, R. H., Braun, G. L., and Elliott, M. C.: The location of the cardinal anatomical orientation planes passing through the center of weight in young adult women, Am. J. Physiol. **121**:465, 1938.

Hellebrandt, F. A., and Waterland, J. C.: The influence of athetoid cerebral palsy on the execution of sport skills: tennis and golf, Phys. Ther. Rev. **41**:257, 1961.

Hellebrandt, F. A., Waterland, J. C., and Walters, C. E.: The influence of athetoid cerebral palsy on the execution of sport skills: bowling, Phys. Ther. Rev. **41**:106, 1961.

Henry, F. M.: Force-time characteristics of the sprint starts, Res. Q. Am. Assoc. Health Phys. Educ. **23**:301, 1952.

Henry, F. M.: Dynamic kinesthetic perception and adjustment, Res. Q. Am. Assoc. Health Phys. Educ. **24**:176, 1953.

Hess, E.: Imprinting in animals, Sci. Am. **198**:81, March, 1958.

Hildebrand, M.: How animals run, Sci. Am. **202**:148, May, 1960.

Hill, A. V.: Living machinery, New York, 1927, Harcourt Brace Jovanovich, Inc.

Hill, A. V.: Muscular movement in man, New York, 1927, McGraw-Hill Book Co.

Hill, A. V.: The mechanics of voluntary muscle, Lancet **2**:947, 1951.

Hirt, S.: What is kinesiology? Phys. Ther. Rev. **35**:419, 1955.

Hirt, S., Fries, E. C., and Hellebrandt, F. A.: Center of gravity of the human body, Arch. Phys. Ther. **25**:280, 1944.

Hollinshead, H. W.: Functional anatomy of the limbs and back, ed. 2, Philadelphia, 1960, W. B. Saunders Co.

Hooton, E. A.: An anthropologist looks at medicine, Science **83**:271, 1936.

Hopper, B. J.: The mechanics of human movement, New York, 1973, American Elsevier Publishing Co., Inc.

Howell, A. B.: Speed in animals, Chicago, 1944, University of Chicago Press.

Howells, W.: Mankind so far, Garden City, N. Y., 1950, Doubleday & Co., Inc.

Hubbard, A. W.: Experimental analysis of running and of certain fundamental differences between trained and untrained runners, Res. Q. Am. Assoc. Health Phys. Educ. **10** (3):28, 1939.

Hubbard, A. W.: Muscular force in reciprocal movements, J. Gen. Physiol. **20**:315, 1939.

Hubbard, A. W.: Homokinetics: muscular function in human movement. In Johnson, W., editor: Science and medicine of exercise and sports, New York, 1960, Harper & Row, Publishers.

Hunsicker, P. A., and Donnelly, R. J.: Instruments to measure strength, Res. Q. Am. Assoc. Health Phys. Educ. **26**:408, 1955.

Huxley, H. E.: The contraction of muscle, Sci. Am. **199**:67, Nov., 1958.

Huxley, H. E.: The mechanics of muscular contraction, Sci. Am. **213**:6, Dec., 1965.

Jensen, C., and Schultz, G.: Applied kinesiology: the scientific study of human performance, New York, 1970, McGraw-Hill Book Co.

Johl, E., and Reich, J.: Guillaume Benjamin Armand Duchenne de Boulogne, J. Phys. Ment. Rehabil. **10**:154, 1956.

Johnson, B. P.: An analysis of the mechanics of the takeoff in the standing broad jump, thesis, University of Wisconsin, 1958.

Johnson, W., editor: Science and medicine of exercise and sports, New York, 1960, Harper & Row, Publishers.

Joseph, J.: Man's posture—electromyographic studies, Springfield, Ill., 1960, Charles C Thomas, Publisher.

Joseph, L.: Gymnastics (symposium), Summit, N. J., 1949, Ciba Pharmaceutical Co.

Karas, V., and Stapleton, A.: Application of the theory of the motion system in the analysis of gymnastic motions, New York, 1968, S. Karger, AG.

Karger's Biomechanics I, First International Seminar, Zurich, Switzerland, 1967.

Karpovich, P. V.: Swimming speed analyzed, Sci. Am. **142**:224, March, 1930.

Karpovich, P. V.: Water resistance in swimming, Res. Q. Am. Assoc. Health Phys. Educ. **4** (3):21, 1933.

Karpovich, P. V.: Analysis of the propelling force in the crawl stroke, Res. Q. Am. Assoc. Health Phys. Educ. **6**(2) (supp.):49, 1935.

Keith, A.: Man's posture: its evolution and disorders. II. The evolution of the orthograde spine, Br. Med. J. **1**:499, 1923.

Kelly, D.: Descriptive kinesiology, Englewood Cliffs, N. J., 1971, Prentice-Hall, Inc.

Kenedi, R. M.: Perspectives in biomedical engineering, Baltimore, 1973, University Park Press.

Ketlinski, R.: How is a curve ball thrown? Athletic J. **51**:5, 1971.

Kinesiology Review, Washington, D. C., 1968 and 1971, AAHPER.

Kinesiology Review, Washington, D. C., 1973 and 1974, AAHPER.

Kleinman, S.: Movement notation systems, Quest, p. 33, Jan., 1975.

Koch, J. C.: The laws of bone architecture, Am. J. Anat. **21**:177, 1917.

Kranz, L. G.: Kinesiology laboratory manual, St. Louis, 1948, The C. V. Mosby Co.

Krause, J. V., and Barham, Jerry N.: Mechanical foundations of human motion, St. Louis, 1975, The C. V. Mosby Co.

Krogman, W. M.: The scars of human evolution, Sci. Am. **185**:54, Dec., 1951.

Krogman, W. M., and Johnston, F. E.: Human mechanics—four monographs, Technical Documentary Report. No. AMRL-TDR-63-123, Wright-Patterson AFB, Ohio, 1963, Behavioral Sciences Laboratory.

Lanoune, F.: Analysis of the basic factors involved in fancy diving, Res. Q. Am. Assoc. Health Phys. Educ. **11** (1):102, 1940.

Lascari, A. T.: The felge handstand—a comparative kinetic analysis of a gymnastic skill, dissertation, University of Wisconsin, 1970.

Lewillie, L., and Clarys, J. P., editors: First International Symposium on "Biomechanics in Swimming," Brussels, 1971, Universite Libre de Bruxelles, Laboratoire de l'Effort.

Lipovetz, F. L.: Medical physical education, Minneapolis, 1946, Burgess Publishing Co.

Locke, L. F.: Kinesiology and the profession, JOHPER **36**:69, Sept., 1965.

Logan, G. A., and McKinney, W. C.: Kinesiology, Dubuque, Iowa, 1970, William C. Brown Co., Publishers.

Loken, N. C., and Willoughby, R. J.: Complete book of gymnastics, Englewood Cliffs, N. J., 1959, Prentice-Hall, Inc.

Lorenz, K. Z.: The comparative method in studying innate behaviour patterns. In Danielli, J. F., and Brown, R., editors: Symposia of the Society for Experimental Biology, No. 4: Physiological mechanisms in animal behaviour, Cambridge, England, 1950, Cambridge University Press.

Lorenz, K. Z.: The evolution of behavior, Sci. Am. **199**:67, Dec., 1958.

Lowman, C. L.: Faulty posture in relation to performance, JOHPER **29**:14, 1958.

MacConaill, M. A., and Basmajian, J. V.: Muscles and movements—a basis for human kinesiology, Baltimore, 1969, The Williams & Wilkins Co.

Magnus, R.: Some results of studies in the physiology of posture, Lancet **1**:531, 1926.

Marey, E. J.: The history of chronophotography, Washington, D. C., 1902, Smithsonian Institute.

Marshall, S.: Factors affecting place-kicking in football, Res. Q. Am. Assoc. Health Phys. Educ. **29**:302, 1958.

Massey, B., et al.: The kinesiology of weight-lifting, Dubuque, Iowa, 1959, William C. Brown Co., Publishers.

Mastropaolo, J. A.: Analysis of fundamentals of fencing, Res. Q. Am. Assoc. Health Phys. Educ. **30**:285, 1959.

Matsui, H.: Review of our researches, 1970-1973, Department of Physical Education, School of General Education, University of Nagoya, Nagoya, Japan.

Mautner, H. E.: The relationship of function to the microscopic structure of striated muscle: a review, Arch. Phys. Med. Rehabil. **37**:286, 1956.

McGraw, M.: The neuromuscular maturation of the human infant, New York, 1943, Columbia University Press.

McKenzie, C.: The action of muscles, New York, 1933, Paul B. Hoeber, Inc.

Merriman, J. S.: Stroboscopic photography as a research instrument, Res. Q. Am. Assoc. Health Phys. Educ. **46**:256, May, 1975.

Metheny, E.: Body dynamics, New York, 1952, McGraw-Hill Book Co.

Miller, D. I.: A computer simulation of the airborne phase of diving. In Cooper, J. M., editor: Proceedings of the C.I.C. Symposium on Biomechanics, Chicago, 1971, The Athletic Institute.

Miller, D. I., and Nelson, R. C.: Biomechanics of sport, Philadelphia, 1973, Lea & Febiger.

Miller, D. I., and Petak, K. L.: Three-dimensional cinematography. In Kinesiology III, Washington, D. C., 1973, AAHPER, p. 14.

Mills, L. N.: Kicking the American football, New York, 1939, G. P. Putnam's Sons.

Monpetit, R., and Boulonne, G.: Biomechanical analysis of the backward swing on the parallel bars, Movement **4**:135, 1969.

Moore, J. C.: Neuroanatomy simplified, Dubuque, Iowa, 1969, Kendall/Hunt Publishing Co.

Morehouse, L. E., and Cooper, J. M.: Kinesiology, St. Louis, 1950, The C. V. Mosby Co.

Morris, H. H.: The effects of starting block length, angle, and position upon sprint performance, unpublished doctoral dissertation, Indiana University, Nov., 1971.

Morris, R.: Coordination of muscles in action: correlation of basic sciences with kinesiology, New York, 1955, American Physical Therapy Association.

Mortensen, J. P., and Cooper, J. M.: Track and field, Englewood Cliffs, N. J., 1959, Prentice-Hall, Inc.

Mortimer, E.: Basketball shooting, Res. Q. Am. Assoc. Health Phys. Educ. **22**:234, 1951.

Morton, D. J.: The human foot, New York, 1942, Columbia University Press.

Morton, D. J., and Fuller, D. D.: Human locomotion and body form, Baltimore, 1952, The Williams & Wilkins Co.

Mountcastle, V. B., editor: Medical physiology, ed. 13, St. Louis, 1974, The C. V. Mosby Co.

Mumby, H. H.: Kinesthetic acuity and balance related to wrestling ability, Res. Q. Am. Assoc. Health Phys. Educ. **24**:327, 1953.

Muybridge, E.: The human figure in motion, New York, 1955, Dover Publications, Inc.

Napier, J.: The antiquity of human walking, Sci. Am. **216**:56, April, 1967.

Nelson, R. A.: The new world of biomechanics of sport, paper presented at the 75th annual Convention of the National College Physical Education Association for Men, New Orleans, Jan. 10, 1972.

Nelson, R. C.: Proceedings, Biomechanics Conference, Pennsylvania State University, 1971.

Nelson, R. C., and Morehouse, C. A.: Biomechanics IV, Baltimore, 1974, University Park Press.

Noble, M. L., and Kelley, D.: Accuracy of tri-axial cinematographic analysis determining parameters of curvilinear motion, Res. Q. Am. Assoc. Health Phys. Educ. **40**:643, 1969.

Northrip, J. W., Logan, G. A., and McKinney, W. C.: Biomechanic analysis of sport, Dubuque, Iowa, 1974, William C. Brown Co., Publishers.

O'Connell, A. L., and Gardner, E. B.: Understanding the scientific bases of human movement, Baltimore, 1972, The Williams & Wilkins Co.

O'Malley, C. D., and Saunders, J. B., de C. M.: Leonardo da Vinci on the human body, New York, 1952, Henry Schuman, Inc.

Palmer, C. E.: Studies of the center of gravity in the human body, Child Dev. **15**:99, 1944.

Pear, T. H.: Skill in work and play, New York, 1924, E. P. Dutton & Co., Inc.

Perrone, N., editor: Dynamic response of biomechanical systems, New York, 1970, The American Society of Mechanical Engineers.

Plagenhoef, S. C.: Computer program for obtaining kinetic data on human movement, J. Biomech. 1:221, 1968.

Plagenhoef, S. C.: Fundamentals of tennis, Englewood Cliffs, N. J., 1970, Prentice-Hall, Inc.

Plagenhoef, S. C.: Patterns of human movement: a cinematographic analysis, Englewood Cliffs, N. J., 1971, Prentice-Hall, Inc.

Posse, N.: The special kinesiology of educational gymnastics, Boston, 1890, Lothrop, Lee & Shepard Co., Inc.

Price, J.: Time as a measure of swinging ability in golf, thesis, University of Wisconsin, 1955.

Proceedings of the C.I.C. Symposium on Biomechanics, Chicago, 1971, The Athletic Institute.

Ralston, H. J., and Libet, B.: The question of tonus in skeletal muscle, Am. J. Phys. Med. 32:85, 1953.

Ramey, M. R.: The use of angular momentum in the study of long-jump take-offs. In Nelson, R. C., and Morehouse, C. A., editors: Biomechanics IV, Baltimore, 1974, University Park Press.

Rasch, P. J., and Burke, R. K.: Kinesiology and applied anatomy, Philadelphia, 1963, Lea & Febiger.

Reuschlein, P.: An analysis of the forward somersault in the pike position, seminar paper, University of Wisconsin, 1962.

Reuschlein, P.: Analysis of levers contributing to the force in the delivery of a bowling ball, seminar paper, University of Wisconsin, 1962.

Reynolds, E., and Lovett, R. W.: Method of determining the position of the center of gravity in relation to certain bony landmarks in the erect position, Am. J. Physiol. 24:286, 1909.

Ricci, B., and Karpovich, P. V.: Effect of height of heel upon the foot, Springfield, Mass., 1962, Springfield College.

Riesen, A.: Arrested vision, Sci. Am. 183:16, July, 1950.

Roberts, E. M.: Cinematography in biomechanical investigation. In Cooper, J. M., editor: Proceedings of the C. I. C. Symposium on Biomechanics, Chicago, 1971, The Athletic Institute.

Rork, R., and Hellebrandt, F. A.: The floating ability of college women, Res. Q. Am. Assoc. Health Phys. Educ. 8 (4):19, 1937.

Roy, B.: Kinematics and kinetics of the standing long jump in seven, ten, thirteen and sixteen year old boys, dissertation, University of Wisconsin, 1971.

Ruch, T. C., and Patton, H. D., editors: Physiology and biophysics, Philadelphia, 1965, W. B. Saunders Co.

Sabol, B.: A study of relationships among anthropometric, strength, and performance measures of college women bowlers, thesis, University of Wisconsin, 1962.

Sanders, J. A.: A practical application of the segmental method of analysis to determine throwing ability, unpublished doctoral dissertation, Indiana University, 1976.

Sanner, J. E.: Stroboscopic photography as an instrument for investigating human movement, unpublished doctoral dissertation, Indiana University, Aug. 1973.

Saunders, J. B., de C. M., and O'Malley, C. D.: Andreas Vesalius, Cleveland, 1950, World Publishing Co.

Scheuchenzuber, H. J. Jr.: Kinetic and kinematic characteristics in the performance of tethered and non-tethered swimming of the front crawl arm stroke, unpublished doctoral dissertation, Indiana University, Aug., 1974.

Schotellius, B. A., and Schotellius, D. D.: Textbook of physiology, ed. 17, St. Louis, 1973, The C. V. Mosby Co.

Schwartz, P., and Heath, A. L.: The definition of human locomotion on the basis of measurement, J. Bone Joint Surg. 29:203, 1947.

Scott, M. G.: Analysis of human movement: a textbook in kinesiology, ed. 2, New York, 1963, Appleton-Century-Crofts.

Sherrington, C.: The brain and its mechanism, Cambridge, England, 1933, Cambridge University Press.

Sherrington, C.: Man on his nature, ed. 2, Garden City, N. Y., 1953, Doubleday & Co., Inc.

Sherrington, C.: The integrative action of the nervous system, New Haven, Conn., 1961, Yale University Press.

Siebert, W.: Investigation of hypertrophy of muscle, J. Phys. Ment. Rehabil. **14:**153, 1960.

Sigerseth, P. O., and Grinaker, V. F.: Effect of foot spacing on velocity in sprints, Res. Ç. Am. Assoc. Health Phys. Educ. **33:**599, 1962.

Singer, C.: A short history of medicine, London, 1928, Oxford University Press.

Skarstrom, W.: Gymnastic kinesiology, Springfield, Mass., 1909, F. A. Bassette Co.

Slater-Hammel, A. T., and Andres, E. H.: Velocity measurement of fast balls and curve balls, Res. Q. Am. Assoc. Health Phys. Educ. **23:**95, 1952.

Slocum, D. B., and Bowerman, W.: The biomechanics of running, Clin. Orthop. **23:**39, 1962.

Snider, R. S.: The cerebellum, Sci. Am. **199:**2, Aug., 1958.

Sparks, K. E.: Physiological and mechanical alterations due to fatigue while running a four-minute-mile on a treadmill, unpublished doctoral dissertation, Indiana University, May, 1975.

Sperry, R. W.: Action current study in movement coordination, J. Gen. Physiol. **20:**295, 1939.

Sperry, R. W.: The eye and the brain, Sci. Am. **194:**48, May, 1956.

Sperry, R. W.: The growth of nerve circuits, Sci. Am. **201:**68, Nov., 1959.

Spray, J.: Three-dimensional film data validation procedures: a vector approach, unpublished thesis, University of Arizona, 1973.

Steindler, A.: Kinesiology of the human body under normal and pathological conditions, Springfield, Ill., 1955, Charles C Thomas, Publisher.

Steinhaus, A. H.: Strength from Morpurgo to Muller—a half century of research, J. Phys. Ment. Rehabil. **9:**147, 1955.

Stetson, R. H., and Bouman, H. D.: The action current as measure of muscular contraction, Science **77:**219, 1933.

Stetson, R. H., and Bouman, H. D.: The coordination of simple skilled movements, Arch. neerl. physiol. **20:**177, 1935.

Stetson, R. H., and McDill, J. A.: Mechanism of different types of movements, Psychol. Monogr. **32:**18, 1923.

Stillwell, G. K.: Physiology of skeletal muscular contraction: a review, Arch. Phys. Med. **38:**682, 1957.

Strauss, E.: The upright posture, Psychiatr. Q. **26:**529, 1953.

Sukop, J., Petak, K. L., and Nelson, R. C.: An on-line computer system for recording biomechanical data, Res. Q. Am. Assoc. Health Phys. Educ. **42:**101, 1971.

Sweigard, L. E.: Human movement potential: its ideokinetic facilitation, New York, 1974, Dodd, Mead & Co.

Szent-Gyorgyi, A.: Chemistry of muscular contraction, New York, 1947, Academic Press, Inc.

Takemoto, M., and Hamaido, S.: Gymnastics illustrated, Tokyo, 1961, Ban-Yu Shuppan Co., Ltd.

Tarbell, T.: Some mechanical aspects of the overarm throw. In Cooper, J. M., editor; Proceedings of the C. I. C. Symposium on Biomechanics, Chicago, 1971, The Athletic Institute.

Tarbell, T.: Unpublished material on throwing, Biomechanics Laboratory, Indiana University, 1972.

Tarrant, G. T. P.: Mechanics of human and animal activity, School Science Rev. **78:**246, 1938.

Taylor, F. S.: A short history of science and scientific thought, New York, 1949, W. W. Norton & Co., Inc.

Taylor, J., editor: Selected writings of John Hughlings Jackson, vol. 1, London, 1931, Hodder & Stoughton, Ltd.

Taylor, P. R.: The relationship among mechanical characteristics, running efficiency and performance of varsity track men, dissertation, Indiana University, 1971.

Thompson, C. W.: Manual of structural kinesiology, ed. 6, St. Louis, 1969, The C. V. Mosby Co.

Tobin, W. J.: The internal architecture of the femur and its clinical signification, J. Bone Joint Surg. **37:**57, 1955.

Tolsma, B.: Quadriceps flexibility: a key to sprinting speed, unpublished paper, Indiana University, April, 1975.

Travis, L. E.: The relation of voluntary movements to tremors, J. Exp. Psychol. **12:**515, 1929.

Travis, L. E., and Hunter, T. A.: Muscular rhythms and action currents, Am. J. Physiol. **81:**355, 1927.

Tricker, R. A. R., and Trickler, B. J. K.: The science of movement, New York, 1967, American Elsevier Publishing Co., Inc.

Tuttle, W. G.: Women who work for victory, Mechanical Engineering **65**:657, 1943.

Tuttle, W. W.: Physiological automatisms in athletics, Athletic J. **24**:6, 1944.

Vallière, A.: Kinetic and kinematic analysis of the backward giant swing on the still rings in gymnastics, unpublished doctoral dissertation, Indiana University, Aug., 1973.

Van der Berg, J. H.: The human body and the significance of human movement, Philosophy Phenomenological Res. **13**:159, 1952.

Van der Stok, A. A.: Practice situations and equipment for indoor teaching of beginning skiing, thesis, University of Wisconsin, 1954.

Verwiebe, F. L.: Does a ball curve? Am. J. Physics **10**:119, 1942.

Vredenbregt, E., and Wartenweiler, J., editors: Biomechanics II—medicine and sport, vol. 6, Basel, Switzerland, 1971, S. Karger, AG.

Wakefield, F., Harkins, D., and Cooper, J. M.: Track and field fundamentals for girls and women, ed. 2, St. Louis, 1973, The C. V. Mosby Co.

Ward, P.: An analysis of kinetic and kinematic factors of the standup and the preferred crouch starting techniques with respect to sprint performance, unpublished doctoral dissertation, Indiana University, Aug., 1973.

Ward, R. D.: An investigation into the use of computer integration of kinematics, kinetics, and cinematography data in motion analysis, dissertation, Indiana University, Aug., 1971.

Wartenweiler, J., Jokl, E., and Hebbelinck, M., editors: Biomechanics—medicine and sport, Basel, Switzerland, 1968, S. Karger, AG.

Wartenweiler, J., editor: Biomechanics, Proceedings of the First International Seminar on Biomechanics, Basel, Switzerland, 1968, S. Karger, AG.

Warwick, R., and Williams, P. L., editors: Gray's Anatomy of the human body, ed. 35, London, 1973, W. B. Saunders Co., Ltd.

Waterland, J. C., and Shambes, G. M.: Biplant center of gravity procedures, Percept. Mot. Skills **30**:511, 1970.

Webster, F. A. M.: Why? The science of athletics, London, 1936, John F. Shaw & Co., Ltd.

Weiner, N.: Cybernetics, Garden City, N. Y., 1953, Doubleday & Co., Inc.

Wells, K. F.: What we don't know about posture, JOHPER **29**:31, May, 1958.

Wells, K. F.: Kinesiology, ed. 5, Philadelphia, 1971, W. B. Saunders Co.

Wickstrom, R. L.: Fundamentals of motor patterns, Philadelphia, 1970, Lea & Febiger.

Widule, C. J.: A study of anthropometric strength, and performance characteristics of men and women league bowlers, dissertation, University of Wisconsin, 1966.

Widule, C. J.: Analysis of human motion, LaFayette, Ind., 1974, Balt Publishers.

Widule, C. J., and Gossard, E. C.: Data modeling techniques in cinematographic research, Res. Q. Am. Assoc. Health Phys. Educ. **42**:103, 1971.

Williams, M., and Lissner, H. R.: Biomechanics of human motion, Philadelphia, 1962, W. B. Saunders Co.

Wooten, E. P.: The structural base of human movement, JOHPER **36**:59, Oct., 1965.

Wright, W.: Muscle function, New York, 1928, Paul B. Hoeber, Inc.

Youm, Y., Roberts, E. M., and Atwater, A. E.: Three-dimensional cinematographic data analysis by computer, abstracts research papers presented at the Houston Convention of the American Association for Health, Physical Education and Recreation, 1972.

Zebas, C. J.: Reward and visual feedback relative to the performance and mechanical efficiency of high school girls in the standing broad jump, unpublished doctoral dissertation, Indiana University, Aug., 1974.

Index